The Doctors Book of
Home
Remedies®
for
Women

The Doctors Book of
Home
Remedies®
for
Women

Women Doctors Reveal Over 2,000 Self-Help Tips on
the Health Problems That Concern Women the Most

By the Editors of **PREVENTION** Magazine Health Books
Edited by Sharon Faelten

Rodale Press, Inc.
Emmaus, Pennsylvania

Library of Congress Cataloging-in-Publication Data

The Doctors book of home remedies for women: women doctors
    reveal over 2,000 self-help tips on the health problems that concern
    women the most / edited by Sharon Faelten and the editors of
    Prevention Magazine Health Books
        p.   cm.
    Includes index
    ISBN 0–87596–343–9 hardcover
    1. Women—Health and hygiene. 2.   Self care, Health,
I   Faelten,   II. Prevention Magazine Health Books.
RA778.D65 1996
613'.04244—dc20   96–22163

Distributed in the book trade by St. Martin's Press

    4   6   8   10   9   7   5   3   hardcover

The Doctors Book of Home Remedies for Women
Editorial Staff

MANAGING EDITOR: **Sharon Faelten**

WRITERS: **Michelle Bisson, Barbara Loecher, Gale Maleskey, Ellen Michaud, Peggy Morgan, Sara Altshul O'Donnell, Caroline Saucer**

CONTRIBUTORS: **Betsy Bates, Judy Lin Eftekhar, Cheryl Sacra, Maureen Sangiorgio, Andrea Warren**

ASSISTANT RESEARCH MANAGER: **Carol Svec**

HEAD RESEARCHER: **Susan E. Burdick**

RESEARCHERS AND FACT-CHECKERS: **Valerie Edwards-Paulik, Carol J. Gilmore, Jane Unger Hahn, Sandra Salera-Lloyd, Anita Small, Bernadette Sukley, Margo Trott**

COVER AND INTERIOR DESIGNER: **Kristen Morgan Downey**

COVER AND INTERIOR CALLIGRAPHER: **Jeri Lyn Anderson**

COVER ILLUSTRATOR: **Michele Manning**

INTERIOR ILLUSTRATOR: **Michael Crampton**

STUDIO MANAGER: **Joe Golden**

TECHNICAL ARTISTS: **William L. Allen, J. Andrew Brubaker**

COPY EDITORS: **Kathy D. Everleth, Amy K. Fisher**

BOOK MANUFACTURING DIRECTOR: **Helen Clogston**

MANUFACTURING COORDINATOR: **Patrick T. Smith**

OFFICE STAFF: **Roberta Mulliner, Julie Kehs, Bernadette Sauerwine, Mary Lou Stephen**

RODALE HEALTH AND FITNESS BOOKS

VICE-PRESIDENT AND EDITORIAL DIRECTOR: **Debora T. Yost**

ART DIRECTOR: **Jane Colby Knutila**

RESEARCH MANAGER: **Ann Gossy Yermish**

COPY MANAGER: **Lisa D. Andruscavage**

Contents

Acknowledgments

We wish to thank the many women physicians, psychologists, nurses and other health professionals who contributed their expertise to this book. In particular, we wish to acknowledge the cooperation of the following members of the American Medical Women's Association (AMWA).

ELIZABETH ABEL, M.D.
Clinical associate professor of dermatology at Stanford University School of Medicine

ROSEMARY AGOSTINI, M.D.
Clinical assistant professor of orthopedics at the University of Washington School of Medicine and a sports medicine and family practice physician at the Virginia Mason Medical Center, both in Seattle

ELIZABETH ARENDT, M.D.
Associate professor of orthopedic surgery at the University of Minnesota in Minneapolis

JEANNE F. ARNOLD, M.D.
Clinical assistant professor of medicine at Boston University School of Medicine

BARBARA BARTLIK, M.D.
Psychiatrist and sex therapist with the Human Sexuality Program at New York Hospital–Cornell Medical Center in New York City

DORIS GORKA BARTUSKA, M.D.
Director of endocrinology, diabetes and metabolism clinical services at Allegheny Universtiy of the Health Sciences in Philadelphia

TAMARA G. BAVENDAM, M.D.
Director of the Female Urology Clinic at the University of Washington Medical Center in Seattle

WILMA BERGFELD, M.D.
Head of clinical research in the Department of Dermatology at the Cleveland Clinic Foundation

SUSAN BLACK, M.D.
Board member of the American Academy of Family Physicians

MARIE L. BORUM, M.D.
Assistant professor of medicine in the Division of Gastroenterology and Nutrition at George Washington University Medical Center in Washington, D.C.

WILLA BROWN, M.D.
Director of Personal Health Services at the Howard County Health Department in Columbia, Maryland

MARY RUTH BUCHNESS, M.D.
Chief of dermatology at St. Vincent's Hospital and Medical Center in New York City

KAREN J. CARLSON, M.D.
Instructor at Harvard Medical School and director of Women's Health Associates at Massachusetts General Hospital in Boston

DIANA CARR, M.D.
Orthopedic surgeon in private practice in Sebring, Florida

SHERYL CLARK, M.D.
Assistant clinical professor of dermatology at Cornell Medical Center and an assistant attending physician in medicine at the New York Hospital, both in New York City

LEAH J. DICKSTEIN, M.D.
Professor and associate chair for academic affairs in the Department of Psychiatry and Behavioral Sciences and associate dean for faculty and student advocacy at the University of Louisville School of Medicine and past president of the American Medical Women's Association

ELAINE FELDMAN, M.D.
Professor emeritus of medicine at the Medical College of Georgia School of Medicine in Augusta

CAROL FLEISCHMAN, M.D.
Staff physician at Allegheny University of the Health Sciences MCP–Hahnemann School of Medicine and at the Center for Women's Health, both in Philadelphia

JEAN L. FOURCROY, M.D., PH.D.
Past president of the American Medical Women's Association and the National Council of Women's Health

NICOLETTE FRANCEY, M.D.
Professor of medicine at New York Medical College in Valhalla and a medical consultant for primary care at the Doctor's Consultants, a physicians' organization in New York City

ERICA FRANK, M.D.
Assistant professor in the Department of Family and Preventive Medicine at Emory University School of Medicine in Atlanta

SUSAN FUCHS, M.D.
Associate professor of pediatrics at the University of Pittsburgh School of Medicine and attending physician in the emergency room at Children's Hospital of Pittsburgh

MARJORIE GASS, M.D.
Director of the University Hospital Menopause and Osteoporosis Center at the University of Cincinnati

LILIANA GAYNOR, M.D., D.D.S.
Clinical assistant professor in the Department of Obstetrics and Gynecology at
Northwestern University Medical School in Chicago

ANNE GELLER, M.D.
Neurologist and chief of the Smithers Alcoholism Treatment and Training Center at St.
Luke's-Roosevelt Hospital Center in New York City and past president of the American
Society of Addiction Medicine

LINDA L. COLLE GERROND, M.D.
Director of the Center for Women's Health at the Shawnee Mission Medical Center near
Kansas City, Kansas

DEE ANNA GLASER, M.D.
Assistant professor of dermatology at St. Louis University School of Medicine

LETHA GRIFFIN, M.D.
Orthopaedic surgeon at the Peachtree Orthopaedic Clinic in Atlanta

NAOMI GROBSTEIN, M.D.
Family physician in private practice in Montclair, New Jersey

TINA HIEKEN, M.D.
Surgical oncologist at the University of Illinois at Chicago Medical Center

ANN HONEBRINK, M.D.
Co-director of the Center for Women's Health at Allegheny University of the Health Sciences MCP–Hahnemann School of Medicine in Philadelphia

DEBRA R. JUDELSON, M.D.
Senior partner with the Cardiovascular Medical Group of Southern California in
Beverly Hills, fellow of the American College of Cardiology and president of the
American Medical Women's Association

LOIS ANNE KATZ, M.D.
Professor of clinical medicine at New York University School of Medicine and associate
chief of nephrology and associate chief of staff for ambulatory care at New York
Veterans Affairs Medical Center, both in New York City

FRANCINE RATNER KAUFMAN, M.D.
Associate professor of pediatrics at the University of Southern California School of Medicine in Los Angeles, director of the Comprehensive Diabetes Program at Children's Hospital of Los Angeles and a member of the American Diabetes Association Board of Directors

MARY ANN KEENAN, M.D.
Chairman of the Department of Orthopedic Surgery at the Albert Einstein Medical
Center in Philadelphia

EVELYN KLUKA, M.D.
Director of pediatric otolaryngology at Children's Hospital in New Orleans

ESTA KRONBERG, M.D.
Dermatologist in private practice in Houston

MERLE S. KROOP, M.D.
Psychiatrist and sex therapist in New York City

VALERY LANYI, M.D.
Physiatrist at Rusk Institute of Rehabilitation Medicine, New York University Medical Center, in New York City

RUTH LAWRENCE, M.D.
Professor of pediatrics in the Division of Neonatology at the University of Rochester School of Medicine and Dentistry

ELIZABETH LIVINGSTON, M.D.
Assistant professor of obstetrics and gynecology at Duke University Medical Center in Durham, North Carolina

MARGARET LYTTON, M.D.
Family practitioner at Thomas Jefferson University Hospital in Philadelphia

KATHLEEN MCINTYRE-SELTMAN, M.D.
Professor of medicine in the Department of Obstetrics/Gynecology at the University of Pittsburgh School of Medicine

MARILYNNE MCKAY, M.D.
Professor of dermatology and obstetrics/gynecology at Emory University School of Medicine in Atlanta

EILEEN MURPHY, M.D.
Clinical instructor in obstetrics and gynecology at Northwestern University Medical School in Chicago

AUDRY NELSON, M.D.
Consulting rheumatologist at the Mayo Clinic in Rochester, Minnesota

SILVIA ORENGO-NANIA, M.D.
Assistant clinical professor of ophthalmology at Baylor College of Medicine in Houston

MELISSA PALMER, M.D.
Gastroenterologist in private practice in New York City

JODY PILTZ, M.D.
Assistant professor of ophthalmology at the University of Pennsylvania School of Medicine in Philadelphia

VERONICA RAVNIKAR, M.D.
Professor of obstetrics and gynecology and director of the Reproductive Endocrinology and Infertility Unit at the University of Massachusetts Medical Center in Boston

PHOEBE RICH, M.D.
Clinical assistant professor of dermatology at Oregon Health Sciences Center in Portland

JO-ELLYN RYALL, M.D.
Psychiatrist in private practice in St. Louis

Jo Shapiro, M.D.
Instructor of otology and laryngology at Harvard Medical School and associate surgeon of otolaryngology at Beth Israel Deaconess Medical Center and Brigham and Women's Hospital, both in Boston

Penelope Shar, M.D.
Internist in private practice in Bangor, Maine

Sheryl Siegel, M.D.
Assistant professor of neurology at New York Medical College in Valhalla, New York

Vesna Skul, M.D.
Assistant professor of medicine at Rush Medical College of Rush University and medical director of Rush Center for Women's Medicine, both in Chicago

Diane Solomon, M.D.
Chief of the cytopathology section of the National Cancer Institute in Bethesda, Maryland

Leonora Stephens, M.D.
Family systems psychiatrist and clinical associate professor of psychiatry at the University of Texas Southwestern Medical School in Dallas

Marla Tobin, M.D.
Family physician in private practice in Higginsville, Missouri

Lila A. Wallis, M.D.
Clinical professor of medicine and director of "Update Your Medicine," a series of continuing medical educational programs for physicians, at Cornell University Medical College in New York City

Judith N. Wasserheit, M.D.
Director of the Division of Sexually Transmitted Diseases Prevention of the National Center for HIV/STD and TB Prevention at the Centers for Disease Control and Prevention in Atlanta

Kristene E. Whitmore, M.D.
Chief of urology and director of the Incontinence Center at Graduate Hospital in Philadelphia

Jacqueline Wolf, M.D.
Gastroenterologist, assistant professor of medicine at Harvard Medical School and co-director of the Inflammatory Bowel Disease Center at Brigham and Women's Hospital in Boston

Kimberly A. Workowski, M.D.
Assistant professor of medicine in the Division of Infectious Diseases at Emory University in Atlanta

Ellen Yankauskas, M.D.
Director of the Women's Center for Family Health in Atascadero, California

Barbara P. Yawn, M.D.
Associate professor of clinical family medicine and community health at the University of Minnesota in Minneapolis and director of research at the Olmsted Medical Center in Rochester, Minnesota

Introduction

If you seem to be noticing more women physicians among the ranks of doctors listed in your local phone directory, you're not imagining things. At some medical schools half the graduates are women.

"By the year 2050 the majority of physicians will be women," predicts Eileen McGrath, executive director of the American Medical Women's Association, a highly respected national organization that you will be hearing more about as women play a more visible role in practicing medicine.

And it can't come soon enough. The *Wall Street Journal* reports that demand for female doctors is outstripping supply as more women choose doctors of the same gender, especially when selecting a gynecologist. And women are often willing to wait longer than usual for an appointment with a woman doctor—up to three or four months, in some cases.

Observers offer various theories about the reasons for a heightened demand for women in medicine. Some say that women doctors have an edge when it comes to communication skills, empathy and compassion—that women listen better than men. Well, maybe they do, and maybe they don't. As with any profession, some people are just better listeners than others, regardless of gender.

My theory is that because women physicians experience the same biological traits, hormonal changes and lifestyle factors as their female patients, they can discuss women's health from a uniquely female point of view—they can relate to their patients. And many women just feel more comfortable talking to a woman physician about uniquely female problems, such as premenstrual syndrome, bikini-line irritation, breastfeeding or gynecological exam jitters than they would be consulting even the most trusted and skilled male doctor. Male and female physicians alike can prescribe the right treatment for these problems, but a woman who has had firsthand experience knows exactly how it feels to experience them.

Women physicians also share some of the same stresses and time pressures that tend to face all working women: taking care of home and family, juggling responsibilities at work and home, deciding whether or not to call in sick when they or their children aren't well.

That's why we wrote this book—to tap into the collective wisdom of women doctors. We attended medical conferences conducted by the

American Medical Women's Association and other professional groups dedicated to women's health. We telephoned hundreds of women doctors in various specialties, from gynecology and urology to dentistry and family practice. We consulted the board of advisers for Rodale Women's Health Books. The result is *The Doctors Book of Home Remedies for Women*, a unique volume packed with women doctors' practical advice for solving health problems at home.

You'll find out what women gynecologists and obstetricians tell women to do to ease menstrual cramps, tender breasts, morning sickness, labor pain, breastfeeding problems, endometriosis, vaginitis and other "women only" problems. Learn what women dermatologists advise for blemishes, rashes, age spots, crow's-feet, lip lines, stretch marks and more. Find out what women psychologists have to say about overcoming depression, anxiety, boredom, low self-esteem and other negative emotions, plus problems with inhibited sexual desire and other relationship issues. In addition, you'll discover hundreds of secrets for managing annoyances such as contact lens problems, bad hair days, perm disasters and saggy upper arms. You'll even find solutions to rarely addressed problems such as sports widowhood, difficulty getting out of bed in the morning and the birthday blues, among others.

All in all, women doctors offer their best advice for relieving more than 200 physical and emotional concerns. We wish all our readers the best of health. But when everyday health problems do arise, we think you'll find yourself turning to this resourceful one-of-a-kind guide again and again.

Sharon Faelten
Managing Editor

Abdominal Fat

Flatten Your Tummy

*T*ime was, the worst thing about a potbelly was that you couldn't wear a bikini anymore. (Some of us never could.) No big deal—just throw on a tunic or a cover-up. Or trade in pencil-thin jeans for a pair of relaxed-fit denims.

But even if carrying a little more weight around your middle doesn't bother you cosmetically, you might want to get rid of it for health reasons. Research indicates that if you tend to gain weight around your middle, so that your body looks like a McIntosh apple—bowing at the middle—you're at higher risk for high blood pressure, heart disease, fatal heart attack, stroke and diabetes than women who are pear-shaped—bowing at the hips, says Jan McBarron, M.D., a weight-control specialist and director of Georgia Bariatrics in Columbus, Georgia.

KEEPING YOUR HOURGLASS FIGURE

Whatever the cause, women doctors say that exercise and weight reduction can help you slim down and firm up your abdomen.

Walk, walk and walk. The best way to permanently lose abdominal fat is to walk, says Dr. McBarron. "Walking will increase your metabolism—the rate at which your body uses up calories stored as fat—burning off abdominal and other body fat."

"Even five minutes a day is a good start," says Marion Nestle, Ph.D., professor and chairperson of the Department of Nutrition and Food Studies at New York University in New York City. "Anything is better than nothing, and more is better than less. Walk around the block, then two blocks, or take short walks several times a day."

If you can, aim to walk briskly at least 30 to 45 minutes three to five times a week, Dr. McBarron says. If you're already walking regularly, add 5 or 10 minutes to your sojourn.

Firm those muscles. You may not be able to flatten your tummy completely, but you can firm up your abdominal muscles. In addition to aerobic exercise like walking, which increases your respiratory and heart rates, try sit-ups and abdominal crunches, says Kathleen Little, Ph.D., ex-

1

ercise physiologist and professor at the University of North Carolina at Chapel Hill.

To do sit-ups, lie on your back with your legs bent at the knees, your feet flat on the floor and your arms flat at your sides, says Margot Putukian, M.D., team physician at Pennsylvania State University in University Park and assistant professor of orthopedic surgery and internal medicine at the Milton S. Hershey Medical Center in Hershey. Raise your head and shoulders from the floor, curling your trunk as much as possible until you reach an angle of about 45 degrees from the floor. Return to the starting position. To start, do at least 4 or 5 repetitions three times a week. Then, as you feel stronger, do at least 10 to 12 repetitions three to five times a week. Slowly progress to 20 repetitions five times a week.

To do abdominal crunches, lie down with your feet propped on a padded weight bench or chair and your arms crossed over your chest or at your sides. Raise your head and shoulders to form a 20 to 30 degree angle with the floor (about 6 to 12 inches off the floor), explains Dr. Putukian. Then lower yourself all the way to the floor. Do at least 4 or 5 repetitions three to five times a week, and as you get stronger, slowly advance to 20 repetitions five times a week.

Working your abs will work only when combined with fat-burning aerobic exercise. Otherwise, you'll still have a layer of fat over your abs.

Eat your veggies (and other ab-friendly foods). "As a rule, ounce-for-ounce, healthy, low-fat foods such as fresh fruits and vegetables always contain fewer calories than high-fat foods," says Elizabeth Somer, R.D., author of *Nutrition for Women.* Try to eat five to nine servings of fresh fruits and vegetables (a serving is about a half-cup cooked or one cup raw); lots of whole grains, such as whole-wheat pasta, multi-grain bread and cooked grains like bulgur; and a couple of servings of low-fat or nonfat milk every day.

Skip the fries, gravy and sweets. If you're bound and determined to keep pounds off your tummy—and everywhere else—skip the fried chicken, high-calorie salad dressings, creamy fettuccine sauces and sugar-filled desserts. That includes "nonfat" desserts. "They are full of sugar and often contain as many or more calories than high-fat desserts," says Dr. McBarron. "And when your body digests excess sugar, it's converted to fat."

Acne

Clearer Skin Can Be Yours

*S*ome women get an occasional pimple or blackhead. Others experience frequent or ongoing bouts of pimples, blackheads and whiteheads beginning in puberty. Some women notice that acne tends to flare up at the time of ovulation and fade after the menstrual period begins.

The woman who is most likely to get acne will generally have both overproducing oil glands and a tendency for cells lining the pores to clog. These two problems work together to trap and incubate bacteria on the skin. The result is a chronic formation of the whiteheads (called closed comedones), blackheads (open comedones), pimples and even cysts.

A DAY-AND-NIGHT REGIMEN

Women doctors recommend the following steps to control mild to moderate acne and keep zits from returning.

Wash with benzoyl peroxide liquid. To reduce the numbers of bacteria that can cause acne, gently wash your face with a benzoyl peroxide cleanser or a mild salicylic acid liquid every morning, says Susan C. Taylor, M.D., assistant clinical professor of medicine in the Department of Dermatology at the University of Pennsylvania School of Medicine in Philadelphia.

If you also break out on your back and chest, use the liquid to wash these areas as well, says D'Anne Kleinsmith, M.D., a staff dermatologist at William Beaumont Hospital in Royal Oak, Michigan.

Employ glycolic acid. Pat your face completely dry, then smooth on a gel, cream or lotion containing 8 percent glycolic acid over your entire face, says Dr. Taylor. Available at drugstores under a variety of brand names, glycolic acid gels, creams and lotions prevent the clogged pores characteristic of acne by preventing older cells from piling up on the skin and blocking pores. In addition, these products leave skin soft and smooth and may decrease discolorations and fine wrinkles.

Use a gel or a noncomedogenic (non-acne-forming) cream or lotion, says Dr. Kleinsmith.

3

WHEN TO SEE A DOCTOR

If you take birth control pills and develop acne before your menstrual periods, consult your doctor. She may be able to adjust the combination of estrogen and progesterone (two hormones in birth control pills) in your pills to prevent monthly outbreaks of acne, says D'Anne Kleinsmith, M.D., a staff dermatologist at William Beaumont Hospital in Royal Oak, Michigan.

You may also want to consider seeing a doctor if your acne is severe—say, if your entire face has broken out, says Susan C. Taylor, M.D., assistant clinical professor of medicine in the Department of Dermatology at the University of Pennsylvania School of Medicine in Philadelphia. A dermatologist may prescribe medications such as antibiotics or tretinoin (Retin-A). If acne is accompanied by the appearance of dark facial hairs, your doctor will examine you to rule out a hormonal abnormality, a rare cause of acne.

Add OTC medication. After a week use medication containing benzoyl peroxide to kill acne-causing bacteria, says Dr. Kleinsmith.

If your skin is either sensitive or dry, start with a 5 percent solution of benzoyl peroxide medication and dab it on problem areas after you've washed your face. If your skin is oily, start with a 10 percent solution and spread it over your entire face, except for the eyelids and area within an eyelash length of your eyes.

Use an oil-free moisturizer. Although many women who have acne will never need a moisturizer, says Dr. Kleinsmith, there is a small group of women who have oily skin only on their foreheads and noses, while their cheeks and jaws are actually dry. These women should apply an oil-free, noncomedogenic moisturizer to the dry areas of the face.

Look for oil-free makeup. If you wear makeup, use only oil-free products that are labeled "noncomedogenic" or "non-acne-forming," so that they won't clog your pores, says Dr. Kleinsmith.

Bleach leftover marks. If you have dark marks left on your skin from zits that have finally healed, try a bleaching cream, such as Porcelana, that contains hydroquinone, says Dr. Taylor. Follow package directions. (For practical ways to camouflage scars left by acne, see page 478.)

Do not squeeze, pop, prick or pick. In other words, keep your mitts off any pimple, blackhead or whitehead that appears on your face, says Dr. Taylor. You'll only make the area more inflamed and the bump larger.

Afternoon Slump
Beat the Four O'clock Fade

*L*unchtime is long past, quitting time is a while away and there's still plenty to cross off your to-do list. But there you sit, too pooped to pick up a pencil.

Sound familiar? Welcome to the afternoon slump.

If you slept poorly the night before or worked through lunch, it's no mystery why your energy evaporates. But sometimes energy flags for no obvious reason. Either way, you want to pull out of it fast.

A GRAB BAG OF PICK-ME-UPS

Here's what experts suggest that you try when you find yourself doing a fast fade.

See the light. "If your afternoon fatigue is worse in winter, and especially if it seems to be part of a general pattern of winter weariness, you may be troubled by seasonal affective disorder (SAD), says Brenda Byrne, Ph.D., director of the SAD Clinic of the Jefferson Light Research Program at Jefferson Medical College of Thomas Jefferson University in Philadelphia. SAD is a mood disorder triggered by the reduced daylight of winter and is responsive to treatment with light. So for your afternoon slump, try natural light treatment by bundling up and taking a brisk midday walk. Especially if done regularly, this combination of light and exercise is likely to boost your energy and alertness. (For more on seasonal affective disorder, see page 483.)

Take an exercise break. "When I need to be revived after sitting and working at my desk for some time, I get up and move around or go for a brief walk," says Tracy Horton, Ph.D., research instructor at the University of Colorado Health Sciences Center, Center for Human Nutrition in Denver. "Exercise is good for renewing energy and spirit."

Roll your shoulders. "Shoulder rolls are a great way to revitalize yourself and relieve tension while you're at your desk," says Peggy Norwood-Keating, director of fitness at Duke University Diet and Fitness Center in Durham, North Carolina. First, inhale and push your shoulders forward as if you're collapsing your chest. Then, lift your shoulders up toward your ears. Next, squeeze your shoulder blades together as you begin to exhale. Finally, drop your shoulders and release the tension, exhaling completely. Repeat once or twice.

Breathe deeply. Norwood-Keating advocates deep, cleansing breaths for afternoon restoration. "Take a very deep breath, pulling air in through your nose as deeply as you can. Hold it in for a few seconds, then breathe it out slowly and deliberately. Do this several times until you feel refreshed and renewed."

Sniff some essential oil. Inhaling certain scents can give you an instant lift, says Jeanne Rose, president of the National Association for Holistic Aromatherapy and author of *The Aromatherapy Book*. "Put a drop or two of the essential oil of rosemary, peppermint or orange peel oil on a hanky," she suggests. "Keep it close to you to feel quickly renewed." Look for essential oils at the Body Shop, health food stores and other stores that sell aromatic soaps and lotions.

Plan for peaks and valleys. Be aware of your own personal body clock. "Some people have a natural downtime that hits at mid-afternoon," says Nancy Clark, R.D., a nutritionist at SportsMedicine Brookline in Brookline, Massachusetts. "If this happens to you, try to schedule easy activities for that time—go for a wake-me-up walk or take a short nap."

SLUMP-BUSTING SNACKS

"If you haven't eaten for the past three to four hours, your blood levels of glucose—the essential fuel for your brain—are probably dropping slightly," says Franca Alphin, R.D., nutrition director at Duke University Diet and Fitness Center. So eating healthfully—small quantities of nutrient-dense foods at regularly spaced intervals—can help restore your zip by providing your blood and brain with an infusion of fuel.

Try some of these tips from experts to pull out of your slump.

Graze, don't gorge. "A big meal full of carbohydrates and fat can tire you out," says Alphin. "With fat being much more calorically dense than carbohydrates and protein, and the large load of carbohydrates prompting a significant rise in blood sugar, this type of meal can require quite a bit of work on the part of your metabolism. Instead, eat small low-fat meals four or five times a day."

Try yogurt. "The ideal snack strikes a balance between carbohydrates, protein and yes, even a little fat," says Kathy Duran, R.D., director of nutrition at the Cooper Wellness Program, a division of the Cooper Aerobic Center in Dallas. This gives you a sense of fullness and well-being. An eight-ounce serving of low-fat yogurt with fruit will do.

Age Spots
Fend Off Unfriendly Freckles

Some people might think that age spots are really just mini-suntans spattered over your face, hands, chest and hands, but they're not.

"Age spots are the result of sun exposure," explains Eileen Lambroza, M.D., clinical instructor of dermatology at New York Hospital–Cornell Medical Center in New York City. "They have nothing to do with age." And they're more permanent than a suntan. They're pigmented spots that represent an increased number of melanocytes, which contain melanin, a natural coloring pigment in skin that tends to darken after the skin has been repeatedly bombarded with ultraviolet rays.

TURN OFF THE MELANIN MACHINE

There are ways that you can minimize any existing spots and give yourself a spotless future. Here's what Dr. Lambroza and other women doctors recommend.

Lighten spots. If an age spot isn't too dark, you may be able to lighten it with an over-the-counter bleaching preparation—a so-called fade cream—containing a 2 percent solution of hydroquinone, says Dr. Lambroza. Darker age spots need a 3 percent solution, which is available only by prescription.

So go ahead and try a fade cream like Porcelana. But be very careful to follow package directions exactly, adds Dr. Lambroza. Any bleaching preparation can irritate your skin, particularly if left on too long.

Opt for an alpha hydroxy acid lotion. If you want to lighten age spots and even out skin texture and tone, Dr. Lambroza suggests making alpha hydroxy acids (AHAs) a part of your daily skin-care regimen. These mild natural acids are derived from sugarcane, fruit and milk. Glycolic acid, made from sugarcane, and the most commonly used AHA, loosens old dead cells on the skin's surface and accelerates the skin's ability to swap them for the new, fresher ones underneath. And they get rid of age spots by exfoliating superficial pigmentation.

To start using AHAs, smear a drop of a 5 percent AHA preparation

A Daily Anti-aging Routine

Eileen Lambroza, M.D.

The first face that Eileen Lambroza, M.D., treats every morning is her own. A clinical instructor of dermatology at New York Hospital–Cornell Medical Center in New York City, her goal is to have glowing, healthy skin that resists the signs of aging—including those little brown blotches called age spots. Here's her regimen.

Every morning, Dr. Lambroza washes her face with a foaming face wash. Next, she smooths on an alpha hydroxy acid lotion that increases cell turnover—a 5 percent lotion in the morning and a 10 percent solution at night. Then she applies a sunscreen with a sun protection factor, or SPF, of 15.

So far, Dr. Lambroza's anti-aging efforts are paying off. At 33 she's a walking advertisement for what an intelligent, knowledgeable approach to skin care can do. Her skin is as sweetly soft and smooth as a baby's. And there is not one age spot in sight.

on a small section of skin under your jaw, says Dr. Lambroza. If there is no sign of redness or irritation by the next day, wash your face, pat it dry, apply your usual sunscreen, then apply the AHA preparation. Smooth it over your entire face, but no closer to your eyes than the length of your eyelashes. Give your face time to dry, then apply your regular moisturizer and follow with your favorite makeup.

If no redness or irritation occurs, begin using the preparation once a day, says Dr. Lambroza. You may experience some tingling as the AHAs begin their work, but the tingling should subside within a few minutes. If there is no sign of any redness or irritation after two to three weeks, you may increase your use of AHAs to twice a day: once in the morning and once at night.

AHAs with a higher percentage of acids must be obtained through your dermatologist, says Dr. Lambroza.

Use camouflage. Some women who use AHA lotions see results in as little as 60 days, while others may have to wait up to a year to see improvement. While you wait for fade creams or AHAs to work, you may want to cover up your spots. Anita Cela, M.D., clinical assistant professor of dermatology at New York Hospital–Cornell Medical Center suggests using Dermablend, a heavy foundation sold at major department stores. For best results, she suggests that you ask a salesperson to help you pick the right shade and show you how to sponge it on and coordinate it with the rest of your makeup.

Block the sun. To prevent age spots from enlarging or multiplying, make sure that you wear a sunscreen on your face every day of your life, says Debra Price, M.D., clinical assistant professor of dermatology at the University of Miami School of Medicine and a dermatologist in South Miami.

"If I could have only one skin-care product, it would be a sunscreen," says Dr. Price. It should go on right after you wash your face in the morning and before you apply anything else. She recommends nonchemical sunscreen containing titanium dioxide, which reflects all the sun's harmful rays—both ultraviolet A and B.

Allergies
Natural Relief for Itching and Sneezing

Hazel and Harriet are sisters. Hazel spends the day spring cleaning and dusting her knickknacks. She takes her dog for a walk, enjoying the breezes that waft from the neighboring fields and woods. Then she comes home and curls up in bed with a pile of dusty mementos from college and her two cats, Pinky and Percy.

Meanwhile, Harriet is miserable. Getting within striking distance of a dusty quilt sends her into fits of wheezing and sneezing. Walking through the park leaves her eyes red and itchy. She misses her dog and two cats—they live with Hazel.

One thing that these sisters don't share is allergies. In women like Harriet, the immune system releases histamines and other irritating substances in response to perfectly normal (and otherwise harmless) airborne particles like dust, mold, tree pollen and animal dander (dandruff).

Typical allergy symptoms include sneezing, nasal itching and a dripping nose, along with congestion and red, swollen, itchy eyes.

9

Dogs She Can Live With

Kathy L. Lampl, M.D.

She has two bouncing Yorkshire terriers running around her house, but that doesn't mean that Kathy L. Lampl, M.D., instructor in the Department of Medicine in the Clinical Immunology Division at Johns Hopkins University School of Medicine in Baltimore, lets her allergies get the better of her.

"I'm probably the only allergist in the world with two dogs," jokes Dr. Lampl, who has allergies to dust mites and pet dander. But she says it's okay—she takes steps to make sure that she'll be sneeze-free.

"I pulled up all the carpeting in the house, and now we only have hardwood floors. Our dogs no longer sleep in the bedroom—they sleep in the kitchen—and they're bathed at least monthly."

To avoid dust mite exposure, Dr. Lampl encased her mattress and pillows in plastic, and she makes sure that her family's books and papers are kept in enclosed shelving instead of on night stands and dressers, since clutter invites troublesome buildup of dust.

Whether or not you'll develop an allergy is part genetics and part environment. A child with one allergic parent has about a 30 to 50 percent chance of getting allergies, while odds rise to approximately 60 to 80 percent if both parents have allergies. Also, exposure to a high level of allergens early on puts you at increased risk of developing allergic symptoms later.

GOOD RIDDANCE

The key to allergy relief, say women doctors, is managing your symptoms and avoiding common allergy triggers. Here are some basic strategies that can help women with allergies breathe easier. (For practical ways to manage asthma, which can be triggered by allergies, see page 27.)

Salt your nose. Over-the-counter saline nasal sprays are a safe way of loosening mucus, notes Carol Wiggins, M.D., clinical instructor of allergy and immunology at Emory University in Atlanta. "It's not a drug, so you can use it as often as you want." To make your own salty solution, take a half-teaspoon of salt dissolved in eight ounces of lukewarm water, put it in a bulb syringe and flush it into your nose while leaning forward over the sink so that it can drip out. Look for bulb syringes at your local drugstore.

Make a cool compress. For itchy, red, swollen eyes, "Take a clean washcloth, run it under cool water, put it over your eyes until it's warm and try again, if you need to," says Helen Hollingsworth, M.D., associate professor of medicine at Boston University School of Medicine and director of allergy and asthma services at Boston University Medical Center Hospital.

Seal your mattress. One of the big problems with dust is dust mites, teeny creatures that live on dust, skin flakes and other bits of microscopic household debris that collects in bedding, furniture and curtains, says Rebecca Gruchalla, M.D., Ph.D., assistant professor of internal medicine and chief of the Division of Allergy and Immunology at the University of Texas Southwestern Medical Center at Dallas. So zipping a plastic cover over your mattress is a good way of limiting dust mite exposure.

Press duct tape into service. Dr. Gruchalla also recommends putting duct tape on the mattress zipper, sealing off the escape route for dust mites.

Dry up. Molds and dust mites thrive in warm, humid conditions, says Dr. Wiggins. So to reduce mold and dust mite levels, keep a dehumidifier in your bedroom and one in your family room.

Clean the dehumidifier. Dehumidifiers should be cleaned out every week, says Dr. Wiggins. Otherwise, molds will proliferate.

WHEN TO SEE A DOCTOR

If you find yourself sneezing, wheezing and coughing even though you take over-the-counter drugs and try to avoid known or suspected allergy triggers, it might be time to visit your doctor, says Carol Wiggins, M.D., clinical instructor of allergy and immunology at Emory University in Atlanta. The same goes if you can't figure out what you're allergic to.

Your doctor may perform a skin-prick test to determine what's bugging you. Women with potentially serious allergies may benefit from prescription medications or allergy shots, in which a tiny portion of the substance that you're allergic to is injected into your system every week for about a year to help desensitize you against troublesome allergens that are impossible to avoid.

Use the exhaust fan. Whenever you take a shower, turn on the fan. A humid, unventilated bathroom makes mold worse, says Kathy L. Lampl, M.D., instructor in the Department of Medicine in the Clinical Immunology Division at Johns Hopkins University School of Medicine in Baltimore.

Simplify. Getting rid of dust mite havens—especially in your bedroom—is a sneeze-free way of coping, notes Dr. Lampl. "Have a clutter-free room with no fabrics or banners on the wall. You shouldn't have carpeting, because vacuuming doesn't clear the dust mites out." Stuffed toys trap dust and should be removed. She also recommends frequent changing of sheets and regular washing of bed linens, pillows and bedspreads.

Anemia
Wake Up Tired Blood

*Y*ou're not tired—you're exhausted. You dragged yourself through the day, doing the bare minimum. And you barely got dinner on the table before collapsing in front of the television like a giant lady slug.

It could be that you're coming down with a bug that's going around. Or maybe you just have too much to do. Or maybe you have anemia.

Diagnosing anemia is a tough call, explains Orah Platt, M.D., a hematologist (a doctor who specializes in blood disorders) at Harvard Medical School and director of laboratory medicine at Children's Hospital in Boston. Some women have no symptoms at all. Others, however, may feel completely drained and have trouble just making it to the end of each day.

Symptoms or no symptoms, women who have anemia tend to have plain and simple iron-deficiency anemia. The body needs iron (and plenty of it) to manufacture red blood cells. These red blood cells contain hemoglobin, the protein responsible for transporting oxygen in the blood. With too little iron, you have less hemoglobin, less oxygen and less energy. In other words, you have tired blood.

"Far and away, the predominant cause of iron-deficiency anemia in women is menstrual blood loss," says Sally S. Harris, M.D., in the Department of Sports Medicine at the Palo Alto Medical Clinic and team physician at Stanford University. "That's why anemia is more common in premenopausal women—-postmenopausal women no longer menstruate. And women with heavy menstrual flow are more prone to anemia, because they lose more blood than women with lighter flow."

Pregnancy and breastfeeding also drain iron stores, contributing to anemia in women. Low dietary intake (or poor iron absorption) also plays a part, says Dr. Harris.

Besides overall fatigue, other symptoms of anemia include shortness of breath, dizziness, light-headedness and fainting, plus apathy (lack of interest), poor resistance to colds or other infections and—not surprising—feeling tired after exercise.

RESTORE YOUR ZIP

If a blood test shows that you have mild anemia, Dr. Harris says that your doctor might recommend over-the-counter supplements that provide up to 18 milligrams of iron a day, the Daily Value for premenopausal women. If your anemia is more severe, your doctor will likely prescribe high-dose iron supplements of up to 180 milligrams a day, adds Dr. Harris. In any case, women doctors advise men and women alike against taking iron supplements without a doctor's supervision, because too much iron can be toxic.

To complement your physician's therapy, here's what women doctors say that you can do on your own to help put the brakes on anemia.

Stock up on iron-rich foods. "The best sources of iron are red meats—especially organ meats, such as liver—because they contain heme iron, the form most completely absorbed by the body," says Dr. Harris. "But organ meats are high in saturated fat and cholesterol, which can contribute to heart disease. So instead, look for lean cuts of steak and extra-lean ground beef."

"The best diet for women who are being treated for anemia is to eat a hamburger or steak two to three times per week," says Dr. Platt.

Help yourself to some wheat germ. "Women with anemia also tend to run low on folate—a B vitamin—and folate deficiency contributes to anemia," says Dr. Platt. "I recommend eating plenty of foods high in folate." You can get your Daily Value of folate—400 micrograms—by eating a bowl of highly fortified grain cereal for breakfast, such as Total, Most or

WHEN TO SEE A DOCTOR

Consult a physician if you have any of these symptoms.
- Extreme fatigue
- Fainting
- Dizziness
- Shortness of breath

If you are treated for iron-deficiency anemia and don't feel better after a month, tell your doctor. You may need another blood test. If the results are still below acceptable levels, your doctor might refer you to a hematologist (a doctor who specializes in blood disorders) to find out what's causing the problem.

Product 19, among others. Other good food sources of folate (as well as nonheme iron) include lentils, pinto beans, lima beans and spinach.

Look for uncoated tablets. "Ask your pharmacist if the iron supplements that you're taking are enteric-coated," says Dorothea Zucker-Franklin, M.D., professor of medicine at New York University Medical Center in New York City and president of the American Society of Hematology. "If they are, try switching to a brand that is not enteric-coated. Uncoated tablets are more completely and quickly absorbed by the body."

Uncoated tablets may upset your stomach, says Dr. Zucker-Franklin. If so, take the tablet after a meal.

Take it right. "You can get the most out of your iron supplement by taking it every day with foods or beverages rich in vitamin C," says Dr. Platt. "Studies have shown that foods high in vitamin C enhance iron absorption." Take your supplement with a glass of orange juice or cranberry juice. Other good food sources of vitamin C include guava (a tropical fruit), red bell peppers, papaya and strawberries.

Stick with the program. "Iron-deficiency anemia is not corrected overnight," notes Dr. Zucker-Franklin. "Women need to know that they should take their supplements for at least six months—a year is best. You may feel better in a few weeks, because your blood level of iron is restored. However, it takes longer to restore your iron stores in your bone marrow."

Anger

Manage Your Temper
before It Manages You

*P*erhaps you've heard or read that women are uncomfortable with anger, find it hard to acknowledge their anger and have more trouble handling it. Researchers, however, are finding otherwise.

"Women are just as able to acknowledge anger as men are," says June Price Tangney, Ph.D., clinical psychologist and associate professor at George Mason University in Fairfax, Virginia, and co-author of *Self-Conscious Emotions*. "We've also found that women are more likely to take constructive approaches to handling anger—like sitting down and talking it over—than men are."

Handling anger constructively is no small feat. As emotions go, anger is pretty intense. Situations that ignite anger—being blamed for something that's not your fault, for example, or being lied to—trigger the flight-or-fight-response, a complex reaction to stress that results in a release of adrenaline, increased heartbeat and other physiological reactions. When angered, our bodies are primed to either duke it out or run for our lives.

HANDLE HOSTILITY

"Most often, anger is functional—a sign that something needs to be changed. It's not a bad emotion; there is nothing wrong with feeling anger."

There are right and wrong ways to handle anger, say researchers. Here's what to do.

First, do nothing. If you don't feel as effective at diffusing anger as you would like, stop the moment that you feel your pulse quicken with anger, and do nothing until you've had some time to think, says Dr. Heitler.

Waiting a moment isn't the same as stuffing anger. "Stuffing is ignoring the problem," she says. "I'm saying stop and think, and then address the problem."

Admit that you're angry. Don't bottle up your anger; you'll feel resentful, says Renana Brooks, Ph.D., a family and clinical psychologist and director of the Sommet Institute in Washington, D.C. Don't blow up, either. That usually escalates tension and leads to more anger.

15

The ideal approach is to express anger in a reasoned way that leads to change, not to hold it in or explode. Studies suggest that people who habitually suppress or vent their anger run a greater risk of heart disease, chronic aches and pains, suppressed immunity and other health problems.

Leave the scene, mentally or physically. If you overhear your co-workers saying something nasty about you in the cafeteria, head for the women's room or the parking lot for a few minutes, suggests Dr. Brooks. If your boss criticizes you in the middle of a meeting—when you can't very well get up and leave—envision yourself leaving the room for a calmer setting.

Get perspective. Ask yourself exactly what made you angry, says Dr. Tangney. "Consider the other person's intentions, what extraneous variables might have figured into the situation at hand and what your contribution (if any) may have been." This alone may diffuse your anger.

If someone cuts you off on the highway, for instance, consider the possibility that she might be rushing home to care for a sick child, or that you might have been driving too slowly.

Speak up. After you've taken some time to get some perspective, talk it out, says Susan Heitler, Ph.D., a clinical psychologist in Denver and author of the audiotape *Conflict Resolution*. Speak calmly and choose your words carefully. Avoid statements like "You made me angry." Blaming remarks like this put the other person on the defensive, which only makes resolution more difficult.

Reason with yourself. Sometimes you can't tell the other person whom you're angry with that you're angry with her. You can't hash it out with the driver who cut you off, or with your elderly mother who is ill with Alzheimer's disease or with your temperamental boss who just chewed you out in public.

When it comes to your mother, reason may be the best balm. "Reminding yourself that she really doesn't have control over what she's saying can help diffuse the anger," says Dr. Brooks.

How can you get past your angry feelings toward your boss?

"If someone dumps on you inappropriately, it helps to realize that there's something wrong with her, and not you," says Dr. Heitler. "You may have been making some mistake, but that's not a reason for her to dump anger—she could politely inform you."

Sweat it. Since situations that anger us trigger a powerful physical reaction, getting out and moving your muscles with brisk exercise can do much to help alleviate angry feelings. When researchers at two California universities asked 308 men and women what they did to improve bad moods, the most popular answer was "Exercise."

Angina

De-cramp Your Heart Muscle

*T*he pain fleetingly brushes the left side of your jaw and disappears. A few days later, it flutters along your collarbone, then drifts down into your left arm. A month after that, it resurfaces as a pressing sensation near the center of your chest.

The problem? Angina, says your doctor. And although you're not even 50 years old—too young for heart trouble, right?—angina means that your heart is not getting enough oxygen to do its job, no matter what your age.

Angina is generally caused by one of three things, says Deborah L. Keefe, M.D., professor of medicine at Cornell Medical Center and a cardiologist at Memorial Sloan-Kettering Cancer Center, both in New York City. Angina can result from a spasm in the wall of the coronary artery that temporarily constricts the artery and cuts off the heart's blood supply for a moment or two. Or a heart wall that has been thickened by high blood pressure can demand more oxygen than the red blood cells in your blood can supply. Or a wandering blood clot can momentarily lodge in an artery that has been narrowed by a lifelong passion for eggs sunny-side up.

"Angina is rare in premenopausal women," says Dr. Keefe. When it does occur before menopause, more than likely it's caused by arterial spasm. After menopause it is more than likely caused by narrowed arteries.

Whatever your age or the cause, though, the real danger isn't angina itself but a shutdown that lasts more than a few minutes, according to Vera Bittner, M.D., associate professor of medicine at the University of Alabama School of Medicine in Birmingham. A complete shutdown in delivery of blood to the heart will lead to a full-blown heart attack.

Fortunately, "not everyone who has angina goes on to have a heart attack," says Pamela Ouyang, M.D., associate professor of medicine at Johns Hopkins University School of Medicine and a cardiologist at Johns Hopkins Bayview Medical Center, both in Baltimore. "In fact, in women angina seems less likely to lead to heart attack than in men."

WHEN TO SEE A DOCTOR

If angina lasts for 20 minutes, you should either call an ambulance or go immediately to a hospital emergency room.

Don't bother calling your doctor and waiting for a return call, she adds. If you're having a heart attack, and not angina, the faster you get medical treatment (say, with clot-busting drugs), the less likely you'll be to suffer permanent heart damage.

OXYGENATE YOUR HEART

If you have angina, your doctor will probably give you a prescription for nitroglycerin (such as Nitrostat), medication that dilates the heart's arteries, says Dr. Ouyang. Follow your doctor's directions carefully. She'll probably suggest that you take one tablet at the first twinge of pain and wait five minutes to see if the pain goes away. If it doesn't, she'll probably tell you to take a second tablet and wait another five minutes. And if that doesn't do the trick, your doctor will probably suggest that you take a third tablet.

To help relieve angina and avoid repeat episodes, doctors also recommend the following measures.

Sit down. Medication or no, your first response to angina should be to sit down and relax, says Dr. Ouyang. If you're having an arterial spasm, it will subside in a minute or two and release its grip on your artery. If clogged arteries are to blame, relief upon resting may suggest that whatever you were doing when the pain hit required more oxygen than your clogged arteries could deliver. Sitting down reduces the workload on your heart and should relieve the pain.

Target cholesterol. Following a program aimed at lowering cholesterol can also head off angina triggered by arterial spasms, says Dr. Bittner, because accumulations of cholesterol can interfere with the smooth operation of the endothelium, the lining of your blood vessels.

Leave smoking to the woodstove. Cigarette smoke sucks oxygen out of your blood and constricts blood vessels, triggering angina rooted in either arterial spasm or narrowed arteries, says Dr. Keefe. If you're not a smoker, don't start. And if you do smoke, try your best to quit.

Slim down. Carrying extra pounds exacerbates high blood pressure, and high blood pressure can exacerbate angina, says Dr. Bittner. So losing excess weight can minimize angina.

De-stress. Anything that adds to your heart's workload requires additional oxygen, which in turn can lead to angina if you are already susceptible. So any steps that you can take to help minimize stress—like delegating what you don't have time to do or learning not to overreact—can help.

Get an exercise prescription. Even though the first response to angina is rest, that doesn't mean that you should sit around when you're not actually having pain, says Dr. Bittner. Like most other muscles, the heart is a workhorse; it needs exercise to stay in shape. A well-conditioned heart uses oxygen more efficiently and is less prone to angina.

If you have angina, your cardiologist will probably order a treadmill test to determine what kind of exercise (and how much) you should get to put your heart in peak condition.

Anxiety
Dissipate Tension and Unease

As unpleasant emotions go, anxiety is the sketchiest. It's a vague, pit-of-the-stomach dread that sneaks up on you—that unease you get when your boss says that she needs to talk to you right away, when the phone rings at 4:00 A.M. or when your dentist looks into your mouth and says "Hmmmm" for the third time.

Anxiety is often confused with fear, says Sharon Greenburg, Ph.D., a clinical psychologist in private practice in Chicago. The difference is that with fear, you know what's scaring you—something specific like an angry dog or some other clear and present danger.

Anxiety is dread of the not-yet known: You don't know precisely what you'll face when you show up in the boss's office, when you pick up the ringing phone or when the dentist finishes probing your gums. But you don't expect good news.

With fear, you can take action—like staying away from angry dogs. But when anxiety is vague and hasn't been traced to a particular prob-

WHEN TO SEE A DOCTOR

If you feel intense anxiety, consult a therapist. You should also consider counseling if:
- Anxiety is interfering with your ability to work or establish and maintain relationships.
- You are always on edge or expecting the worst.

Various combinations of therapy—including behavioral, cognitive or supportive or medication, if necessary—can help relieve chronic anxiety.

lem, immediate solutions don't come to mind, and the anxiety tends to linger, says Susan Heitler, Ph.D., a clinical psychologist in Denver and author of the audiotape *Anxiety: Friend or Foe?*.

DITCH THE JITTERS

Anxiety can be harder to shake than an appliance salesman pitching an extended warranty. What's more, lingering anxiety can keep you up at night, make you irritable, undermine your ability to concentrate and either ruin your appetite or precipitate Olympian eating binges. And the constant state of readiness generated by anxiety—adrenaline pumping, heart racing, palms sweating—may contribute to high blood pressure and heart disease, says Dr. Heitler.

Odds are that you can learn to handle anxiety better, says Irene S. Vogel, Ph.D., a psychologist and director of Vogel Psychology Associates in the Washington, D.C., metropolitan area. Here's how.

Remember to breathe. When you're anxious, you tend to hold your breath or breathe too shallowly, says Dr. Greenburg. That makes you feel more anxious. Breathing slowly and deeply can have a calming effect. To make sure that you're breathing correctly, place your hand on your diaphragm, just below your rib cage. Feel it rise with each inhalation and fall with each exhalation.

Analyze and act. The antidote to anxiety is analysis and action. To rid yourself of that vague sense of dread, you have to figure out exactly what it is that you dread. Then you can map a plan of action to do something about it, says Dr. Heitler. Usually, the first step in this action plan is to find out more about the problem.

Let's say that you are anxious about your competence on the job.

Ask yourself, "What, in particular, am I afraid that I'll muff?" Maybe you're afraid that you'll get further behind and miss your deadlines. Or maybe you're worried that you're blowing it whenever you present your ideas in meetings. Are your worries founded? Have you had several near misses with deadlines? Are your suggestions routinely vetoed? If not, the anxiety is needless, says Dr. Vogel. If there is a real problem, work on a solution: Pace yourself to better meet deadlines or join a public speaking class.

Meditate. Maybe you're just high-strung. If so, meditation is worth a try. It cultivates a calmness that eases anxious feelings and offers a sense of control. A study at the University of Massachusetts found that volunteers who took an eight-week meditation course were considerably less anxious afterward.

"People who are high-strung find that they are dramatically calmer with 20 minutes of meditation in the morning and another 20 minutes after dinner," says Dr. Heitler.

If you've never done meditation, try this technique: Sit quietly in a comfortable position and take a few deep, cleansing breaths to relax your muscles. Then choose a calming word or phrase. (Experts suggest either a word or short phrase with religious significance or the word *one*.) Silently repeat the word or phrase for 20 minutes. As you find your thoughts straying, gently return your focus to your repeated word and continue to breathe deeply.

Jog, walk, swim or cycle. If you can't make time for meditation, be sure to make time for regular exercise, says Dr. Heitler. "Exercise can have the same calming effect as meditation, particularly if it's something repetitive like running or swimming laps."

Arm Flab

Firm Up the Slack

ave you been wondering if surgeons do liposuction on arms as well as thighs? And where did this arm flab come from, anyway? It certainly wasn't there when you starred on the college tennis team.

"As we age, our skin loses elastin and collagen—the connective tissues that hold everything together," says Anita Cela, M.D., clinical assistant professor of dermatology at New York Hospital–Cornell Medical Center in New York City. Elastin and collagen also keep skin flexible enough to stretch and contract through multiple pregnancies, weight gains, diets and smiles. But when your body starts to produce less collagen and elastin, your skin starts to sag. The overall result is loose, flabby skin that, under your arms, just hangs.

Sagging underarm skin also contains fat, accentuating the problem, says Debra Price, M.D., clinical assistant professor of dermatology at the University of Miami School of Medicine and a dermatologist in South Miami. Losing extra pounds is always a good idea in terms of general all-around health. But weight loss is generally not the most effective way to beat underarm flab, since no one can predict whether the fat will be taken from your hips, thighs, abdomen or under your arms. Even normal weight or underweight women can have flabby arms.

What's more, says Dr. Cela, since the skin is no longer able to snap back into shape once it has been stretched by even a few extra pounds, weight loss can actually make underarm sag even worse.

TONE AT HOME

Until someone invents control-top panty hose for arms, women bothered by jiggly skin between their armpits and elbows will have to investigate other options, like toning.

"If you can build up your biceps and triceps muscles—the biceps run along the front of your upper arm, while the triceps run along the back of it—you'll fill the empty, sagging skin with muscle, creating the illusion of firm skin," says Dr. Price.

Experts advise women who want to get rid of arm flab to try these simple exercises, some of which use light hand-held weights available at sporting goods stores.

Push forward. Sit on the floor with your knees bent, feet flat or heels resting on the floor and palms flat on the floor beside your hips with your fingers pointing forward, says Peggy Norwood-Keating, director of fitness at Duke University Diet and Fitness Center in Durham, North Carolina. Bend your elbows and lean back, supporting your upper-body weight with your arms and keeping your hands in place by your hips. Then, using your hands, press yourself forward, straightening your arms until you're sitting upright once again.

This works the triceps muscle running along the back of your upper arm, says Norwood-Keating. Do three sets of 15 repetitions twice a week.

Bend your elbows. To further build your triceps muscles, pick up a one- to three-pound dumbbell in your right hand, then sit up straight on a bench or chair, holding the weight at your right shoulder, says Norwood-Keating. Put your left hand under your right elbow to help you steady the weight-bearing arm. Then gently lift the bent arm upward from the front until your right elbow is above your right shoulder. Your arm remains bent, and your weight is behind your head. This is the starting position. Hold that position for about one second, then—leaving your left hand in place—slowly extend your right elbow and raise the weight above your right shoulder. Hold that position for another second, then slowly lower the weight back to the starting position. Repeat the exercise 12 to 15 times. That's a set.

Switch the dumbbell to your left hand and repeat the exercise. When you've finished, switch back to the right, then repeat the entire 12 to 15 repetitions a second time on the right side. Switch to the left and repeat the entire 12 to 15 repetitions a second time.

Try two to three sets of 12 to 15 repetitions twice a week, suggests Norwood-Keating. You may choose to progress to three sets or, as you become stronger and the exercise becomes easier (when you can do 15 repetitions without straining), switch to a heavier weight and decrease the number of repetitions to 8 to 10.

Arthritis

Self-Help for Joint Pain

*I*f you think that only snowy-haired grandmothers get arthritis, your vision needs revision. The same goes if you think that the first inklings of arthritis mean the beginning of the end to playing golf, cooking gourmet meals from scratch or doing everything else that you love.

"Today, women with arthritis can lead full, satisfying lives," says Teresa Brady, Ph.D., national medical adviser for the Arthritis Foundation. And Dr. Brady should know: At the age of 21, she was diagnosed with rheumatoid arthritis. But at 41, she's still enjoying an active, happy life.

WHY JOINTS FREEZE UP

Though there are more than 100 forms of arthritis, the two most prevalent are osteoarthritis and rheumatoid arthritis.

Osteoarthritis, or "wear-and-tear" arthritis, is a degenerative joint disease that usually affects people over the age of 45.

Rheumatoid arthritis is an inflammatory autoimmune disease that often occurs in people ages 30 to 40, but it occurs most frequently in people between the ages of 40 and 60. (Autoimmune means that your body turns against itself.) A disease with a decided sexual bias, rheumatoid arthritis is two to three times more common in women than men. And pregnancy can change its course: Symptoms often decrease, only to flare up again after delivery. Rheumatoid arthritis is more sinister than osteoarthritis, because it can affect virtually every tissue in the body.

HELP FOR CRICKS AND CREAKS

No matter which form of arthritis you have, women doctors offer this advice for minimizing aches, pains, swelling and stiffness.

Nuke a sockful of rice. "One of my patients swears by her home-made rice pack for warming painful joints," says Dr. Brady. "She fills a little cotton bag (about five by eight inches) with rice and heats it in the microwave oven for two minutes."

You can make your own pouch using a fluffy white tube sock right out of the package. Either way, make sure that you test the temperature of the rice pouch before placing it on your skin. Leave the pouch in place until it cools down.

Pass the peas. Heat isn't the answer for everyone, says Dr. Brady. "Many women prefer using heat for pain, but some find cold more comfortable." When pain flares up, grab a bag of frozen peas. "Drape the bag around the joint to ease pain and swelling."

Cream yourself with hot pepper. "Applying capsaicin cream, made with the active ingredient from hot peppers, can ease arthritis pain," says Geraldine M. McCarthy, M.D., assistant professor of medicine in the Division of Rheumatology at the Medical College of Wisconsin in Milwaukee. "In our study, people applied a 0.075 percent capsaicin cream four times a day with good results. There is a 2.5 percent cream available that may work more quickly.

"Capsaicin has an effect on substance P, which nerve endings release to mediate pain," adds Dr. McCarthy. Capsaicin cream doesn't work instantly; regular applications are the key. Also, the cream burns, but this side effect diminishes over time. You can buy capsaicin cream in drugstores.

Support swollen wrists. Splinting a joint with a simple store-bought wrist splint can ease pain, says Mary Moore, M.D., director of the Ein-

WHAT WOMEN DOCTORS DO

A Daily Bike Ride

Teresa Brady, Ph.D.

The Arthritis Foundation's national medical adviser, Teresa Brady, Ph.D., has had rheumatoid arthritis for 20 years. Here's how she takes care of herself.

"For me, feeling good means following a daily routine. I take my medication regularly. (It's easy to forget, and then you start hurting.) I wear wrist splints to bed at night. I loosen morning stiffness in a long, hot shower. And I ride my exercise bike daily, even when I don't feel like it.

"When I really don't feel like riding my bike, I tell myself that I only have to ride for two minutes. That gets me over the hump of starting—and once I've started, I'm usually able to keep on going for a complete workout."

WHEN TO SEE A DOCTOR

Women doctors say that the key to living well with any form of arthritis is getting an early, accurate diagnosis.

"If you have arthritis, your doctor can refer you to a physical therapist right away," says Nadine M. Fisher, Ed.D., assistant professor of rehabilitation medicine at the State University of New York at Buffalo School of Medicine and Biomedical Sciences. "Getting therapy early helps you head off the pain that can reduce your activity level—and the quality of your life."

stein-Moss Arthritis Center and professor of medicine and rheumatology at Temple University School of Medicine in Philadelphia. "Sleeping with flexed wrists causes wrist pain. To keep your wrists from curling as you sleep, wear wrist splints sold at drug and department stores."

Go to bed gloved. "If you wake with stiff, swollen hands, it's because body fluids resettle at night, causing swelling in fingers that may already be swollen," says Dr. Moore. "To reduce swelling—and pain—get a snug-fitting pair of stretch gloves like Isotoners and wear them to bed."

Lubricate for lovemaking. "Sex can be painful for some women who have arthritis," says Leslie Schover, Ph.D., staff psychologist at the Center for Sexual Function at the Cleveland Clinic Foundation. "Some kinds of arthritis cause vaginal dryness. Get Replens—a vaginal moisturizer available over the counter—follow the directions and use it regularly as suggested."

ANOTHER VITAL INGREDIENT

Women doctors agree that to get the best of arthritis, some type of exercise is, well, just what the doctor ordered.

"You want to strengthen the muscles that support the joints," says Nadine M. Fisher, Ed.D., assistant professor of rehabilitation medicine at the State University of New York at Buffalo School of Medicine and Biomedical Sciences. "If arthritis affects your knees, walking up or down stairs may be painfully hard. If you strengthen your knee muscles, then those stairs won't be so hard to manage."

Take an indoor ski trip. "The ideal exercise program should combine range-of-motion exercises with aerobics," says Dr. Brady. For example, a cross-country ski machine accomplishes both. "The gliding lower-body motion of cross-country skiing is good for knee and hip problems. Take it easy if you have wrist pain, though—pressure from the poling motion may hurt if you have arthritis in your hands and wrists."

Everyone, into the pool! If you have access to a pool—especially a heated indoor pool—count yourself lucky. "Water exercise benefits almost everyone with arthritis," says Dr. Brady.

Ride a bike. "Riding an exercise bike for 20 to 30 minutes three times a week improves function and reduces pain," says Bevra H. Hahn, M.D., chief of rheumatology in the Department of Medicine at the University of California, Los Angeles, UCLA School of Medicine. If you're not the most coordinated person on Earth, or if you're afraid of crashing or getting lost out on the road, a stationary bike is perfect.

Asthma
Tame Twitchy Airways

Some women describe asthma as feeling like they're trying to breathe through a straw. The description fits perfectly, because during an attack, airways in the lungs squeeze shut, making it difficult to draw in air. At the same time, the narrowed airways become inflamed and filled with mucus, stifling the airways still further.

A family history of asthma and exposure to viruses or allergens set the stage for asthma, says Sally Wenzel, M.D., associate professor at the University of Colorado School of Medicine and a pulmonary specialist at the National Jewish Center for Immunology and Respiratory Medicine, both in Denver. "Men are just as likely to develop asthma as women," says Dr. Wenzel, "although women seem to react to irritants at lower concentrations."

Asthma can be serious—even fatal. Experts speculate that the people who succumb to asthma tend to smoke cigarettes, abuse drugs and misuse their asthma medications. But if you take care of yourself, asthma isn't cause for alarm.

WHEN TO SEE A DOCTOR

If you're having attacks more easily than in the past, if your attacks seem more severe than usual or if you're waking up at night with attacks more than twice a week, it means that your asthma is no longer under control. See your doctor as soon as possible. She may need to adjust your medication.

"Women who get proper medical care, stop smoking and use their medications correctly are unlikely to die from asthma," says Susan Pingleton, M.D., director of the Pulmonary and Critical Care Division at the University of Kansas Medical Center in Kansas City.

SELF-RESCUE FOR ASTHMA ATTACKS

Here is what doctors recommend that people with asthma do for themselves—starting with knowing how to use their medicine correctly.

Mark quick-action inhalers "rescue medicine." Most people being treated for asthma use two different kinds of prescription inhalant drugs: long-acting and short-acting, says Dr. Wenzel. If you're having an attack, you should use *only* a short-acting drug such as albuterol (Proventil), metaproterenol (Ventolin) or pirbuterol (Maxair) and others. These drugs kick in almost immediately.

The long-acting drug salmeterol (Serevent) can take 20 to 30 minutes to work—that's long enough to die from an asthma attack, says Dr. Wenzel. According to the U.S. Food and Drug Administration, up to 20 deaths have been associated with inappropriate use of this drug.

Don't leave home without it. You should have a fast-acting inhaler with you at all times—at home, in your purse, in your pocket, in your car—anywhere you could have an attack. "It doesn't do any good if it's not right there when you need it," Dr. Wenzel says.

Ask for a spacer. For most people it's easier to get the medicine where it needs to go—deep into your lungs—by using a metered-dose inhaler with a holding chamber, also called a spacer.

This is a tubelike device that you attach to the inhaler. Sprayed medicine goes first into this chamber, allowing you to then inhale it slowly over a period of five seconds, says Dr. Wenzel. If you inhale the medicine too quickly, it hits the back of your throat and sticks there. Spacers also reduce medication side effects such as tremors or shakes.

DAY-TO-DAY CONTROL MEASURES

Once you have an attack under control, women doctors say that it's a good idea to take steps to prevent future episodes. To defend yourself on all fronts, heed these recommendations.

Max out on magnesium. This essential mineral helps relax the smooth muscles that line airways. In a study by British researchers, people who were getting the most magnesium from foods were the least likely to have wheezing and supersensitive airways.

Choose whole grains, beans, nuts and seeds as your best magnesium sources. Some women may still need to take magnesium supplements to reach the Daily Value of 400 milligrams, says Nan Kathryn Fuchs, Ph.D., a nutritionist in Sebastopal, California, and nutrition editor of the *Women's Health Letter*.

Consider antioxidant protection. Vitamins C and E, the trace mineral selenium and beta-carotene, a pigment found in orange and dark-green leafy vegetables, all seem to offer some protection to sensitive lungs.

"I always tell people first to start eating better, with lots of fresh fruits and vegetables, whole grains and beans, and then to add nutritional supplements as necessary," says Dr. Fuchs. You may want to consider consuming 1,000 to 2,000 milligrams of vitamin C, 400 international units of vitamin E and up to 200 micrograms of selenium a day through diet and supplements, she suggests. (Vitamin C levels above 1,200 milligrams daily may cause diarrhea in some people.)

Declare war on insects. Two kinds of bugs—dust mites and cockroaches—are well-known asthma aggravators, says Marianne Frieri, M.D., Ph.D., associate professor of medicine and pathology at the State University of New York at Stony Brook and director of the Allergy Immunology Training Program at Nassau County Medical Center in East Meadow, New York. "People actually inhale microscopic cockroach parts and dust mite feces, which sets off attacks."

It's impossible to get rid of dust mites, which are in every house and are kicked up through normal household activity. So minimize their presence by encasing mattresses and pillows in plastic covers and washing your bed linens frequently in hot water.

Banishing cockroaches can be a real hassle, too, as any urban dweller can attest. Get in a professional exterminator, Dr. Frieri advises, and then, be obsessive about putting food away. Keep food in bug-proof tins or the refrigerator, clean up crumbs immediately and never leave cat or dog food out. Fix leaks so that there are no damp spots in your house, since mites require high humidity to live.

Stop the acid. The same backflow of stomach acid into the esophagus that causes heartburn can bring on asthma, especially if you're lying down, experts say.

"People who do a lot of coughing at night are most likely to have this problem," Dr. Wenzel says. This is most likely to be an asthma trigger in adult nonsmokers with no history of lung disease or allergies. "We can do tests to determine the extent of their reflux and see if it correlates with symptoms they are having."

To avoid acid-induced asthma, you can take acid-suppressing drugs (such as Pepcid AC), forgo late-night foraging and shed excess weight, Dr. Wenzel says.

Relax with massage. In one study people with asthma who got weekly 15-minute upper body massages reported drops in chest tightness, wheezing, pain and fatigue. "Massage may make you more aware of the stress in your life, and awareness is, for most people, the first step toward reducing stress," explains Mary Malinski, R.N., of Allergy Associates in Portland, Oregon, and a licensed massage therapist. "Stress often makes asthma symptoms worse."

Breathe better with yoga. Try exhaling for twice as long as you inhale. This is a yoga breathing technique, and in one experiment, it helped reduce the number of attacks in people with asthma.

To do this easily, breathe in normally, then exhale normally, but as you come to what seems like the end of your exhalation, continue for a bit longer without forcing out the breath, says Mary Pullig Schatz, M.D., a pathologist in Nashville, a yoga instructor and author of *Back Care Basics*.

Turn off the fireplace. As cozy as fireplaces and woodstoves may be, they spew pollutants into indoor air. "If you're having trouble controlling your asthma, you're better off not using either of these in your house," Dr. Frieri says.

Cover up to avoid cold. Sucking in cold, dry air can set off twitchy lungs. So wrap a scarf around your mouth and nose to help warm the air before you inhale, suggests Dr. Frieri.

Because people with asthma are accustomed to feeling winded, they don't always recognize when they are having serious breathing problems. So these days, doctors have their patients measure the amount of air that their lungs can blow out—in the morning, at night and before and after they use their short-acting inhalers. They use a simple tubelike device, called a peak flow meter, that measures exhaled air.

"National guidelines on asthma recommend that if your airflow falls below 80 percent of your peak flow, you may need to take an additional dose of a short-acting inhaler and call your doctor," Dr. Wenzel says. Airflow below 50 percent of your peak flow usually warrants a prompt trip to the emergency room.

If you have noticed your symptoms worsening soon after you start taking a new drug or after increasing the dosage of a drug, check with your doctor about a possible connection, says Dr. Wenzel. Aspirin, ibuprofen and other nonsteroidal anti-inflammatory medications—both prescription and over-the-counter—and beta-blockers (used to control high blood pressure) can aggravate asthma, says Dr. Frieri.

Athlete's Foot
Stop the Infernal Itching

*D*on't make the mistake of thinking that athlete's foot is some sweaty, smelly guy problem. The fungi that cause trouble (there are about six of them) are equal-opportunity organisms whose idea of a great place to hang out is in the damp skin between toes and on the bottom and sides of feet, male or female. Worse yet, these fungi can get around and possibly give you—surprise!—a vaginal infection, says Teresa G. Conroy, D.P.M., a podiatrist in private practice in Philadelphia. Taking a bath instead of a shower can increase your risk of developing this problem.

FIRST, TACKLE THE FEET

Women pick up athlete's foot the same way men do: in swimming pools, locker rooms and showers—even in their own bathrooms if a family member has it. The unsightly white flakes, cracked and peeling skin and stubborn itch can drive you crazy. So athlete or not, you'll want relief. And that calls for an all-out effort—to eradicate the fungus on your feet and banish it from your footwear and house, permanently. Here's what to do.

WHEN TO SEE A DOCTOR

If you've done everything by the book, but your feet still itch and burn after 10 to 14 days of at-home treatment, see a podiatrist (a doctor specializing in foot care) or your family physician.

A skin culture can determine the type of fungus and the proper antifungal medication to use. Or you may not have a fungus at all, but a bacterial infection that can only be beat with an antibiotic cream. Sometimes, say doctors, allergic skin reactions are mistaken for athlete's foot.

Powder up and dry out. Athlete's foot fungi can't survive without moisture, so the best thing that you can do is keep your feet desert-dry, says Cheryl Weiner, D.P.M., a podiatrist in Columbus, Ohio, and president of the American Association for Women Podiatrists. She recommends an over-the-counter medicated powder—Zeasorb-AF—applied twice daily directly to your feet. "This is the most absorbent foot powder available without a prescription."

Cream the germs and don't quit. Used properly, over-the-counter fungus-killing creams such as tolnaftate (Aftate or Tinactin) and miconazole nitrate (in Micatin products) can work, says Dr. Weiner.

"Most people stop using a cream as soon as all the white, flaky areas on their feet clear up," she says. "But to permanently eradicate fungus, you must continue using the cream for 50 percent longer than it took to clear up the problem." If it takes a month to knock out an entrenched fungus, for example, use the cream faithfully for an additional two weeks to really get the last of it.

The drier, the better. Fungus-ridden feet may crack, peel and look dry. But you'll want to avoid using moisturizing creams or petroleum jelly on your feet, since these products trap moisture and can actually promote fungus growth, says Dr. Weiner. Stick with antifungal creams.

Wear cotton when you can. "When it comes to the proliferation of athlete's foot, nylon panty hose are the biggest offenders," says Dr. Weiner. "Wear cotton socks or all-cotton tights instead."

Nylon seals moisture in, while cotton absorbs it. If your job dictates that you wear stockings and pumps during work hours, Dr. Weiner suggests wearing cotton socks instead of stockings to and from work.

Or buy polypro socks and tights. Wicking fibers—polypropylene, Capilene and the like—that draw moisture away from the skin and release it into the air also keep the feet dry, even more so than cotton, says Phyllis Ragley, D.P.M., vice president of the American Academy of Podiatric Sports Medicine who practices in Lawrence, Kansas. "And unlike cotton, these fabrics air-dry quickly." Look for polypropylene socks and other foot-friendly fiber socks at sporting goods stores.

Change your socks. It's important to change your socks once a day, says Dr. Conroy. Otherwise, you re-expose your feet to trapped moisture and fungus.

Wash socks with disinfectant. When laundering socks and hose, add a capful of liquid Lysol disinfectant to the final rinse to help destroy fungus, says Dr. Conroy. Or soak them in a disinfectant solution for a few minutes before drying them.

Crank up the heat. Drying your socks on a hot setting will also help destroy fungus, says Dr. Conroy.

Socks first, then undies. Antifungal strategies don't stop with your socks. "If your feet are actively infected, pulling your undies on over your bare feet is a sure way to transfer the fungus to your groin," says Dr. Conroy. Avoid this potentially maddening problem by getting dressed socks-first. If you wear pantyhose: (1) Shield your feet with socks, (2) pull on your panties, (3) remove the socks and (4) put on your hose.

Fumigate your footwear. The same fungi that enjoy nibbling away at your tootsies also find refuge in your footwear. The best way to destroy them, once and for all? Blast the insides of your shoes with a disinfectant spray, such as Lysol, Dr. Conroy says. Let your shoes dry overnight before wearing them. If you have an active infection, do this every day with whatever shoes you wear. Don't forget to treat your bedroom slippers, too.

Air out your shoes. "If it's a nice sunny day, I tell people to loosen the laces and put their shoes out to air-dry," Dr. Conroy says.

If it's not a sunny day, stuff your shoes with newspaper, which will absorb moisture, and let them dry indoors, says Dr. Weiner. She also recommends alternating shoes so that at no time would you be wearing wet ones.

Back Pain

Advice for Desk Workers, Moms and Others

*W*omen and men suffer from about the same amount of back pain, but while men most often get long-lasting back pain from lifting too much, women often ache from sitting too much.

"The second highest incidence of back pain is reported by sedentary workers, most of whom are women who sit at desks—often in front of computers all day," says Sheila Reid, P.T., coordinator of rehabilitation services at The Spine Institute of New England in Williston, Vermont.

Most commonly, people suffer from lower-back pain, which is generally caused by straining or spraining muscles and tissues that connect bones and cartilage. A sudden action in which you use muscles that are tired or out of condition is particularly likely to cause sudden pain.

Childbearing and child rearing also put a heavy load on women's backs, say women doctors. During the last two trimesters of pregnancy, the fetus literally can shift the center of gravity of your back, increasing the curve of your spine, so that your back may really hurt, says Deborah Caplan, P.T., a teacher of the Alexander Technique for posture and back pain in New York. Afterward, it can get worse.

"Soon after pregnancy and when children are toddlers, women experience back pain from bending and lifting," says Caplan. Women have two-thirds the muscle mass of men who are otherwise the same size as they are, says Rose Hayes, Ph.D., an ergonomist (specializing in the study of technology design and people's needs) for the United States Postal Service. "They need more muscle power to do the same work."

While most women would think carefully before lifting a 50-pound weight in a gym, they think nothing of picking up a toddler and a 10-pound bag of groceries while still carrying a briefcase crammed with books and papers, says Dr. Hayes. And that can cause back-muscle strain.

SUFFER NO MORE

If your doctor has confirmed that what you're experiencing is from muscle spasms or chronic lower-back ache, and not a herniated disk, you'll be relieved to hear that there's plenty you can do.

Yoga Works

Judith Lasater, P.T., Ph.D.

As a yoga instructor and physical therapist in San Francisco, Judith Lasater, P.T., Ph.D., says that she twists her body into all kinds of unusual positions and always feels fine. Here's what the author of Relax and Renew: Restful Yoga for Stressful Times *has to say.*

"Yoga not only works to stretch and strengthen muscles, but it can also help women be aware of their bodies and emotions. It can help you lessen back pain by making you aware of what brings it on," she says.

Other remedies for back pain include hot-water bottles, ice or a heating pad applied to the side of pain; gentle stretching; and sitting with a pillow supporting the small of your back. To prevent back pain at work, move around every half-hour.

Stay calm. Most lower-back pain goes away within a few days or a week, even if you do nothing, says Mary Ann Keenan, M.D., chairman of the Department of Orthopedic Surgery at Albert Einstein Medical Center in Philadelphia. Take a deep breath and calm down as much as you can. It'll help ease the distress, and it may speed your healing.

Take the day off. If your back hurts, you won't feel up to doing much of anything. So don't try. Go to bed and give yourself some much needed respite, says Carol Walker, M.D., an orthopedic surgeon in private practice in Atlanta.

Rest for a day or two, but no more. Too much rest, however, can do more harm than good, say back care experts. "Even if you don't feel A-OK, you need to get active within a day or so," says Dr. Walker. "If you stay in bed for longer than two days, your circulation will slow down, your muscles and joints will stiffen and you'll actually increase your chances of another back injury."

Turn on the heat. To soothe the ache, apply a hot-water bottle or heating pad to the site of the pain, says Reid.

Or ice it. "Sometimes women find that ice is the best way to relieve inflammation," Dr. Walker says. Put an ice pack on the site of the pain for five to ten minutes at a time—say, every hour—for a day or so.

Go OTC. Any over-the-counter pain reliever containing aspirin, ibuprofen, acetaminophen or ketoprofen can ease back pain, says Dr. Walker.

Try gentle stretches. "Gentle stretches can actually help you heal more quickly," says Dr. Walker.

While lying down, try bringing up your knees to your chest, suggests Reid. Then, put a little pressure on your knees. Stretch, then relax. Repeat a few times unless you feel pain. If you do, stop.

Stop smoking. If you smoke, quit. Studies have shown that people who don't smoke are more likely to experience long-lasting relief from back pain, including less persistent problems overall than those who do smoke, says Carol Hartigan, M.D., a physiatrist who specializes in spine rehabilitation at the Boston Back Center of New England Baptist Hospital and the New England Spine Center, also in Boston. What's more, smoking makes the disks in your back age faster and stiffen up, because it keeps oxygen and blood from getting to your back, says Dr. Walker.

FOR PREGNANT OR NURSING WOMEN

Back pain is a common complaint among pregnant women and new mothers. Here's what to do.

Ask your obstetrician for an exercise prescription. Exercise is key to supporting your back, says Dr. Walker. "The stronger your muscles,

---

WHAT WOMEN DOCTORS DO

Comfortable Clothes = Less Pain

Barbara A. Stuart, M.D.

After spending long days as medical director of a family planning and sexually transmitted diseases clinic in Bremerton, Washington, Barbara Stuart, M.D., noticed that bending forward all day to examine patients put a strain on her lower back. Here's how she solved the problem.

"I bought a slew of loose slacks and comfortable below-the-knee dresses to wear to work," she says. "That way, when I need to examine a patient, I don't have to worry about keeping my knees together, and I can pull my office stool right up to the patient. The closer to my patients that I sit, the less I have to bend forward, lessening the strain on my back."

The lesson for women in other professions: Get close to your work—your back will thank you. And wear low heels. Anything higher than 1½ inches is hard on your back.

the more likely they'll be able to support the weight of the fetus," Dr. Walker says. Walk, run, swim—any aerobic exercise that you can do as often as is comfortable—can help your back.

Support your back. When you're nursing, put pillows behind your back for comfort and bring your baby to your breast rather than strain your back by bending over your infant, says Caplan. "If you're nursing in a chair, make sure that it's a chair with good back support."

Use a glider. To help your back while nursing, try a gliding or platform rocker with arm support—available from the same store where you bought your baby's crib. "It will take the pressure off your back and let your arms rest while you nurse your baby," says Dr. Hartigan.

Use a footrest. While you're shopping, pick up a small footstool to use at home. Propping up your feet gives them a rest and keeps your back in a comfortable, supported position, says Dr. Hartigan.

BACK CARE AT HOME AND AT WORK

Once you've had an episode of back pain, chances are that it's not an experience that you would care to repeat. Here's what women doctors say that you can and should do to protect your back against future attacks.

Stay close to your loads. Think about it: The closer you stand to whatever you're picking up—be it a child, a bag of groceries or a box of office supplies—the less strain you put on your muscles, says Dr. Hayes. Here's the right technique.

Beginning in a standing position, squat from your knees rather than bending from the waist to pick up the load. Plant your feet firmly in front of you, one foot slightly ahead.

Once you have your arms around it, keep the load as close to your abdomen as possible while lifting and lowering. And use both hands so that you lift symmetrically.

Lift first, turn second. It seems natural: You grab a bag of groceries and turn to load them into the car—or lift an infant up and out of a crib—in one quick movement. Don't do it, says Dr. Hayes. Over time, twisting can lead to herniated disks. Instead, lift your load, hold it close to your abdomen, and *then* turn, using your feet to get you where you want to go instead of swiveling your hips.

Wear free-flowing clothing. "If you need to lift things, wearing long, full skirts or roomy slacks gives you much more freedom of movement than tights skirts that cram your knees together," says Caplan.

Wheel your belongings. Briefcases are heavy. So are big purses slung on shoulder straps. "Dangling from one shoulder, those big loads

WHEN TO SEE A DOCTOR

If back pain lasts a week or more, or if pain strikes intermittently every day, see a doctor, says Carol Walker, M.D., an orthopedic surgeon in private practice in Atlanta. And see your doctor immediately if you experience pain radiating down your leg, or if your leg feels weak or numb.

create an unequal stress on your spine, which can hurt your back," Dr. Hayes says.

Just carry the minimum in a purse, she says. For the rest of your belongings, try switching to a fanny pack or backpack or cart your belongings in a suitcase on wheels, as do many travelers and flight attendants, says Dr. Keenan.

Or buy a luggage cart (a lightweight metal frame with wheels) from a discount store.

Adjust your work station. "A good chair should be fully adjustable and fit the person who sits in it as well as the tasks that she performs," says Annie Pivarski, ergonomics and injury prevention program supervisor at Saint Francis Memorial Hospital in San Francisco.

To get the best back support, your feet should be flat on the floor and your lower back supported by the back of the chair. Your knees should be slightly lower than your hips or level with them, and you shouldn't have to crane to see your computer, says Reid.

Move around. Every half hour, move around to keep your muscles and spine from stiffening, says Reid.

Try a lumbar pillow. Buy one at a medical supply store or just roll up a towel behind your waist for greater lower-back support while you sit at your desk, says Caplan.

Wear low heels. Low-heeled shoes can sometimes help with arch support, but more than 1½ inches will misalign the curvature of your back, which can lead to back pain, Dr. Walker says. If you must wear heels, save them for special occasions.

(For practical ways to prevent osteoporosis, another possible cause of back pain, see page 407.)

Bad Breath
Help for Stubborn Halitosis

Even women who aren't normally concerned about their breath worry when they reach for a wedge of garlic bread, a dollop of onion dip or a helping of their favorite curry.

Contrary to what you might think, popping a breath mint or swishing mouthwash may not always be the best answer. Used too often—several times a day—mints and rinses mask the problem and don't get to the cause, says Mahvash Navazesh, D.M.D., associate professor and vice-chair in the Department of Dental Medicine and Public Health at the University of Southern California School of Dentistry in Los Angeles.

Just as you would hunt for the source of an odor in your kitchen, your best bet is to figure out what's causing your bad breath, Dr. Navazesh advises. Smoking and drinking alcohol are common—but obvious—causes.

Researchers have always suspected that the true culprit behind ordinary bad breath may live on your tongue. This hypothesis gained support in a study by Erika H. DeBoever, D.D.S., conducted at the Department of Biologic Materials Sciences at the University of Michigan in Ann Arbor. Dr. DeBoever studied 16 men and women with bad breath, most of whom had already tried regular mouthwash, mints and gum. She found that the problem was most noticeable in those whose tongues were naturally coated with a film of bacteria and whose tongues also contained deep fissures in which organisms could hide.

SCIENCE AND FOLK REMEDIES BOTH WORK

If you have bad breath more than just occasionally and you don't smoke, and your doctor has ruled out an underlying medical cause, such as gastrointestinal upset, medications, gum disease, infected or decayed teeth or a respiratory tract infection, try these tactics suggested by women doctors.

Start with the basics. Occasional use of odor-masking rinses can help, but it's also important for women to pay strict attention to good dental hygiene, says Geraldine Morrow, D.M.D., past president of the

WHEN TO SEE A DOCTOR

Since bad breath can arise from a variety of causes—some minor and some serious—you should schedule an appointment with a dentist if the problem isn't resolved with home care in a few weeks.

American Dental Association, a member of the American Association of Women Dentists and a dentist in Anchorage, Alaska. Start by brushing and flossing your teeth and scrubbing your tongue.

Brush with mouth rinse. A study by Dr. DeBoever found that people who brushed their tongues and rinsed with mouth rinse after breakfast and before going to bed reduced foul mouth odor. Specifically, people in the study followed these steps: They brushed their teeth with a toothpaste of their choice. Then they dipped their toothbrushes in a mouth rinse with 0.12 percent chlorhexidine gluconate (such as Peridex, a mouth rinse made by Proctor and Gamble) and brushed their tongues. Then they rinsed for 60 seconds with the same rinse. Last, they refrained from eating, drinking or rinsing with water for at least a half hour.

When the men and women in Dr. DeBoever's study followed this ritual for seven days, the suspect organisms in their mouths were significantly reduced, and so was their bad breath.

Switch to a rubber-tipped brush. Use a toothbrush with a rubber pick on the end to do a little housecleaning when you say "ah," says Penelope Shar, M.D., an internist in private practice in Bangor, Maine. Food can gather not only in your teeth and gums but also in hidden folds near your tonsils—"anywhere in the little pockets in the back of your mouth," she says. Left there, it can cause bad breath. A Water Pik–type device works, too.

Snack on a sprig. For basic food-related odors, munching on some parsley—a folk remedy of sorts—really does clear the air, says Dr. Shar.

Make water your after-dinner drink. Merely swishing your mouth with good old H_2O will freshen your mouth after a meal or a coffee break. As an added bonus, it also helps remove plaque—the sticky buildup of bacteria and tartar that leads to tooth decay, gum disease and bad breath, says Dr. Navazesh.

Bad Hair Days
Tame the Tress Mess

*Y*ou know the feeling: Up until yesterday, your hair looked fine. Well-behaved, no big surprises. Today, your formerly poufed hair is flat. Or boinking out in new directions. Or so staticky that you're afraid you'll electrocute yourself if you touch it.

You're having a classic bad hair day, and your knee-jerk reaction is to dunk your head in a bucket of water and start over. What happened?

WHEN GOOD HAIR GOES BAD

Your environment—internal and external—can affect the way your hair looks. So can using too many hair-styling products.

Whatever the cause, here are some instant ways to fix various causes of bad hair, recommended by hair-care experts from Los Angeles to New York.

Soak your head. Dunking your head in the sink might not be a bad idea, says Yohini Appa, Ph.D., director of product efficacy at the Neutrogena Corporation in Los Angeles.

"More often than not, bad hair is caused by residue left by various products," explains Dr. Appa. Leave-in conditioners, styling gels and hair sunscreens all leave a residue on hair that builds up and eventually causes it to do something other than what you intend. Use a clarifying shampoo—a mild cleansing shampoo with no conditioners—to strip all the gunk from your hair. Lather and rinse thoroughly.

Condition it. Follow shampooing with a lightweight conditioner that's intended to detangle hair, says Dr. Appa. Look for one that's labeled "detangling conditioner" and follow the label directions. This type of conditioner is designed to keep hair smooth and shiny without leaving a heavy residue.

Go for the gel. If your hair is limp and flat, a small dab of gel can give it a lift, says Elizabeth Hartley, the West Coast creative director for Vidal Sassoon in San Francisco. When your hair is still damp, smear a dime-size dollop of gel into your hand, rub your hands together, then lean over from your waist and flip your hair forward. Smudge the gel through your roots. Stand up, flip your hair back, shake your hair and forget it. You should have all the volume you need.

Moisten ends only. If your hair tends to be a little dry on the ends, squeeze a half-teaspoon of a leave-in moisturizer on your hands, Hartley adds. Then smudge it through your hair from mid-shaft to the ends of each strand. Shake or comb your hair into place and be on your way.

Fix frizzies. If humidity gives short or medium hair a bad case of the frizzies, tame it with styling gel and protective moisturizer, such as a spray-on, leave-in conditioner, says Liz Cunnane, a consultant trichologist (a hair-care specialist) at Philip Kingsley Trichological Centre in New York City. Shampoo and condition first, towel dry, then put a teaspoon of gel in your palm, rub your hands together and work the gel through your hair. Apply the moisturizer, style as usual and go.

Snip and trim. When frizzies are caused by a perm gone bad, the only remedy is a trim, says Rebecca Caserio, M.D., clinical associate professor of dermatology at the University of Pittsburgh.

Spray, roll, then blow-dry. To tame staticky, flyaway hair, spray a thermal styling conditioner such as HeatSafe on your hair after shampooing and conditioning with your regular daily products, says Dr. Appa. HeatSafe has four different moisturizers that penetrate the surface of each hair, allowing you to style, condition and protect your hair as you dry it. You can find HeatSafe in most drugstores.

Then pop a few Velcro rollers into your hair and use your dryer on its lowest setting to set the curl. Or simply blow-dry, without rollers. To prevent damaging your hair, hold the dryer at least 6 to 12 inches away from your head, says Dr. Appa. Let your hair cool, then style as necessary.

Curl with steam. If your normally wavy or curly hair has lost its bounce, a curling iron can help, says Dr. Caserio. Before curling, cool the iron by curling it around a wet towel. The result is a cooler treatment less likely to cause split ends.

Plug in your hot rollers. You can bring almost any hair under control by applying a thermal styling conditioner and using a set of electrically heated hair rollers, says Wendy Resin, hair-care manager at Neutrogena. Wash and condition as usual, spray in the thermal styling conditioner, then roll your hair. Wait ten minutes, remove the rollers, let your hair cool, then style as usual.

Get it shaped. For preventing bad hair days, nothing beats a great haircut, says Hartley. The cut is the foundation of every style. A professional stylist can structure your hair into a shape that will emphasize your hair's strengths—texture, line, color and shine, for instance—to prevent many of the problems that trigger bad hair days.

Baggy Knees
A Lift-and-Shape Routine

*B*aggy panty hose are easily remedied: Pull them up or buy a new pair. Baggy knees are another matter. Who wants to walk around looking as though the skin around your knees is one size too big, saggy and wrinkled like an elephant instead of smooth and taut like a French dinner roll? Yet as years pass, the skin over your knees can start to look like it needs a face-lift.

Why does the skin sag?

Baggy knees are caused by the natural reduction of two supporting substances in the skin as you age—collagen and elastin, says Anita Cela, M.D., clinical assistant professor of dermatology at New York Hospital–Cornell Medical Center in New York City.

WORK YOUR KNEES—GENTLY

Once your skin's natural elasticity starts to fade, there's no way skin can regain its ability to snap back into shape. Luckily, say women doctors, you can firm up the neighboring muscles—namely, the four quadriceps that form the front of your thigh—to tone the skin around the knees and improve their appearance.

"Exercise makes a big difference," says Dr. Cela. Here's how to get started.

Do shallow knee bends. Use squats to build up the quadriceps muscle that runs along the front of your thigh above the knee, says Peggy Norwood-Keating, director of fitness at Duke University Diet and Fitness Center in Durham, North Carolina. Properly developed, the quadriceps can fill out the sagging skin that leads to baggy knees.

To begin the exercise, stand up straight and hold on to the back of a chair directly in front of you, says Norwood-Keating. It's helpful if you can work with a full-length mirror, so that you can study your movements and make sure that you're doing the exercise correctly. Now, bend your knees and move your rear end away from your body as though you were about to sit down. Look in the mirror—if you have one—to make sure that your knees are directly in line with—that is, directly above—your ankles or the tops of your feet. Do not allow your knees to move

43

forward past your toes, as this defeats the exercise and can hurt your knees, says Norwood-Keating.

Squat down as far as you can, but—keeping an eye on your body in the mirror—don't let the angle formed by your lower legs and thighs exceed 90 degrees, says Norwood-Keating. Then, again watching your body in the mirror to keep your knees and ankles aligned, slowly stand up straight. Again, look down to see that your knees are over your feet and not pointing inward or outward.

Begin with two sets of 12 to 15 squats each (or less if this is too difficult at first), she suggests. When the squats begin to get easy, add a third set.

Put some weight into it. When the third set of squats seems easy, begin trying to let go of the chair and balance on your own, suggests Norwood-Keating. When you can squat unassisted, hold a pair of three- to five-pound dumbbells in each hand down by your sides. Then add two or three pounds each time the squats become easy once again.

If you do this exercise two to three times a week, you'll not only keep the skin over your knees nice and tight, you'll also be bouncing out of chairs at age 80 the way you did at 20.

Tuck some sunscreen in your golf bag. Since ultraviolet rays from the sun can speed destruction of elastin in the skin, Dr. Cela strongly encourages women to wear a sun protection factor, or SPF, 25 sunscreen on their legs when wearing shorts or a bathing suit, to prevent further sagging around the knees. Apply (and reapply) regularly, according to package instructions.

Bags under the Eyes
Vanquish Permanent Puffiness

Women and women doctors alike often talk about puffy eyes and baggy eyes interchangeably. But there is a difference. Puffy eyes primarily stem from fluid retention—they're temporary. Bags under the eyes develop over the years, as fat accumulates in the eye area.

Not everyone develops baggy eyes. But unfortunately, once bags form, there's no diet or workout to reduce them.

MINIMIZATION TACTIC

"Short of cosmetic surgery, there's not much that you can do about bags under your eyes," says Marianne O'Donoghue, M.D., associate professor of dermatology at Rush-Presbyterian–St. Luke's Medical Center in Chicago, except the following:

Pat on concealer. A concealer is more opaque than a foundation and meant to be used sparingly, says Fatima Olive, product developer for Aveda Corporation, a cosmetics and health products manufacturer in Blaine, Minnesota. For best results select a concealer that's just one tone lighter than your foundation. Or, if you're wearing concealer alone, match the concealer to your shade of skin. Since baggy skin tends to be darker, you want to blend it correctly, says Olive.

Using an eyeliner brush, apply concealer to the dark areas, then blend with your pinky finger, patting very lightly. Finish with foundation and with light powder, or powder alone, to set the concealer.

Bee Stings
Ease the Zing from Winged Things

*W*hether you've been stung by a honeybee, hornet, wasp or yellow jacket (or bitten by a fire ant, which also belongs to the same venomous class of insects), in most cases the symptoms are pretty much the same: pain, redness, swelling and itching at the site.

Bee stings smart because the bee has injected venom into your skin. Only females sting, by the way, says insect expert May R. Berenbaum, Ph.D., head of the Department of Entomology at the University of Illinois at Urbana-Champaign.

KAMIKAZE ATTACKS

The honeybee is the only one of these critters who commits suicide when she stings. That's because her stinger is barbed, and she can't extract it from your skin. So when she pulls away, she leaves behind her stinger—and also the stinger sac, which contains venom. The good news: She dies. The bad news: The stinger sac keeps pumping venom into your skin if you don't remove it, making the sting worse, says Saralyn R. Williams, M.D., a toxicologist and emergency physician at the San Diego Regional Poison Center.

All of the others—hornets, wasps and yellow jackets—are able to remove their stingers. The problem is, they don't die, so they can sting you repeatedly if you don't get away from them, says Dr. Williams.

TAKE THE STING OUT OF STINGS

"Once you've been stung, there's no antidote for bee venom and no way to draw the venom out of your skin," says Dr. Williams. "So what you're looking for are ways to relieve the symptoms." Here's what women doctors suggest for taking the sting out of stings.

First, remove the stinger. You must properly remove a honeybee's stinger and venom sac from your skin promptly. "If you get it out right away, very little venom will be released. But if you wait, you'll have a much worse reaction," says Leslie Boyer, M.D., medical director of the Arizona Poison and Drug Information Center in Tucson.

The best way to remove the stinger and sac? Use the back of your thumbnail or a credit card or a dull knife blade to scrape along your skin underneath the barb and flick it out, without squeezing the venom sac, suggests Dr. Williams

Don't use your fingers or tweezers to pinch the fuzzy part sticking out, says Dr. Williams. "That's the venom sac. If you squeeze it, you'll inject more venom into yourself."

Ice the sore spot. Put an ice cube on the sting site to keep the swelling and pain down. "Use ice on and off for about the first ten minutes—put it on for a few minutes, leave it off a few minutes, and so on," suggests Dr. Boyer. But don't leave ice on your skin for an hour at a time, or you'll freeze your skin and get frostbite.

Apply baking-soda paste. "Some people find relief by making a paste from baking soda and water and putting it on the sting," says Dr. Boyer.

Comfort the sting with a compress. To ease soreness and itching,

WHEN TO SEE A DOCTOR

People who are allergic to bee venom can develop serious life-threatening reactions to a sting. "Their airways swell shut, which could be fatal," says Saralyn R. Williams, M.D., a toxicologist and emergency physician at the San Diego Regional Poison Center.

If you're stung by a bee (or another winged venomous creature such as a hornet, wasp, yellow jacket or fire ant) and you develop hives that travel up your arm, leg or body, or if you start having trouble breathing, call your local emergency medical number or go to a hospital *immediately*.

If you know that you're allergic to stings, says Constance Nichols, M.D., an emergency physician and associate residency director in the Department of Emergency Medicine at the University of Massachusetts Medical Center in Amherst, you should carry an Epipen—a prescription device that looks like a big Magic Marker—to quickly and easily inject yourself with a dose of epinephrine if you're stung. "Your physician will train you how to use it."

"Keep one Epipen in your purse, briefcase or backpack, one in your car and one at home," says Dr. Nichols. And even if you use an Epipen, you still need to get emergency help, says Dr. Williams. "There may not be enough epinephrine in the pen to save your life—just enough to buy you time to get to the hospital."

You should also get to a hospital if you've been badly stung by hundreds of bees, even if you're not allergic.

And see a doctor if a sting becomes infected. If redness increases, if you start getting red streaks around the sting or if there is drainage or crusting from the sting, these are signs of infection.

apply a compress made from a washcloth soaked in cool water. Or soak a mini-compress in Burow's Solution (available in drugstores as Domeboro Astringent Solution powder packets) and hold it on the itchy site, suggests Dr. Williams.

Soothe the itch. More itch relief can come from dabbing calamine lotion on the sting or from soaking in a soothing bath prepared with a powdered oatmeal, such as Aveeno, says Dr. Williams.

Go anti-itch with an antihistamine. Some people develop a severe local allergic reaction to a sting, which is very uncomfortable but not life-threatening, as long as it is contained to the sting site. "Instead of having an inch or two of swelling around the sting, these people might find that half of their arm is swollen," says Dr. Boyer. If you experience a lot of itching, and the sting is swelling rapidly, try taking one dose of an over-the-counter antihistamine, such as Benadryl (the active ingredient is diphenhydramine), she suggests.

Elevate the area. If a sting becomes so swollen that it actually aches, elevate the stung arm, leg or other body part so that gravity helps fluid leave the area, reducing swelling and the soreness that comes with it, says Constance Nichols, M.D., an emergency physician and associate residency director in the Department of Emergency Medicine at the University of Massachusetts Medical Center in Amherst.

Belching
Burst Your Bubbles

A belch is swallowed air that comes back up—usually, with a noisy, embarrassing vengeance.

In fact, 70 percent of air in the gastrointestinal tract is swallowed air, says Ernestine Hambrick, M.D., a colon and rectal surgeon at Michael Reese Hospital in Chicago.

You gulp in air because you eat too fast, drink carbonated drinks or chew gum or sometimes because you're nervous. Perhaps most commonly, you swallow air when you talk and eat simultaneously. "Along with the peas goes in air," says Robyn Karlstadt, M.D., a gastroenterologist at Graduate Hospital in Philadelphia.

SILENT DIGESTION

A few simple tricks can minimize belching, say doctors.

Try simethicone. Available over-the-counter as Gas-X or Phazyme, this enables you to belch, so the bloating goes down, says Dr. Karlstadt.

Skip the bubbly stuff—and bubble gum. Certain foods and drinks are particularly gas-producing. Stay away from carbonated beverages and chewing gum, says Dr. Karlstadt.

Drink from a straw. Drinking through a straw results in less air-swallowing, says Ann Ouyang, M.B., B.S. (the British equivalent of an M.D.), professor of medicine and chief of the Division of Gastroenterology at the Milton S. Hershey Medical Center of the Pennsylvania State University College of Medicine in Hershey.

And, yes, chew your food. The more quickly you eat, the more likely you are take in air, says Dr. Hambrick. If you chew your food thoroughly before you swallow it, air is less likely to enter your digestive tract.

Put a few morsels in your tummy. Haven't eaten all day? If your stomach gets too empty, says Dr. Karlstadt, it'll fill up with gassy air.

Problem is, the air doesn't stay put, but sooner or later comes out as gas—and you can't control when.

Switch to relaxed-fit jeans. Sometimes, wearing tight girdles or belts or too-snug pants and skirts can force air up and out, says Linda Lee, M.D., assistant professor of medicine in the Division of Gastroenterology at Johns Hopkins University School of Medicine in Baltimore. To keep the belching down to a minimum, wear loose, comfortable clothes.

Bikini Bottom

Banish Itchy Rump Bumps

Whether you favor a serious swimmer's tank suit, a sensible skirted number or a revealing thong, if you sit around the pool too long in a wet suit, your backside may break out in little itchy red bumps. When that happens, you have a classic case of folliculitis—in other words, bikini bottom.

"When you sit around in a wet suit, bacteria gets embedded in the hair follicles in your skin and they become inflamed—that's what makes those red bumps," says Toby Shaw, M.D., associate professor of dermatology at Allegheny University of the Health Sciences MCP–Hahnemann School of Medicine in Philadelphia. (The skin on your buttocks may seem too smooth to contain any kind of hair. But most of the skin on your body actually supports tiny or invisible hairs growing out of follicles in skin cells.)

Bikini bottom isn't confined to bathing suits, say doctors. "Women who wear panty hose can get it when they sweat and they can't dry off and their skin can't breathe," says Diane L. Kallgren, M.D., a dermatologist in private practice in Boulder, Colorado.

Wearing tight jeans can produce the same damp conditions that foster bikini bottom, says Jane M. Grant-Kels, professor and chief of the Division of Dermatology at the University of Connecticut Health Center in Farmington. Pedaling an exercise bike for two hours in tight spandex shorts can cause friction and increased moisture, leading to bikini bottom.

DON'T JUST SIT THERE

Women doctors well-versed in bikini bottom offer this simple strategy for relief.

Grab an antibacterial soap. Whenever you come off an afternoon at the swim club or the swimming hole with a jumpy, bumpy butt, strip off that suit, leap in the shower and wash your backside with antibacterial soap, like Dial, says Dr. Shaw. That will eliminate the microorganisms that flourish on the damp playing fields of your swaddled buttocks and help dry out the rash.

Use antibacterial soap on the affected area every time you wash until the bumps disappear—about a day or two.

Scrub and rub. When you soap up with your antibacterial bar, use a washcloth, says Dr. Kallgren, and rub your bottom for about 15 to 30 seconds. That will exfoliate—remove—dead skin cells that accumulate and aggravate bikini bottom. (A damp bathing suit or bicycle shorts holds those cells tightly.) One exfoliation should be all you need.

Try a vinegar compress. "You might smell like a salad, but a good way of calming down bikini bottom, especially if it's weepy and infected, is to apply an acetic acid—vinegar— compress," says Karen S. Harkaway, M.D., clinical instructor of dermatology at the University of Pennsylvania School of Medicine and a dermatologist at Pennsylvania Hospital, both in Philadelphia.

To make your compress, mix one part plain white vinegar to four parts lukewarm water in a one-quart bowl or basin. Dip a clean hand towel into the mixture, soak it, then wring it out. Lie on your belly on your bed, then apply the compress to your itchy bottom and let it soak into your skin for 20 minutes. One or two applications should help.

Reach for cortisone cream. Before you put your clothes back on, Dr. Harkaway suggests applying a film of over-the-counter hydrocortisone cream (such as Bactine or Cortaid) to your buttocks.

Bikini-Line Problems
Get Rid of Unwanted Hair Down There

*E*ven if you have the figure and self-confidence to wear a swimsuit with high-cut legs, you still have one problem: pubic hair that peeks out from behind an abbreviated front panel.

A depilatory (chemical hair-remover) isn't necessarily the answer. The skin along your lower abdominal area adjoining your upper thigh is especially sensitive. "Some depilatories can cause irritant reactions," says Allison Vidimos, M.D., a staff dermatologist at the Cleveland Clinic Foundation. The same goes for waxing (stripping away the hair, often used for legs) and electrolysis (where tiny needles zap hair shafts, often on the upper lip.)

A GENTLER ROUTE

When it comes down to it, women doctors say that shaving is the best way to get rid of unwanted hair along the bikini line. Perhaps you've already tried shaving, only to end up with a nasty outbreak of little bumps and a red rash—signs of a classic bikini-line infection.

"The skin in the bikini area harbors a lot of bacteria that your razor can pick up and drag into hair follicles (the pores from which the hair shaft grows)," explains Dr. Vidimos. The infected follicles erupt into little bumps, a condition that doctors call folliculitis.

51

NO MORE LITTLE RED BUMPS

Here's how to remove pubic hair safely.

Scrub it. "Before you shave, scrub your bikini-line area with an antibacterial soap such as Zest, Coast, Dial, Lever 2000 or Safeguard, says Dr. Vidimos. That will reduce the amount of bacteria on your skin.

Scrub again. When you've finished shaving, rinse off the shaving foam or gel, then use a washcloth to once again scrub your entire bikini area with an antibacterial soap, says Dr. Vidimos. Doing so removes some of the bacteria left after shaving. Pat the area dry with a clean, dry towel.

Wash twice a day. If, despite using the correct technique, you develop a bumpy rash, Dr. Vidimos advises using the antibacterial soap to thoroughly wash the area twice a day.

Apply an astringent. After you wash, dab an over-the-counter astringent such as Phisoderm on the affected area, suggests Dr. Vidimos.

Dab on some cortisone. Pick up an over-the-counter hydrocortisone preparation such as Cortaid and smooth it over the affected area according to package directions, says Dr. Vidimos. It will soothe any irritation and help it heal.

Binge Eating
Stop Out-of-Control Eating

*Y*ou've just had a fight with your husband about how much you spent on your new wardrobe. You head for the refrigerator and stick your spoon into a half-gallon of ice cream. Next thing you know, the ice cream is gone, and so is the cake that went with it—the one you baked for Saturday-night company.

And so is everything else in the fridge. You've even licked the jar of chutney clean. Suddenly, you find yourself en route to the supermarket for more. What's going on?

You're having an episode of binge eating—a bout of uncontrollable consumption driven by at least three emotions: depression, anger and anxiety.

MORE THAN JUST A MEGA-CRAVING

"Binge eating is a psychological disorder that usually has much deeper roots than a simple food craving," says Mary Ellen Sweeney, M.D., obesity researcher at Emory University School of Medicine and an endocrinologist and director of the Lipid Metabolism Clinics at the Veterans Affairs Medical Center, both in Atlanta.

"Binge eating is literally stuffing feelings down," says Mary Froning, Psy.D., a clinical psychologist in private practice in Washington, D.C. As long as we're eating, we don't have to deal with feelings such as anger, anxiety or depression, say women doctors.

"When you're bingeing, you're out of control," says Dori Winchell, Ph.D., a psychologist in private practice in Encinitas, California. "It's not so much the amount or what you eat, but what it feels like. Is the food in control? After the first bite, can you stop?"

If the answer is no, you're on an eating binge.

It's a vicious cycle. You feel depressed, anxious and angry, so you binge. Then you feel depressed, anxious and angry about bingeing—and despair of ever being able to stop. So you binge again, Dr. Winchell says.

Bingeing also can be triggered by starvation diets, says Jan McBarron, M.D., a weight-control specialist and director of Georgia Bariatrics in Columbus, Georgia. Living on small salads and water during the day, deprived physically and psychologically of sustenance, some women run amok in the kitchen at night. They try to fill the nutrition gap by eating everything in the house.

HELP FOR HOME-ALONE BINGERS

To stop the bingeing cycle and take control of what and how you eat, women doctors suggest these methods. (For information on how to handle cravings, which can and often do lead to binges, see page 225.)

Stop while you're ahead. You couldn't help yourself. You stopped at the mall and bought a five-pound box of chocolates. Now, you and the chocolates are home alone.

"Throw them out," says Elizabeth Somer, R.D., author of *Food and Mood* and *Nutrition for Women*. And while you're at it, take a walk or call a friend so that you can think about something else.

WHEN TO SEE A DOCTOR

If you feel that you are a binge-eater who can't stop, see a doctor or counselor trained in eating disorders. To locate qualified professional help in your area, contact either the American Society of Bariatric Physicians, 5600 South Quebec Street, Suite 109A, Englewood, CO 80111; the National Association of Anorexia Nervosa and Associated Disorders, Box 7, Highland Park, Illinois 60035 or the Center for the Study of Anorexia and Bulimia at 1 West 91st Street, New York, NY 10024.

Toss the goodies. "Too late? Already ate half the box? Throw out the rest," says Somer.

Record your indulgences. Even if you've just eaten the whole box of goodies, it's not too late to do something about the binge, says Somer. Write down what triggered the binge, so that you can figure out what to do differently next time.

Stave off nighttime binges. On its simplest level, binge eating at night is often brought on by starving all day, says Susan Zelitch Yanovski, M.D., director of the Obesity and Eating Disorders Program at the National Institute of Diabetes and Digestive and Kidney Diseases at the National Institutes of Health in Bethesda, Maryland. "Eat a sensible breakfast and lunch, and you're less likely to clean out your refrigerator at night," Dr. Yanovski says.

Savor something spicy. "Hard as you try, you just can't binge on chili peppers and Tabasco sauce," says Maria Simonson, Sc.D., Ph.D., director of the Health, Weight and Stress Clinic at the Johns Hopkins Medical Institutions in Baltimore. In fact, spicy foods fill you up faster than bland or sweet foods, and they may even help burn calories faster.

Do something complicated—and constructive. "Take your mind away from your forbidden food by focusing on something that takes all your concentration, like the Sunday crossword puzzle," Dr. Winchell says. "Once your mind is engaged in a task that you enjoy and must pay attention to, you're less likely to be fixated on food."

Wait. If you feel the urge to binge, set the kitchen timer for 15 minutes and try to figure out what's going on, Dr. Froning says. "Is anger or depression or anxiety making you want to stuff yourself with candy bars? If so, try to figure out why you feel so upset."

Ask for help. Women almost always binge alone. With friends, you'd be able to talk out your feelings instead of eating them away.

"So if you're feeling down, and you're about to raid the refrigerator, call a friend first," Dr. Froning says.

Forgive yourself. You didn't start bingeing overnight, and you won't be able to stop that quickly, either, says Dr. Froning. Each small step that you take away from bingeing will help you feel better about yourself, but it can take a few years to change your behavior completely.

"Forgive yourself in advance for slip-ups. And just remember, to succeed, the trick is to try and try again," Dr. Froning says.

Biological Clock Anxiety
Think through All Your Options

Should you have a baby? If so, why and when? To women in their thirties and forties, these questions loom large. If you're 35 or 40 and single, you may also ask how. While the odds vary from woman to woman, the likelihood of conceiving and delivering a healthy child declines appreciably after 35 and more so after 40.

Some of us hear our biological clocks ticking loudly and still aren't sure whether motherhood is for us. Others know that it is but don't have willing partners. Still others are trying to conceive and having trouble.

The resulting anxiety can be so intense that we're distracted from other things that matter, like our jobs and relationships, says Vicki Rachlin, Ph.D., a child and family psychologist in private practice in Concord, New Hampshire. Sometimes there is an accompanying fear that, under pressure, we'll decide to have a baby when we shouldn't, or with someone who isn't right.

WHEN TO SEE A DOCTOR

Worrying about whether you can or should have a child can take over your life if you let it. Therapy and support groups can help you cope with these difficulties, says psychologist Laura Barbanel, Ed.D., head of the graduate program at the Brooklyn College School of Psychology. You may benefit from therapy or outside support if:

- Anxiety is interfering with your job or relationships.
- Your partner doesn't want a child, you do and you're torn apart by the choice you face.
- You've thought about becoming pregnant despite your partner's objections or misgivings.
- Unsuccessful efforts to conceive are leaving you extremely depressed or burned out.

To find a support group near you, write to RESOLVE, an organization for women contemplating motherhood, at 130 Broadway, Somerville, MA 02145.

PRACTICE THOUGHT CONTROL

You can't slow down your biological clock, but you can manage the stress while pondering your options. Here's what the experts suggest.

Go ahead and worry—once a day. To keep the anxiety from taking over your life, confine your worry to a 30-minute block of time once a day or once a week, suggests Susan G. Mikesell, Ph.D., a psychologist in Washington, D.C., and a consulting psychologist for the Montgomery Fertility Institute in Bethesda, Maryland. Devote this half-hour to mulling over the consequences of your decisions. "This helps you contain the anxiety," she says. "It gives you some control."

Reflect, don't obsess. "Don't get stuck trying to catalog all the pros and cons of parenthood—'We can find day care, but we'll have less money'—that sort of thing," Dr. Rachlin says. "If you do, you'll go crazy, because the pros and cons balance each other out. Instead, think about parenthood at a deeper, emotional level. Ask yourself, 'How much do I want to have the experience of being a parent?'"

This isn't the same as asking, "How much do I want to be pregnant?" cautions Dr. Mikesell. Some women want to experience pregnancy but aren't excited by the prospect of 20 years of feeding, clothing, disciplining, teaching, comforting and nurturing a child.

"You may want to ask yourself, 'When I get to menopause, will I feel complete even if I never had a pregnancy or if I never had a child?'" says Dr. Mikesell. "The way you answer these questions tells you different things."

Ride out the ambivalent moments. Even women with intense baby lust—the ones who gaze longingly at every child they see—have ambivalent moments. That's natural, says Dr. Rachlin. "If you think about the startling responsibility that being a parent entails and the dramatic ways that it changes your life, a certain degree of ambivalence is healthy."

Ask your partner what he really wants. Make certain that the prospective father has realistic expectations, advises Dr. Rachlin. Face it: Once you have a baby, you'll no longer be able to take off for the weekend or go to the movies at a moment's notice. And you'll have less money to spend on yourselves. "Talk about those scenarios," she says.

Above all, realize that a child is *not* the prescription for an ailing relationship. In fact, a baby can sound the death knell for a sickly relationship, because parenting can be so stressful.

Give it time. If your partner is dead set against having children, don't force the issue, says Dr. Mikesell. "I try to steer people away from hoping or trying to convince the other person. Sometimes that happens, but usually, he has to make that shift of his own accord."

If you're holding out for a change of heart, she suggests giving yourself a deadline. When the deadline arrives, though, be prepared for a truly heart-wrenching decision. You may have to decide what's more important to you—the baby or the relationship.

Whatever you do, says Dr. Mikesell, don't get pregnant "accidentally"—it may be tempting, but it's a bad idea.

If you've suffered a loss, wait. The desire for a baby can be most intense after suffering a loss—the end of a relationship or a job, says psychologist Laura Barbanel, Ed.D., head of the graduate program at the Brooklyn College School of Psychology. So you have to distinguish between wanting to be a parent and wanting something to make up for the loss.

Look forward, not back. Trying to conceive without success can be one of the most stressful, heartbreaking experiences in a woman's life, says Dr. Mikesell. Some women blame themselves or their partners for not starting earlier. Women who had abortions when they were younger may feel overcome with regret.

It's important to remember that you had good reasons for making the decisions you made, Dr. Mikesell says. Your circumstances were different. Maybe you and your partner decided to wait because you weren't able to support a baby. Don't lose sight of that.

Birthday Blues

Forget Regrets and Forge Ahead

Someone once quipped that considering the alternative, birthdays aren't so bad. Still, many women find their birthdays bittersweet—or downright upsetting.

There's no denying it: A birthday means that we're one year older. In a culture that seems to worship youth, we can all be affected at some time in our lives.

Surprisingly, our first brush with the birthday blues may come as early as age 18—childhood's end, says Marion Hart, M.D., assistant professor of psychiatry at Cornell Medical Center and an adult and child psychiatrist and psychoanalyst in Scarsdale, New York. We may run into them again at 21, as an "official grown-up." But as they say, old is a state of mind. Dr. Hart recalls one woman who arrived for an appointment feeling blue and explained that she'd just hit "The Big 2-3."

Though 30 is still relatively young, Dr. Hart and others say that it's the birthday many women mind the most. By the time we've reached 30, we've already made some of life's big decisions—about careers and relationships—and sometimes, those plans haven't panned out.

On our fortieth birthdays we begin to anticipate the end of fertility, says Dr. Hart. For many women birthdays from age 45 through 50 or so coincide with physical and emotional changes associated with premenopause. And midlife is yet another natural time for taking stock and making choices.

COMMISERATE OR CELEBRATE?

Just about any birthday can nudge us into taking stock, says Carol Goldberg, Ph.D., a clinical psychologist specializing in stress management in New York City. We compare where we are with where we thought we'd be at whatever age we've reached. If we haven't accomplished what we'd hoped, we may feel disappointed.

Women doctors offer these suggestions for seeing birthdays in a rosier hue.

Count yourself in good company. "It helps to remind yourself that the birthday blues aren't at all unusual," says Dr. Hart. "Most people celebrate with a bit of sadness." So if you're sad, that's okay—let yourself be sad. There is no reason to feel embarrassed or vain.

To party or not to party. If you really don't want a birthday party, give advance warning to the people most likely to try to throw one for you, says Dr. Goldberg. Thank them nicely for their offer and tell them that you appreciate the gesture, but you prefer not to celebrate with a party.

If you didn't get word out in time and your spouse, family, friends or co-workers spring for a birthday bash, be a good sport whether you're delighted or not, says Dr. Goldberg. Focus on the fact that you're with a group of people who really like you and not on the fact that you're a year older.

It could be just what the doctor ordered, says Dr. Hart. "Gathering with supportive people, having a good time and joking about birthdays is part of sharing—a way to get through what can be a difficult time."

If you feel like celebrating, but no one knows that it's your birthday, or if nothing is planned, call an impromptu party. Invite your friends out to dinner or drinks, says Dr. Hart. Say, "Today is my birthday, and I'd love to celebrate with you."

Buy yourself a birthday present. No matter how many years it's been, herald your birthday with a gift to yourself—a compact disc, a massage, a day at a spa, tickets to the opera or that weekend getaway that you've been wanting to take, suggests Dr. Hart.

Rethink your goals. If you're feeling down because you haven't yet accomplished what you expected to by your current age, you can explore a few options, says Dr. Goldberg. One, ask yourself if it really matters after all. Two, ask yourself if your expectations are realistic. If they are realistic and you still care, then figure out what you can do to boost your odds of reaching your goals. To find a soul mate, for example, you may need to get out and meet men who share your interests—on a Sierra Club hike, at the local coffee house or at the baseball stadium. To further your career, you may need to attend night school or learn a new skill. To improve your financial situation, you could bone up on financial planning or investment management.

Have no regrets. Those of us with the most regrets often find birthdays hardest to handle, says Dr. Hart. Some of the decisions that you regret—like leaving an old boyfriend 20 years ago—can't be undone. So forget about it. For other decisions, it's never too late to reconsider. If you regret not finishing your college education, for example, finish it now. "I know several women in their fifties and sixties who just graduated from college," she says.

Count your achievements. Instead of spending your birthday cataloging all the things that you wish you had done, start cataloging all the things that you *have* done, says Dr. Hart. "And recognize that it's not possible to do everything."

Remember: It's only one day. "The birthday blues are usually short-lived," says Dr. Hart. "Many people who feel down on their birthdays find that they feel happier the next day."

Blemishes
Clear Up Clogged Pores

Margaret was way past adolescence. But she wasn't past pimples. They still popped up sometimes—on her chin or her neck, where most adult blemishes make their mark.

"It's not true that people over 20 are no longer prone to blemishes," says Mary P. Sheehan, M.D., chief of pediatric dermatology at Mercy Hospital in Pittsburgh.

In fact, at least half of all adult women suffer occasional breakouts triggered by stress and other things, says Diana Bihova, M.D., a dermatologist in New York City and author of *Beauty from the Inside Out.*

Basically, blemishes are clogged pores consisting of dead skin cells, oil secreted by tiny sebaceous glands in the skin and bacteria that feast on oil the way cats gobble up fish.

"There are three kinds of blemishes: blackheads/whiteheads, papules and cysts," says Esta Kronberg, M.D., a dermatologist in private practice in Houston. Blackheads and whiteheads, which develop close to the surface of the skin, are two versions of the same type of blemish. With a blackhead, the oil and accumulated debris has forced the pore open and the oil has oxidized to black. A whitehead is the same as a blackhead, but closed, so that the oil and debris remain beneath the skin surface. A papule is a red bump that occurs because of an inflammation under the skin at a hair follicle. Cysts occur deeper within the pores in the form of swollen red or white pustules. All three—blackheads/whiteheads, papules or cysts—can last three to four weeks or longer, says Dr. Kronberg.

RESCUES AND REMEDIES

You can shave some time off that unwanted stay. You can also treat the interloper well so that your skin doesn't look abused. And you can conceal it. Here's how.

Cool it. "A good emergency pimple treatment for emerging pimples is to apply ice as soon as you feel it," says Mary Lupo, M.D., associate clinical professor of dermatology at Tulane University School of Medicine in New Orleans.

Wrap an ice cube in a washcloth or dish towel and hold it to the pimple for about five minutes. "Cooling it will decrease some of the inflammation," she says.

Pop an aspirin, not a pimple. "You get a great degree of inflammation and pain with a blemish, so some women benefit by taking an anti-inflammatory like aspirin," says Susan C. Taylor, M.D., assistant clinical professor of medicine in the Department of Dermatology at the University of Pennsylvania School of Medicine in Philadelphia. Popping a pimple, while tempting, only spreads the inflammation, making matters worse.

Take the standard dose of aspirin—one to two 325 milligram tablets four times a day—until the swelling goes down. If you're sensitive to aspirin, use ibuprofen instead, says Dr. Taylor. But discontinue either drug after two days if you see no improvement.

Say benzoyl peroxide. Products with benzoyl peroxide can help get rid of blemishes and prevent new ones from forming, says Mary Ruth Buchness, M.D., chief of dermatology at St. Vincent's Hospital and Medical Center in New York City. Applied in cream, wash or ointment form to your skin, the oxygen in benzoyl peroxide kills the bacteria snacking on your skin's oil.

Benzoyl peroxide is the chief ingredient in anti-acne preparations like Clearasil and Oxy brand products. Make sure that you get a product that contains the mildest percentage of the benzoyl peroxide—2.5 percent. "The biggest mistake that women make is to buy too strong a product; it can burn their skin," says Dr. Kronberg.

"Apply a very tiny amount—the size of a pea—to your entire face once a day, every day, preferably at night," says Dr. Kronberg. If you find the creams too drying, use a benzoyl peroxide cleanser once a day; it kills the bacteria without drying your face too much.

Paint over it. "Virtually every cosmetics company makes a green blemish cover-up that, applied under makeup, neutralizes the red of a blemish and normalizes skin color," says Dr. Buchness. Cover-up cosmetics are available at drug and department stores.

Blemish cover cream is designed to be used with regular cover creams. To apply, says Dee Anna Glaser, M.D., assistant professor of dermatology at St. Louis University School of Medicine, "Cover the red blemish with the green makeup, then let it set for a couple of minutes. Apply a regular flesh-colored cover-up and let that set. After that, apply your foundation. That usually gets you deep coverage," she says.

Blisters

Soothe Those Bubbles of Pain

What do the following activities have in common?
- Dancing in sling-back heels
- Wearing a new pair of sandals for the first time
- Taking a day-long hike with your friends
- Raking a yard full of leaves

All can leave you with painful blisters.

"Most everyday blisters are caused by friction, and the foot is the most frequent site—usually because of shoes that don't fit, combined with an activity like dancing or running or tennis," says Wilma Bergfeld, M.D., head of clinical research in the Department of Dermatology at the Cleveland Clinic Foundation. The hand is the second-most common site of friction blisters, because of activities like raking and sweeping.

Despite the pain, blisters function as natural bandages for irritated skin, says dermatologist Karen E. Burke, M.D., Ph.D., an attending physician at Cabrini Medical Center in New York City and at Greensboro Specialty Surgical Center in North Carolina.

"The fluid sealed inside washes the irritated skin surface and keeps it moist so that the blister will heal quickly," says Dr. Bergfeld. "And if the blister is closed, it is less likely to get infected, since it is not exposed to the open air."

NATURE'S BANDAGE

"Ideally, a blister should be left intact so that nature can take its course in healing," says Dr. Burke.

If a blister does open, that's okay—you just have to give it extra care so that it doesn't get infected, says Dr. Bergfeld.

Here's what women doctors recommend you do to heal these bubbles of pain. (For practical ways to deal with blisters from poison ivy, see page 432.)

Pop it correctly. If a blister is large and uncomfortable, women doctors say that you can carefully prick the bubble with a sterilized needle to release fluid pressure. "Prick the part of the blister that is lowest on your body, so gravity helps drain fluid out of the little hole," suggests Sheryl Clark, M.D., assistant clinical professor of dermatology at Cornell Medical Center and an assistant attending physician in medicine at the New York Hospital, both in New York City.

WHEN TO SEE A DOCTOR

Sometimes even a tiny blister needs to be treated by a physician. Women doctors suggest that you get medical help for the following:

- You develop a severe blister or blisters that are very painful and don't seem to be healing well.
- A blister suddenly shows signs of infection—pain, swelling, redness, weeping or a yellow crust—and you have a fever.
- You develop a wide-scale eruption of blisters.
- Blisters continue to form over time without an obvious cause, such as friction or poison ivy.
- You develop a single or repeated episodes of a cluster of tiny blisters, often with tingling, which may represent herpes simplex.
- You develop blisters while pregnant.

Leave the roof on. If you pricked a blister, or if it has popped on its own, leave the top flap of skin in place. "This roof of tissue will cover and protect the sore so that it heals faster," says Dr. Clark.

Wash with liquid soap. Gently clean the blister with soap and water to eliminate bacteria that could cause infection. "Liquid soap is preferable to bar soap, which may contain bacteria from previous uses," says Dr. Bergfeld.

Fight the germs. If a blister is open, you must apply antimicrobial ointment, such as Bacitracin or Polysporin, to kill bacteria and prevent infection, says Dr. Bergfeld.

Cover it. After you apply ointment, cover the blister with a bandage to cushion it from pressure and keep it clean. "Gauze and surgical tape or a plain old adhesive bandage work fine," says Dr. Clark. The bandage also keeps ointment from ruining your clothes and helps absorb any fluid that leaks out of the blister.

Use a doughnut pad. If you want to protect a small blister from friction and pressure, cover it with a Dr. Scholl's doughnut-shaped pad, called a soft corn cushion, which has a hole in the middle, says Dr. Clark.

Protect with petroleum jelly. If you know that you're prone to blisters in a certain site, prevent future friction by applying a coating of plain petroleum jelly, such as Vaseline. "Vaseline is an excellent lubricant," says Dr. Clark. "It doesn't contain any irritating ingredients, and it helps you avoid friction by keeping skin moist so it doesn't chafe."

Bloating
Deflate the Human Balloon

When was the last time that you saw a guy pull on a pair of snug jeans, look in the mirror and whine that he's bloated? Probably never. Not that guys don't get bloated; when they do, they just shrug it off as the downside of having one too many beers, loosen their belts a notch and figure that it will pass. And it does. Because the main cause of bloating—for either sex—is air swallowed (like when you eat) or air produced by your own body in reaction to high-fiber foods.

If you're feeling bloated and gassy but haven't been drinking any beer or soda, it could be caused by air-containing foods like ice cream. (Think of a pint of Haagen-Dazs as the female counterpart to Budweiser.) And not just any ice cream—*chocolate* ice cream.

You may also experience bloating right before your menstrual period. Some of the discomfort that many women chalk up to fluid retention may actually be abdominal discomfort from bloating, says Barbara Frank, M.D., gastreoenterologist and clinical professor of medicine at Allegheny University of the Health Sciences MCP–Hahnemann School of Medicine in Philadelphia.

GET RID OF GAS *FAST*

Until the National Institutes of Health in Bethesda, Maryland, dedicates multimillion-dollar research grants to the study of bloating in women (don't hold your breath), the following advice from women doctors can help deflate your distended abdomen.

Buy a gas de-bubbler. For quick relief of bloating, head to the nearest drugstore for an over-the-counter gas remedy such as Gas X or Phazyme, which contain simethicone, says Melissa Palmer, M.D., a gastroenterologist in private practice in New York City. Or try Charcoal Plus, which contains activated charcoal. Both compounds break up gas bubbles fast.

Chew your food. "The more slowly you eat, and the better your food is broken down, the less likely you are to suffer from gas caused by swallowing air," says Dr. Frank. And the less likely you are to feel bloated.

Clue in to classic "bloat foods." Raw vegetables, cabbage, beans, bagels and pretzels (which are cooked in boiling, bubbly water) also are big gas—and by extension, bloat—producers, Dr. Palmer says.

Soak your limas and lentils. Beans are full of fiber and good for you, so if you want to keep eating limas, lentils or any other members of the bean crowd, soak them in water overnight, says Dr. Frank. The water will drain out some of the gas. "Then, throw out the water and cook the beans in fresh water."

Neutralize bean gas. Not cooking? Beano, available over the counter in liquid or tablet form, is a liquid enzyme that breaks down the indigestible sugars in beans, says Linda Lee, M.D., assistant professor of medicine in the Division of Gastroenterology at Johns Hopkins University School of Medicine in Baltimore. Just sprinkle several drops right on the beans or take two tablets before you eat.

Shun the sugarless. Sorbitol, a natural sugar used in sugarless gums and candies and many diet sodas, also is hard to digest and causes gas and bloating, Dr. Lee says.

PMS? Skip the chocolate. You want, you crave, you must have chocolate before you menstruate. But do you want it so badly that you're willing to risk getting bloated?

"Be especially sure to monitor symptoms when you eat chocolate, a major cause of that overfull feeling," Dr. Frank says. Why chocolate? Because it contains sugar and dairy, both major sources of gas. And, as it happens, studies have shown that women crave chocolate more than men, especially just before menstruation. If you find that chocolate, or any other food, is a bloating culprit, stop eating it.

Lace up those walking shoes. "If you have bloating from premenstrual syndrome, walking can really help dispel gas," says Dr. Palmer. Light exercise may help relieve that bloated, gassy feeling.

(For practical ways to manage lactose intolerance, which can also cause bloating, see page 336.)

Bloodshot Eyes
Out with the Red

As eye problems go, bloodshot eyes are easy to self-diagnose: The tiny network of blood vessels on the surface of your eyeballs (barely noticeable, most times) are swollen and your eyes are red.

Anything that irritates your eyes can leave them instantly bloodshot: Wind. Crying. A smoke-filled room. An allergic reaction to pets. Mold. Even troublesome makeup.

And, yes, drinking too much alcohol can cause the blood vessels to dilate and redden, says Anne Sumers, M.D., an ophthalmologist in Ridgewood, New Jersey, and a spokeswoman for the American Academy of Ophthalmology. Often when your eyes are red, they are also dry, so they feel and look uncomfortable.

FOR CLEAR EYES, READ THIS

To shrink those blood vessels and get the red out, try following these tips from experts.

Chill. Applying a cold compress to your eyes for 30 minutes will shrink your swollen blood vessels, says Dr. Sumers. "Wrap ice cubes in a clean washcloth or just use a damp washcloth. It brings the swelling way down."

Artificial tears to the rescue. They won't whiten your eyes immediately, but they will lubricate and remoisten, ease that stinging feeling and clear up the underlying irritation that makes your eyes red, says Dr. Sumers. Artificial tears, such as Moisture Drops, Hypotears and Tears Naturale, are available over the counter at your local drugstore.

If you wear contacts, rewetting drops will work. They serve the same function as artificial tears, says Dr. Sumers.

Use medicated eyedrops only in an emergency. Over-the-counter eyedrops, such as Murine and Visine, are medicated; they contain a vasoconstrictive substance that will shrink your blood vessels for about 45 minutes. So if you need to show up at an important meeting with crystal-clear eyes, it's okay to pop in a few drops, says Dr. Sumers. But use medicated drops sparingly. The more you use medicated eyedrops, the more you need them, says Dr. Sumers. "It's a medical situation that we call rebound hyperemia." If your eyes are chronically bloodshot, you need to find out why and not just mask the symptom.

WHEN TO SEE A DOCTOR

If your eyes are still red after a day, see your doctor. Bloodshot eyes may be a sign of a foreign body trapped in your eye, allergies or infection, says Anne Sumers, M.D., an ophthalmologist in Ridgewood, New Jersey, and a spokeswoman for the American Academy of Ophthalmology.

If you get a strong chemical or poison, such as ammonia, in your eye, flush your eye with water and call 911 immediately (or have someone call for you).

If you're in pain or have vision loss from an injury to the eye (like getting whipped in the eye by a branch), call your doctor immediately.

Body Odor

Smell Sweeter, No Sweat

What woman hasn't given a surreptitious sniff to a just-worn sweater before deciding whether to stow it in the closet or the laundry. Her mission, of course, it to detect lingering scents of body odor in the sweater, to avoid offending others when it's worn.

Most people develop a body odor—or B.O., as many of us called it in junior high—sometime around puberty, says Dee Anna Glaser, M.D., assistant professor of dermatology at St. Louis University School of Medicine. It begins when a surge of sex hormones in both men and women cause the apocrine glands—a particular type of sweat gland found in hairy areas under the arm and around the genitals—to secrete an odorless milky goo that, when combined with bacteria on the skin, raises a pungent scent.

Apocrine odors may be particularly intense during ovulation, says Dr. Glaser. And they shift into gear when you're angry, fearful or excited. But the apocrine glands aren't the only glands that play a role in generating sweat. The rest of your body is home to some two million or more eccrine glands, responsible for a salty liquid sweat that cools you down when you get hot. That liquid is odorless, but it creates a moist environment in which bacteria grow and thrive. Once the bacteria mixes with apocrine gland secretions, the resulting liquid creates body odor.

MORE THAN JUST A SHOWER

For most women a daily shower followed by a deodorant is all that's needed to keep body odor in check. For women who need extra help, women doctors offer these suggestions.

Grab a baby wipe. If a tense encounter of some sort gets you so steamed that your apocrine glands start to squirt, step into the bathroom and wipe your odor-prone areas with premoistened towelettes, sold as feminine hygiene wipes or baby wipes, says Dr. Glaser. Then toss your odor problems away.

Wash with two kinds of soap. Since B.O. occurs only when a secretion from the apocrine glands mixes with bacteria under your arms and around your genitals and anus, wash these odor-prone areas with an antibacterial soap once a day, suggests Mary Lupo, M.D., associate clinical professor of dermatology at Tulane University School of Medicine in New Orleans. To avoid the drying side effects of antibacterial soap on other areas of your body, use a milder all-purpose soap like Cetaphil.

Use an antiperspirant. Once you've reduced the numbers of bacteria on your skin, apply an antiperspirant-deodorant that contains aluminum chlorhydrate under your arms, says Karen S. Harkaway, M.D., clinical instructor of dermatology at the University of Pennsylvania School of Medicine and a dermatologist at Pennsylvania Hospital, both in Philadelphia. The antiperspirant will reduce the moisture on which bacteria feeds.

Sprinkle a little cornstarch. You can also reduce the amount of moisture that normally develops over the course of a day by sprinkling odor-prone areas with cornstarch, says Dr. Glaser.

Boils
Mini-Strategies for Mega-Pimples

Boil, boil, soiled and troubled; skin that burns, oh nasty bubble! This mutation of a classic line from *Macbeth* might make Shakespeare turn over in his grave, but it aptly describes the witch's brew of pus, infection, pain and inflammation that make up a boil.

A boil occurs when bacteria—usually *Staphylococcus aureus*—invade a hair follicle in the skin, travel down the follicle and form a collection of infected pus at the base. The boil often comes to a head when the fluid naturally pushes its way to the skin surface.

The result is a swollen, hard red bump on your skin.

"The most common places for boils to form are in blocked hair follicles on the buttocks, inner thighs and under your arms—areas with a lot of moisture," says Sheryl Clark, M.D., assistant clinical professor of dermatology at Cornell Medical Center and an assistant attending physician in medicine at the New York Hospital, both in New York City. Oc-

WHEN TO SEE A DOCTOR

If you have just one boil, you're probably safe treating it at home, says Wilma Bergfeld, M.D., head of clinical research in the Department of Dermatology at the Cleveland Clinic Foundation. But you should see a doctor if:

- The area around a boil becomes red.
- A boil is deep and contains lots of pus. Your doctor may inject it with a steroid to decrease swelling and inflammation.
- You develop multiple boils.
- You develop a boil on your upper lip, nose, cheeks, scalp or forehead. Infection in these areas can gain easy access to the brain.
- You develop a boil on your breast. Also, if you're breast-feeding, stop until the boil has been treated. Otherwise, you could pass highly infectious bacteria on to your infant.
- You get boils frequently. You may be harboring bacteria somewhere in your body.

casionally, boils can also form on the face or neck. A stye on your eyelid is also a type of boil.

FIRST-AID FOR BOILS

Never pop a boil, says Dr. Clark. "A boil drains a large amount of highly infected fluid. If you squeeze it, you will actually spread the infection and make it worse." Instead, try these doctor-recommended steps.

Apply warm compresses. "Warm, moist heat increases blood flow to the area, which may bring the boil to a head and speed healing," says dermatologist Karen E. Burke, M.D., Ph.D., an attending physician at Cabrini Medical Center in New York City and at Greensboro Specialty Surgical Center in North Carolina.

Apply a washcloth soaked in hot water to the boil for 20 to 30 minutes, two or three times a day, until the boil comes to a head. "Sometimes that allows the boil to pop on its own and drain," says Dr. Clark. Once the boil pops naturally, it should feel better immediately, and it should heal in several days.

Reap the benefits of benzoyl peroxide. Especially if a boil is large, the acne preparation benzoyl peroxide may help dry it out. "An over-the-counter benzoyl peroxide agent such as Oxy 10 can be used twice a day to dry out the lesion and reduce its size," says Wilma Bergfeld, M.D., head of clinical research in the Department of Dermatology at the Cleveland Clinic Foundation. "Benzoyl peroxide is also an antiseptic, so it kills bacteria."

Try a saline solution. Once a boil pops, apply saltwater to draw out pus and fluid and dry it out. "In a clean basin or sink, mix a teaspoon of salt for every cup of hot water. Dip in a washcloth, wring it out and hold it on the boil. When it cools, redip it and reapply," suggests Dr. Clark.

Wash away germs. Keep the area clean by washing with a liquid antibacterial soap and water, especially when a boil has started to drain. "Tap water is fine unless it's an open wound; then use sterile bottled water," says Dr. Bergfeld.

Apply antibacterial ointment. Bacitracin or Neosporin can help kill off any bacteria that is inside the boil or on the skin, says Dr. Clark.

Boredom
How to Perk Up Your Interest

The next time you feel bored, consider the daily routine of eighteenth-century gentlewomen, as described in Samuel Richardson's book *Clarissa*: Six hours for rest; three hours for "praying, meditating, reading pious books;" two hours for "domestic management;" five hours for "needle, drawing, music;" an hour for "visits to the neighboring poor" and the rest of the day in conversation, reading aloud and paying and receiving social visits.

It's no wonder that letters written by women who lived at the time refer to the tedium of women's lives.

"When there ceases to be a sense of newness, challenge and excitement, we all get bored," says Susan Heitler, Ph.D., a clinical psychologist in Denver and author of the audiotape *Anxiety: Friend or Foe?*. Our minds need a steady diet of new input the same way that our bodies need fresh and nourishing food, or we feel stressed.

Boredom isn't fatal, says Harriet Braiker, Ph.D., a clinical psychologist in private practice in Los Angeles. "But psychologically, it can be very painful."

Boredom may contribute to depression or erode self-esteem, says Camille Lloyd, Ph.D., professor in the Department of Psychiatry and Behavioral Sciences at the University of Texas Medical School at Houston.

PRESCRIPTIONS FOR BOREDOM

Boredom is curable, say doctors. And you have plenty of options.

Give yourself antiboredom assignments. For generalized boredom, Dr. Braiker prescribes the following remedy: "Every day, do two things that are different from the usual—preferably, activities that you can discuss with others—like reading a news, travel or sports magazine; listening to new music or taking a class."

Make a wish list. Write down new things that you would like to try—see that new Chinese film at the art-movie theater, for example, or check out the espresso bar across the street after the show.

Think ahead. For activities that require advance planning, start now, says Dr. Lloyd. If you've jotted down "learn French," for instance, pick up the phone, call the local community college and ask them to send you a course catalog so that you can sign up for next semester.

Recruit your spouse. If part of your problem is that you're bored with your marriage, part of the solution is to make your antiboredom plan of action a joint effort, says Dr. Heitler. Once a week for three months, do something new together: Go horseback riding, try country line-dancing, visit a local art museum, volunteer at a homeless shelter, picnic with friends or rent mountain bikes, for example. After three months of weekly adventures, single out the activities that you enjoy the most and continue to pursue them together.

Expand your circle of friends. If you're like most people, you need more novelty than one person can provide. That's where friends come in. Others can provide you with new insights, ideas and inspiration, keeping you interested and interesting, says Dr. Lloyd.

Get out of the house. Staying home—to work out of a home office or raise the kids—can be gratifying. But the isolation can lead to boredom, says Dr. Heitler.

If work keeps you cloistered at home, join a local professional association. Or start a dining club—invite neighbors, friends and business acquaintances to get together regularly (once a week or once a month) for meals.

To break out of the child-rearing routine, Dr. Heitler suggests arranging play groups with your friends and their kids. Take day trips with them. Go to the library. Or invite friends to do laundry or cooking together.

Bring novelty to work. If it's the workplace grind that's wearing you down, look for something new to do at the office.

"Ask yourself if there is a new challenge to be had in your current job," says Dr. Lloyd. You might be able to add to your responsibilities or take on a new set altogether.

If you're in phone sales, for example, maybe you could volunteer to train new salespeople part of the time. Or go to night school and take courses in a new but related area. Then let your boss know that you're in the market to try out your new skills. Or take on a volunteer position until you get more experience that can be parlayed into a new, less boring job.

Breast Discomfort
Ease Pain, Tenderness and Distress

*C*heck out the crowd the next time you go to the beach, and you'll see that women's breasts come in all shapes and sizes. Breast problems are equally diverse. Some women's breasts ache just before or during menstruation. Others develop worrisome lumps. Some women have no problems—until they show up for their annual mammograms and wince at the pressure of the x-ray machine.

BLAME IT ON YOUR PERIOD

Breast care specialists say that for most women, breast discomfort waxes and wanes with the menstrual cycle. Right before and during

Easing the Ouch of Mammograms

Doctors say that a mammogram (low-dose x-ray of the breasts) is the single best way to detect breast cancer early, in its most treatable stages. Yet women often skip their appointments or put them off.

The reason: Mammograms hurt. To get a clear picture, the technician needs to compress your breasts between two plastic plates, explains Ellen Yankauskas, M.D., director of the Women's Center for Family Health in Atascadero, California. So if your breasts are at all tender (and even if they're not), the test may be uncomfortable.

Dr. Yankauskas offers women this advice to minimize discomfort.

- Schedule your test for about one week after the last day of your menstrual period, when breast swelling and tenderness is minimal.
- A few weeks before your appointment cut down on your intake of caffeine and start taking 200 to 400 international units of vitamin E daily.
- Immediately before your mammogram take a standard dose of ibuprofen or acetaminophen.
- If pain persists despite these preventive measures, apply an ice compress and take an additional over-the-counter painkiller, if needed.

menstruation, higher-than-usual levels of the female hormone estrogen may cause one or both breasts to swell and become tender. Discomfort ranges from mild tenderness in some women to excruciating pain in others. (Taking oral contraceptives produces similar effects.) For many women monthly bouts of breast discomfort disappear with menopause—unless they undergo estrogen replacement therapy.

Sometimes premenstrual changes foster the development of tender but harmless cysts in the breasts' milk-producing glands. Once labeled fibrocystic disease, these tiny fluid-filled sacs are actually quite normal. Fibrocystic changes are less likely in women over age 35, because with age, glandular tissue—where breast cysts tend to occur—is replaced with fat tissue.

SOMETHING OLD, SOMETHING NEW

Assuming that your doctor has assured you that you have nothing serious to worry about, here is what women physicians and other health professionals advise for breast pain or tenderness.

Warm gently. Holding a warm compress such as a heated towel or a heating pad against the breast for 10 to 15 minutes can give some relief from breast tenderness, says Ellen Yankauskas, M.D., director of the Women's Center for Family Health in Atascadero, California.

Cool down swelling. The uncomfortable swelling of breast tissues that often occurs before and during a menstrual cycle can be relieved with cold compresses, says Dr. Yankauskas. Wrap ice packs or bags of frozen vegetables in towels, mold them around your breasts and keep them there until the packs warm. Repeat as needed. (Never eat food that's been thawed and refrozen. Mark the packages before refreezing.)

Wear a supportive bra. The mere act of not wearing a bra can contribute to breast pain, says Michele A. Gadd, M.D., a participating surgeon at the Comprehensive Breast Health Center Division of Surgical Oncology at Massachusetts General Hospital in Boston. "The weight of the breasts themselves can contribute to discomfort." So many women find it helpful to wear supportive bras.

Be sure that you wear a bra that's constructed in a way that won't add to the irritation, suggests Dr. Yankauskas. Look inside the cups and make sure that there are no seams and nothing pushing up against you. If there is an underwire, make sure that it's very well-padded so that it doesn't add to the friction.

"This might not be the time of the month to wear your Wonderbra," she says. "Try a sports bra instead."

Serve up some soy. In societies where soybeans are a routine part of the diet, women have fewer breast problems, says Dr. Yankauskas. Soybeans, and foods made from soy, contain isoflavones—naturally occurring substances that are converted to hormonelike substances and may block certain unwanted effects of estrogen in the body, thus mitigating breast discomfort.

So the next time you order Chinese food, order an entrée with tofu instead of meat. Pour soy milk on your cereal. Or pick up some soy burgers for your next cookout. You can find soy milk, soy burgers and other soy products in health food stores.

Cut salt. "Salt is a water magnet," says Dr. Yankauskas. "So if breast discomfort is associated with fluid retention, then watching salt intake should help."

Cut caffeine. If you experience breast discomfort, abstain from caffeine in all forms, advises Tina Hieken, M.D., a surgical oncologist at the University of Illinois at Chicago Medical Center. This includes coffee, tea, caffeine-containing soft drinks, chocolate and painkilling medications (such as Excedrin) that contain caffeine. The culprit seems to be a compound called methylxanthine, contained in caffeine, that may stimulate breast tissue and cause pain.

You may feel an improvement if you cut back to just one or two cups of coffee a day, says Dr. Yankauskas. "But some women are very sensitive and really can't have any caffeine at all."

If you cut down, be patient, says Dr. Hieken. It may take a few weeks or even months to notice a difference.

Make yourself a cup of herbal tea. Corn silk, buchu, and uva ursi—herbal teas found at health food stores—act as mild diuretics that can flush out some of the fluid that contributes to breast discomfort, says Dr. Yankauskas.

Ease pain with evening primrose oil. "Though there is no scientific explanation for it, taking evening primrose oil relieves breast pain in about 30 percent of the women I see," says Dr. Gadd. Health food stores sell evening primrose oil in tablet form. Take three tablets nightly before bed when you experience breast discomfort, says Dr. Gadd.

Try some vitamin E. "Some studies have shown that taking slightly larger amounts than the Daily Value of vitamin E is very effective in relieving breast tenderness and discomfort from fibrocycstic breasts," says Dr. Yankauskas. Either start with the Daily Value of 30 international units (IU) and increase it when you experience breast problems or take 200 to 400 IU of vitamin E a day. "That should be safe. But don't take more," she says. Vitamin E is stored in your body fat, so too much could be toxic.

Eat less fat. Women in cultures that customarily consume a low-fat diet have fewer breast complaints than those where women eat high-fat diets, says Dr. Yankauskas. So she advises women who complain of breast problems to eat a diet consisting of less than 30 percent fat. (On a 1,800 calorie-per-day diet, that's no more than 60 grams of fat.)

Lose weight. Women store estrogen in body fat, says Dr. Yankauskas. Losing excess weight can therefore help minimize the hormone's contribution to breast discomfort.

Walk away breast pain. "Women who exercise two or three times a week have fewer breast problems," says Dr. Yankauskas. Exercise helps by reducing body fat and increasing circulating levels of endorphins—natural feel-good chemicals released by the brain. Avoid exer-

WHEN TO SEE A DOCTOR

If you have breast pain every month, without respite, consult your doctor, even if it seems to be related to your menstrual cycle, says Michele A. Gadd, M.D., a participating surgeon at the Comprehensive Breast Health Center Division of Surgical Oncology at Massachusetts General Hospital in Boston. You should also consult your doctor if you notice:

- Breast pain that comes on suddenly, especially when you haven't been experiencing monthly pain
- Breast pain that occurs after starting new medication or hormone replacement therapy
- Bloody or milky discharge from one or both nipples
- Any breast lump or thickening, whether or not it is painful

If you have had breast lumps in the past that your doctor diagnosed as noncancerous, you might choose to wait until your menstrual period passes to see if the lump or thickening disappears, says Dr. Yankauskas.

If you have no symptoms but are worried about your breasts for any reason, go ahead and see a physician, says Frances Marcus Lewis, R.N., Ph.D., professor of family and child nursing at the University of Washington in Seattle. "A woman's feelings about what is happening are as important as what's actually happening."

Also, women over the age of 30 should be sure to see a physician for a breast exam every year. Ask your doctor or nurse to teach you how to do a monthly self-exam. Become familiar with your normal breast anatomy in order to detect any subtle changes, says Dr. Lewis.

cises such as running or aerobic dance that create bounce and tug at your ligaments; that can contribute to breast pain. "A good brisk walk is just as good as any type of running or aerobic dance classes and probably easier on the breast tissue," she says. Be sure to wear a supportive athletic bra with nonelastic straps.

Swimming is also a good exercise choice for that sensitive time of the month.

Don't worry. Fear of breast cancer may make breast pain more noticeable. So if you're worried, get a checkup, advises Dr. Gadd. "In my practice, once most women know that they don't have cancer, the pain seems to be not so much of an issue. At first the pain seems to affect everything—from their jobs to their ability to carry on day-to-day functions—but once we've determined that they don't have cancer, they're not even that interested in taking any pain medication."

LUMPS THAT AREN'T

As it happens, worrisome (but harmless) lumps and thickenings in the breast are pretty common, especially among premenopausal women. Rest assured, though, doctors say that most breast lumps are not cancer, especially in women under the age of 40. Nevertheless, it is important that you become familiar with the normal terrain of your breasts in order to detect any changes in existing lumps or new lumps that warrant medical attention.

Here's what women doctors advise.

Check once a day only. "Many times, a woman finds a lump in her breast and keeps touching it and checking it, and guess what she's doing? She's making it hurt more," says Dr. Yankauskas. If you discover a lump at an "obvious" point in your menstrual cycle—either right before your period or mid-cycle, wait a few days to see if it disappears after your period.

"Go ahead and recheck the lump," says Dr. Yankauskas. "But once a day is enough."

Unplug your milk duct. If you're breastfeeding and find a lump, don't panic: What you feel could simply be a backed-up milk duct, says Dr. Yankauskas. To release the blockage, soften the affected breast with a warm washcloth, express the excess milk and feed your baby.

Breastfeeding Problems

Brush Up on Your Nursing Skills

*B*reastfeeding is as natural as walking. But nursing doesn't always come naturally for mother or child. A newborn doesn't always "get it" right away. Or perhaps your body doesn't seem to produce enough milk to satisfy your child. Or nursing leaves your breasts sore. Don't despair: Women doctors have plenty of helpful advice.

REMEDIES FOR COLIC AND FUSSINESS

Breast milk is ideal nutrition for babies, and breastfeeding can be part of an important emotional relationship between mother and infant, says Ruth Lawrence, M.D., professor of pediatrics in the Division of Neonatology at the University of Rochester School of Medicine and Dentistry. But successful nursing doesn't always come easily. "It is not a reflex, but a skill that must be learned," she says. Here are ways to deal with some of the challenges that can arise when you want to breastfeed, but your baby has other ideas.

Rest, rock, relax. Babies can and do sense any insecurity and tension in their moms, says Dr. Lawrence. "Colic in babies has been associated with maternal tension," she says. "It also interferes with letting down your milk—that is, release by your milk-producing glands." So find somewhere peaceful to feed your baby, somewhere with low lights and maybe some quiet music, especially during the first few weeks of nursing.

Sitting in a rocking chair can be a big help, adds Dr. Lawrence, because the structural design forces you to lean back and relax.

Nurse early, nurse often. Babies' appetites vary widely, says Susan Schulman, M.D., attending physician in the Department of Pediatrics at Maimonides Medical Center in Brooklyn. Little Jimmy may require 6 feedings a day, while Joey needs 16. Not to worry, she says: Frequent feedings actually keep Mom's milk flowing. So the more frequently your baby nurses, the more milk you produce. It's a common misconception that frequent nursing encourages overproduction of milk and a condi-

WHEN TO SEE A DOCTOR

Breastfeeding shouldn't hurt, says Ruth Lawrence, M.D., professor of pediatrics in the Division of Neonatology at the University of Rochester School of Medicine and Dentistry. So if nothing you try seems to relieve pain and discomfort brought on by nursing, consult your doctor, especially if nursing leaves your breasts red, hot, swollen and painful. You may have mastitis, a breast infection that requires attention.

tion called engorgement, but that's not true, says Dr. Schulman. Frequent nursing improves drainage and a healthy flow of milk, she says.

Tilt and switch. Some babies are unsatisfied, because they nurse on just one breast, fall asleep, then wake up hungry an hour later, says Dr. Schulman. Try this: When you notice your baby drifting off to dreamland, gently tilt her up and down until her eyes open—to wake her—then switch her to your other breast. "Don't take no for an answer. Finish feeding on both sides," Dr. Schulman says.

At first, forgo all bottles. Babies who are bottle-fed part-time within the first couple of weeks get confused when prompted to breastfeed, says Dr. Schulman. "They start looking for a rubber nipple on their mother and are unhappy when they don't find it," she says. So wait until your baby is at least three weeks old before you introduce a bottle.

Desalt your milk. Some babies refuse to nurse right after mom has exercised, says Dr. Lawrence. To get rid of sodium that accumulates at your nipples when you work up a sweat, express and discard a teaspoon or two of milk and wash off your breasts after exercise and before nursing.

Drink a glass of water both before and after exercise. When you perspire, your breasts, which are actually modified sweat glands, use up water needed to produce milk, says Dr. Schulman. To stay hydrated, drink up.

PRIME THE PUMP

Sometimes you know you have milk, but it's not flowing. To help nature along, try these suggestions.

Massage yourself. A gentle breast massage stimulates milk flow, says Elaine Stillerman, a licensed massage therapist on the staff of the

Swedish Institute of Massage in New York City and author of *Mother-Massage*. With your fingertips, circle around the base of one breast, then the other. Then place both hands flat on either side of one breast and slowly slide outward from the areola, the dark area surrounding the nipple. Repeat on your other breast.

Warm a clogged duct. It's not unusual for a milk duct to clog, preventing free flow of breast milk. A warm washcloth or shower and some gentle massaging helps unplug a clogged milk duct by increasing blood flow to the area, says Dr. Lawrence. After your breast softens, feed your baby or express excess milk.

Cool engorgement. Dr. Lawrence recommends an ancient folk remedy for tender, engorged breasts the first few days following birth: Place cool, fresh cabbage leaves on your breasts until they fully wilt. (The cabbage leaves, that is, not your breasts.) If you're fresh out of cabbage leaves or prefer a less exotic approach, a cool, moist washcloth may help: Applying a cold compress for 15 to 20 minutes at a time between feedings reduces blood flow and the overfilling of the breasts, says Dr. Lawrence. But don't apply just before feeding, as it will interfere with letdown of your milk.

Quit smoking. Smoking right before breastfeeding interferes with release of milk from milk glands, says Dr. Lawrence. So if you smoke and have been meaning to quit, breastfeeding is a good time to stop.

SORE BREASTS? DO THIS

If your baby is enthusiastic about nursing, but your breasts are the worse for wear, women doctors offer these strategies.

Change your position each time you nurse. Using a variety of positions encourages your baby's mouth to create pressure on different parts of your nipple, which helps prevent soreness as well as clogged ducts, says Dr. Schulman. Two tried-and-true positions include the regular cradle position, where you support your baby's head in the crook of your arm while nursing, or the lying down position, with your baby lying down in the bed next to you. Dr. Schulman also recommends the football position. Hold your baby's head in your hand, and allow her body and legs to rest on your hip, like carrying a football downfield.

Moisten up. If your nipples become dry and cracked—often the case if you live in a dry climate and you breastfeed, says Dr. Lawrence—try between-feeding applications of a form of purified lanolin such as Lansinoh, made especially for nursing mothers. Thoroughly wash off the lotion before baby's next feeding.

Brittle Nails

Put an End to Dry, Fragile Nails

Growing up, many women remember their mothers drinking a daily concoction of gelatin and water or juice, hoping that the gelatin would make their nails stronger. But that beauty aid, popular in the 1950s, probably did little or nothing for Mom's brittle nails.

"There's no scientific evidence that drinking gelatin makes your nails stronger," says Elizabeth Abel, M.D., clinical associate professor of dermatology at Stanford University School of Medicine. Nor has she seen evidence to prove that applying biotin, a B-complex vitamin, to the nails—another traditional belief—helps.

Sooner or later, every woman experiences split or cracked nails, says Dr. Abel. The problem isn't too little protein or too little biotin—it's too little moisture.

"Nails get weak and brittle, then split, because they dry out," explains Dr. Abel. "Exposure to household chemicals and detergents tend to dry out the nails. And some nail dryness is simply a product of aging. Our nails become more brittle and thinner, and they split more easily as we grow older."

NO MORE SPLITS AND CRACKS

Here's what you can do to strengthen brittle nails.

Moisturize to the max. "Petroleum jelly (such as Vaseline) or a thick, water-washable cream acts as an emollient; it holds in moisture around and under your nails," says Dr. Abel.

Wear cotton gloves to bed. Another fan of petroleum jelly is skin-care specialist Lia Schorr, owner of Lia Schorr Skin Care Salon in New York City. She advises her clients to put a thick layer of petroleum jelly on their hands when getting ready for bed, then wear cotton gloves overnight. This is especially helpful in winter, when hands and nails dry out quickly.

"It's a fantastic treatment," Schorr says. "Women love the way it makes their nails look."

Soak 'em in olive oil. Schorr recommends an oil treatment for dry nails. She has learned through years of experience that it's best to use a half-cup of warm olive oil and soak your hands for 15 to 30 minutes. "Olive oil is the best because it's natural," she explains.

Hydrate with bath-oil capsules. Dr. Abel also advises women with brittle nails to soak their hands in diluted bath oil for five minutes once a day. "I like those little bath-oil capsules. I break them into warm water and then apply a moisturizer or a cream with alpha hydroxy in it. The alpha hydroxy is basically a moisturizer that helps hydrate your hands and nails."

Or use other good mositurizers. Phoebe Rich, M.D., clinical assistant professor of dermatology at Oregon Health Sciences Center in Portland, also advises women to use a good moisturizer. She recommends an over-the-counter product called Complex 15 to women with brittle nails.

Beware of nail polish remover. Women doctors also warn that frequent manicures can dry the nails, because polish removers that contain acetone are drying.

"Also, avoid nail products that contain formaldehyde," warns Marianne O'Donoghue, M.D., associate professor of dermatology at

WHAT WOMEN DOCTORS DO

Petroleum Jelly, All Day

Marianne O'Donoghue, M.D.

Women entering the office of dermatologist Marianne O'-Donoghue, M.D., can't help noticing the jar of petroleum jelly prominently visible on her desk. The jar of Vaseline petroleum jelly is a clue as to how the associate professor of dermatology at Rush-Presbyterian–St. Luke's Medical Center in Chicago keeps her nails healthy.

"I think that petroleum jelly is the best thing in the world for dry hands and nails," she says. "I rub it lightly on my nails at least four or five times a day—often in front of patients—and I tell them to do the same. I suggest that they keep several jars on hand—one by the television, one by the telephone and one on the nightstand—and I advise them to rub it on their nails throughout the day."

Dr. O'Donoghue credits this humble product with keeping her nails in great shape.

WHEN TO SEE A DOCTOR

If your nails are chronically brittle, and you don't know what's causing the problem, see your dermatologist for help. Be sure to tell her about any medications that you're currently taking or other symptoms that you're experiencing, says Phoebe Rich, M.D., clinical assistant professor of dermatology at Oregon Health Sciences Center in Portland. She may also want to test you for anemia, another possible cause of brittle nails in women.

Rush-Presbyterian–St. Luke's Medical Center in Chicago. "It can actually cause contact dermatitis, and it also dries out the nails."

Polish, then moisturize. "If you use polish remover often enough to cause drying—frequency varies from woman to woman—then you need to counterbalance the dehydrating effect by putting moisture back into your nails," says Loretta Davis, M.D., associate professor of dermatology at the Medical College of Georgia School of Medicine in Augusta. "So always be sure to moisturize your hands and nails after a manicure."

Let your nails breathe. To stay strong, your nails need to breathe occasionally. So women doctors suggest taking your nail polish off the night before a manicure and then moisturizing them with cream or ointment. Even better, let your nails go a few days at a time without polish to let air reach them.

Keep nails short. Trimming your nails closely is yet another way to minimize problems if you have brittle nails, says Dr. Davis. File or trim them after bathing, when they're damp and soft. They'll cut more easily, minimizing the chance of damage or splitting.

Bronchitis

Silence the Killer Cough

*Y*ou had the flu, that's true, but that was weeks ago, and you're still coughing, hacking and bringing up those disgusting little blobs of mucus that boys in junior high call lungers. (Doctors call this a productive cough.) Sounds like you have bronchitis—inflamed, irritated airways.

Bronchitis can last just a few weeks—the result of a hard-to-shake cold or flu. When bronchitis drags on for more than three months or occurs once a year or more often, it's considered chronic (most likely to happen to smokers or people with other lung problems such as emphysema or cystic fibrosis).

FIRST THINGS FIRST

If you have bronchitis, getting mucus up and out of your lungs is a primary concern, because mucus-filled lungs breed bacteria that can cause pneumonia, says Sally Wenzel, M.D., associate professor at the University of Colorado School of Medicine and a pulmonary specialist at the National Jewish Center for Immunology and Respiratory Medicine, both in Denver. Avoiding inhaled irritants is important, too. And keeping your immunity strong can help prevent the worst complications of bronchitis.

Here's what you can do.

Toss the cigarettes. If you smoke, consider that lingering cough as an early warning signal of lung damage. "Smokers are much more likely to develop bronchitis than nonsmokers," says Dr. Wenzel.

If you stop smoking, you may cough up even more mucus for a time, but that's actually a good sign. "It means that your lungs are working to clear themselves out," she explains. As your lungs heal, the cough will soon fade.

Women who stop smoking may be surprised to notice that they get fewer so-called chest colds—and that goes for their children, too, who will no longer suffer the ill effects of secondhand smoke.

Ask others not to smoke in your vicinity. Breathing someone else's cigarette smoke can make your bronchitis worse, Dr. Wenzel says. "Stay away from secondhand smoke."

85

WHEN TO SEE A DOCTOR

Bronchitis can set the stage for pneumonia, so see a doctor promptly if your cough gets worse, if you feel weak and tired or have a fever or if you're short of breath. The only sure way to determine whether or not you have pneumonia is a chest x-ray. If you have pneumonia, you'll be given antibiotics.

Get misty. "When you breathe in moist air, you help thin out mucus, which makes it easier to clear out the lungs," explains Karen Conyers, a respiratory therapist at the University of Kansas Medical Center in Kansas City. Taking a hot shower or bath, draping a towel over your head and breathing the steam from a bowl of hot water or running a humidifier in your bedroom as you sleep can all provide the moisture that your airways need to stay clear.

Drink your fill. Imbibing water also helps thin mucous secretions in the lungs, Conyers says.

"Eight eight-ounce glasses a day is the minimum," says Dr. Wenzel.

Try a cup of mullein tea. A brew of this herb is said to soothe mucous membranes and help remove mucus from the lungs, reports Nan Kathryn Fuchs, Ph.D., a nutritionist in Sebastopal, California, and nutrition editor of the *Women's Health Letter.*

To make the tea, steep a handful of dried mullein leaves (about two teaspoons per cup) in a pot of freshly boiled water for about ten minutes. Strain and drink up to three cups a day. Check at a health food store for dried mullein leaves.

Blow up balloons. Respiratory therapists sometimes have their patients blow into a device with an adjustable valve that exercises the lungs the same way as blowing up balloons.

"By taking deeper breaths and blowing harder than one would normally, blowing up balloons may help people move mucus up and out of their lungs," Conyers says.

Eat onions. "Onions contain a number of ingredients, including quercetin, a compound in the bioflavonoid family that may help protect the lungs from infection," says Dr. Fuchs. In test-tube experiments, quercetin proved effective against several viruses.

Add some spice to your life. Red peppers, curry and other spicy foods that make your eyes water or nose run can help thin mucous secretions, says Dr. Fuchs.

Bruises

Erase the Black and Blues

*M*ost bruises occur in either of two ways: You hit something hard—a desk, a coffee table or a chair. Or, something hard—a cyclist, a falling carton or a toppling bookshelf—hits you.

"In the process, you break blood vessels, which leak blood into areas under your skin, causing swelling, discoloration and soreness," says Wilma Bergfeld, M.D., head of clinical research in the Department of Dermatology at the Cleveland Clinic Foundation.

Almost a taboo topic, "fingerprint" bruises are also common in women, along their shoulders, wrists, hips or thighs—a result of rough handling by a boyfriend or husband, either during moments of too-rough intimacy or unfortunately, during physical abuse, says Dr. Bergfeld.

Bruises are also common in older women whose skin is thinning with aging, because collagen—the connective tissue that cushions skin—breaks down, leaving underlying blood vessels more vulnerable, says Dr. Bergfeld. Long-term sun damage can also make women's skin more susceptible to repeat bruising. And older women who take multiple medications for diseases, including blood thinners like aspirin, also have an increased risk of bruising.

THE GEOGRAPHY OF BRUISES

Women doctors say that a common bruise should heal on its own within a few weeks. As it progresses through the stages of healing, the bruise evolves through a horrid rainbow of colors—reddish-blue, then purplish-black, then yellowish-green, says Dr. Bergfeld.

As a general rule, bruises tend to heal more slowly as you go down the body, says dermatologist Karen E. Burke, M.D., Ph.D., an attending physician at Cabrini Medical Center in New York City and at Greensboro Specialty Surgical Center in North Carolina. "They heal fastest on your face (usually within a week), slower on your trunk (in one to two weeks) and even slower on your legs. Don't be disconcerted if a leg bruise doesn't completely heal for up to a month."

WHEN TO SEE A DOCTOR

Women doctors say that you should see a physician if:
- You have a large bruise from a collision or injury of some kind (a fall or car accident, for example), especially if the bruise is painful and limits movement in a joint.
- You tend to bruise a lot for no apparent reason.
- You bruise easily and rely heavily on aspirin or other over-the-counter painkillers, such as ibuprofen or acetaminophen, for chronic conditions such as arthritis.
- You develop a large bruiselike clot of blood that is swollen and very painful (known as a hematoma) after surgery. Return to your surgeon, who will be able to treat it so that it will heal faster.

Bruises on the legs are usually the worst, because there is more blood pressure in leg vessels, so they bleed more than blood vessels in the arms, for example, explains Dr. Bergfeld.

BRUISE CONTROL

The next time you bruise yourself, women doctors suggest that you take these measures to help minimize pain and ugliness.

Ice on, ice off. If you apply ice right after you bump your skin, you can limit the size and severity of a bruise and relieve pain, says Sheryl Clark, M.D., assistant clinical professor of dermatology at Cornell Medical Center and an assistant attending physician in medicine at the New York Hospital, both in New York City. "The coldness clamps blood vessels shut so that less blood escapes into surrounding tissue."

Using ice wrapped in cloth, or a cold pack, ice the bruise for 10 to 20 minutes, then take a break. Repeat every two hours. "Try keeping a cold pack in the refrigerator instead of the freezer," Dr. Clark suggests. "It still gets good and cold, but instead of freezing solid, it stays flexible so that you can conform it to your body."

Wrap it. Wrap an elastic bandage around the bruised area immediately (especially if it's on your leg) to apply mild pressure to broken blood vessels. The support might prevent vessels from leaking as much blood, minimizing the severity of the bruise, says Dr. Bergfeld.

Bring in the heat. After 24 hours, when the bruise has fully developed, it's safe to apply heat. "At that point heat actually helps open up the surrounding blood vessels so that they can sweep away fluids and blood cells much more quickly," says Dr. Clark. Soak in a hot bath or apply a heating pad or a washcloth soaked in hot water, for 20 minutes, three times a day, until the bruise resorbs. But don't apply heat immediately.

"Heat causes tissues to swell, and at that early stage it can actually cause more bleeding and make the bruise worse," cautions Dr. Bergfeld.

Knock out a bruise with vitamin K. Look for a brand-name bruise-diminishing cream containing vitamin K, such as Vitamin K Formula Clarifying Cream, at drugstores. "The cream penetrates your skin and provides vitamin K at the bruise site, which your body needs to break down blood and resorb it," says Dr. Clark.

"I've found that vitamin K cream helps resolve bruises faster. A lot of my patients really like it," she says. Rub vitamin K cream into a bruise right away and reapply twice a day until the bruise is dissolved. (Eating foods rich in vitamin K doesn't seem to provide high enough concentrations of the vitamin at the bruise site to be effective.)

Try cosmetic cover-up creams. You can camouflage a bruise with special yellow-tinted cover-up makeups, says Dr. Clark. "Since bruises are a mixture of blue and red, if you apply yellow—the opposite color on the primary color wheel—that cancels out the bruise so that it appears neutral."

"You can usually buy this at the cosmetic counter of a major department store," she says. Estee Lauder, for example, makes Under Cover Tint in yellow. And a company called Physician's Formula sells a less expensive version at drugstores. Look for a waterproof formula so that it won't wash or sweat off.

Boost bruise immunity with vitamin C. Bruises occur more frequently in people who don't get enough vitamin C. So if you notice that you bruise regularly, up your vitamin C intake. "Eating lots of fresh fruits and vegetables should give you all the vitamin C you need, but if you think that you're not getting enough, try a multivitamin," says Dr. Clark.

High doses of vitamin C could increase your risk for kidney stones. To prevent this, make sure that you drink plenty of water if you take extra vitamin C, advises Dr. Bergfeld.

Build collagen with vitamin C cream. As a long-term bruise preventative, try daily applications of vitamin C creams and lotions (available at drugstores or through your dermatologist). "The vitamin C is absorbed into the skin and, over time, helps rebuild collagen, which cushions and supports blood vessels, making bruising less likely," says Dr. Bergfeld.

Bunions

Baby Those Bony Bumps

*D*oes your foot resemble a triangle, with the tip of your big toe angling inward and your joint jutting outward? If so, you have a bunion. And it probably hurts.

The pain of bunions occurs when the knobby lump that forms at the outside of the big-toe joint becomes sore and swollen, irritating nearby nerves. This is most likely to happen when your feet have been encased in shoes that press against the bunion.

Some of us inherit bunions from our parents. And wearing pointy shoes that squeeze our toes together—as many women do—doesn't help.

DO-IT-YOURSELF RELIEF

Here's what to do for immediate relief—and how to help prevent bunions from getting worse.

Try ice. If your bunion feels hot and swollen, it may be inflamed. Cool it down by applying a cloth-covered ice pack, suggests Marika Molnar, P.T., director of West Side Dance Physical Therapy in New York City. "I like to use a Ziploc-type resealable plastic bag half-filled with water and crushed ice and wrapped in a damp cloth," she says. Apply for 10 or 15 minutes, then remove for a few minutes to let your foot warm up before applying again.

If you have circulation problems in your feet or diabetes, you're better off avoiding ice for any foot problems.

Exercise your toes. Work the muscles that control the side-to-side movement of your big toe with the following exercise, says Molnar.

Sit with your feet flat and straight out in front of you. Try to move your big toes toward each other, then bring them back. If you can't manage this at first, use your hand to help move your toes. "The muscle that you are using is under the inside anklebone, about one inch down. You can feel a little bulge at this spot as you contract the muscles."

"This exercise helps properly align the joint by rebalancing muscles and stretching contracted tendons in your foot," Molnar says. "Unless your joint is very deteriorated, it will help keep your bunion from getting worse."

She suggests that when you're sitting, try to do five or six repetitions of the exercise every few hours. "This is a difficult exercise to do," she admits. "It takes time to begin to get it, and this muscle fatigues quickly." Keep at it however, and it will get easier.

Measure your foot. Experts advise selecting footwear that gives bunions plenty of space. "You must get the pressure off your bunions with properly fitted shoes," says Cheryl Weiner, D.P.M., a podiatrist in Columbus, Ohio, and president of the American Association for Women Podiatrists.

To do that, always get your foot measured when you buy shoes, says Nancy Elftman, a certified orthotist/pedorthist (a professional shoe fitter) in La Verne, California. Make sure that the width of your foot is measured at its widest point—from your big toe across to your baby toe—while you're standing barefoot or in socks.

Look for a full or softly rounded toe box. The toe box is the front of the shoe where the toes sit. The toes of any shoes you wear should be round or square, not pointy. Certain sport-shoe makers, such as New Balance and Avia, sell models with lots of toe room. Among dress shoes look for Easy Spirit and Nine West, Elftman recommends.

Stick with flats. Heels shift your weight forward to the ball of your foot, which is something that you don't want if you have bunions, says Kathleen Stone, D.P.M., a podiatrist in private practice in Glendale, Arizona. "You want no more than a 1½ inch heel to distribute your body weight evenly across your foot."

Try men's footwear. If you're having trouble finding shoes wide enough in women's sizes, try men's shoes, which are generally cut wider, says Dr. Weiner.

Get arch support. This also helps distribute your body weight evenly across your entire foot surface, says Dr. Stone. Running shoes usually fit the bill.

WHEN TO SEE A DOCTOR

If your bunions hurt every day, even with properly fitting shoes, or if the pain limits your activities, see a doctor. Specially fitted orthotics (inserts worn inside your shoes) may help relieve bunion pain. Or your podiatrist might recommend surgery to remove the bony overgrowth and help realign the bones in the big-toe joint.

Burnout
Hope for the Hopelessly Exhausted

High in the mountains surrounding majestic Aspen, Colorado, Jackie Farley runs a sleep-away camp for burned-out women.

Campers who sign up for a stay at her retreat—CenterPoint— are treated to four days of relaxation, hikes, meditation, massages, gourmet meals, camaraderie, quiet solitude and bedtime stories.

A one-time burnout herself, Farley knows the territory. In 1992, fresh from divorcing a successful and very demanding CEO of a well-known company, she was simultaneously relocating, starting a business, doing charitable work for a handful of philanthropies, and (in her words) "exercising compulsively," when she found herself utterly exhausted. "I never called it burnout; I called it compulsive bulldozer mode."

THE TELLTALE SIGNS

Too many responsibilities, too few resources, too little control, too little encouragement and no end in sight all add up to burnout, says Susan Brace, R.N., Ph.D., a psychologist in private practice in Los Angeles. Telltale symptoms include exhaustion, sorrow, discouragement, migraines, anxiety, stomachaches, irritability, insomnia, depression, apathy, social withdrawal and—most of all—hopelessness.

"What distinguishes burnout is the feeling of helplessness or powerlessness—the conviction that nothing is going to get better," says Beverly Potter, Ph.D., a psychologist in Berkeley, California, and author of *Beating Job Burnout*.

Women appear to be particularly vulnerable to burnout, Dr. Potter says. "Women aren't conditioned to speak up, grab control and be in charge the way men are. We're more likely to think, 'This always happens to me. What can I do? Nothing.'"

A SELF-RESCUE PLAN

Fortunately, there's plenty that you can do to combat burnout. Here's what experts advise.

Give yourself a break. One of the first things that Farley tells women who find their way to CenterPoint is to make a commitment, without judgment, to set aside 15 minutes for themselves every day.

Do whatever you like, says Farley: Go for a short hike, listen to music, take a bath, read, meditate or sit in a quiet place. The idea is to get out from under all the responsibilities that weigh you down, and find perspective. Farley says that you must honor these rituals to help you reduce stress and gain insight.

Recruit a stand-in. If you have kids or care for an elderly parent, ask your partner or a friend to relieve you during your break, says Camille Lloyd, Ph.D., professor in the Department of Psychiatry and Behavioral Sciences at the University of Texas Medical School at Houston.

Diagnose what ails you. If you feel burned out but don't know why, carefully observe what's going on when you feel distressed and take notes, says Dr. Potter. Get specific: Is your boss dumping a weekend's worth of work on your desk every Friday? Does your husband drop the ball every time he's supposed to cook dinner or put the kids to bed? Are you overwhelmed by the demands of caring for a critically ill parent?

Speak up. Once you've identified the problem, it's time to talk.

"But don't just go to the boss and say, 'I'm feeling burned out,'" says Dr. Potter. It's too vague. Instead, be specific and offer suggestions. Say your boss tells you to do one thing and her supervisor tells you differently. Suggest a meeting so that the three of you can get together and work things out.

By the same token, don't tell your spouse, "You're never there for me," says Dr. Lloyd. Instead, explain that you need extra support while the kids are small or while your mother is sick. Say, "It's tough for me right now; it would be nice if you could spend time with me every Saturday night."

Talk to a sympathetic other. Friends, co-workers or members of a support group can also help, says Dr. Brace. In fact, a study conducted at California State University found that college professors were significantly less likely to suffer burnout if they had a social support network to fall back on.

Take periodic vacations. You don't have to go far or spend a lot of money, says Dr. Lloyd. The idea is to get out from under all your responsibilities and get a clearer view of things. Again, if you take care of an elderly parent, enlist the help of a sibling or ask other family members to help pay for a home health-care aide or a respite-care worker who can fill in for you while you're getting R and R. The Visiting Nurse Association in your area may be able to help with arrangements.

WHEN TO SEE A DOCTOR

Sometimes burnout is easily remedied; sometimes it's not. Consult your local mental health agency, employee counseling service or a mental health professional if:

- Feelings of depression linger for more than two weeks.
- A sense of being burned out interferes with your ability to do your job, interact socially or function in other ways.

Reward yourself for small accomplishments. Don't rely on others to recognize and encourage your efforts, says Dr. Potter. Divide each thing you have to do into manageable parts. Then set a deadline for each part and reward yourself (with, say, a trip to the movies or a cappuccino) as you meet a deadline.

Burns

Beat the Heat and Soothe Your Skin

Even the smallest burn—accidentally grazing a red-hot oven rack with one hand or singeing your neck with a curling iron—can cause big-time pain, redness, throbbing, swelling and even blistering.

"The most common burns that I see on women come from either working in the kitchen (cooking injuries and hot-liquid scalds) and from using curling irons," says D'Anne Kleinsmith, M.D., a staff dermatologist at William Beaumont Hospital in Royal Oak, Michigan.

Despite their convenience, microwave ovens are a surprising source of an increasing number of kitchen burns, says Candy Kuehn, R.N., nurse manager at the Burn Center at St. Paul–Ramsey Medical Center in Minnesota. "People overheat liquids beyond the boiling point in the microwave, then pull out the cup without realizing that the cup is hot, or they spill it and they burn themselves."

Erase Curling Iron Burn Marks

Using a curling iron takes finesse: One false move, and the hot metal rod is apt to graze your ear or neck, leaving you with a reddish welt that blisters. Unless properly cared for, curling iron burns can leave a brownish scar.

To help diminish the unattractive brownish spot left behind after curling iron burns heal, D'Anne Kleinsmith, M.D., a staff dermatologist at William Beaumont Hospital in Royal Oak, Michigan, offers the following tips.

Bleach away the scar. First, says Dr. Kleinsmith, you can apply a mild over-the-counter skin-bleaching cream containing hydroquinone (such as Porcelana) to the scarred area to help lighten it. "Don't use this until after the burn has healed, because it could sting and irritate an open wound and interfere with healing. But if you use a bleaching cream on a healed, closed scar, it's very rare that you would develop a skin irritation."

Reach for glycolic acid. As an alternative, Dr. Kleinsmith suggests trying an over-the-counter glycolic acid product, such as Alpha-Hydrox, which helps peel away the top layer of skin. You'll get fastest scar-fading results if you use the glycolic acid and a bleaching cream, she says.

COOL IT

Major burns require medical attention. But even when a burn is minor, immediate action helps keep pain and skin damage to a minimum, say women doctors and other health care professionals. Here's their advice.

Run it under cool water. Apply cool water immediately to stop the burning process, says Kuehn. "Don't use ice, because it's too cold and could further traumatize already damaged skin."

Milk or soda works, too. If water is not convenient, use whatever you have nearby to cool a burn quickly—even milk or a cold can of soda wrapped in a clean towel, says Dr. Kleinsmith. Then rinse the burn with cool water as soon as possible.

Cool with a compress. Apply a washcloth or towel soaked in cool (not icy) water on and off for several hours. So says Evelyn Placek,

Think Fast

D'Anne Kleinsmith, M.D.

During lunch one day, D'Anne Kleinsmith, M.D., a staff dermatologist at William Beaumont Hospital in Royal Oak, Michigan, spilled boiling-hot coffee on her finger. Fortunately, quick thinking literally saved her skin.

"I immediately dunked my finger in the glass of ice water at my place setting and kept it there until the pain began to subside," says Dr. Kleinsmith.

Other options include:
- Running your finger under cold water
- Dunking it in a glass of cold milk
- Wrapping it in a cold washcloth

Afterward, apply an antibacterial ointment and loosely bandage the burn.

M.D., a dermatologist and doctor of internal medicine in private practice in Scarsdale, New York.

Take aspirin or ibuprofen. If you take an anti-inflammatory medication quickly enough—within the first hour or so after a burn—it will not only ease pain but it might also actually prevent the burn from getting worse, says Dr. Placek. If you do not have a stomach ulcer, she recommends that you continue taking two 200-milligram tablets or capsules every six hours for one to two days to keep inflammation and swelling down and to help decrease the severity of the wound.

Be gentle with blisters. In general, leave a burn blister intact—it's your body's way of providing a protective bandage, says Kuehn. "The collection of fluid in the blister is the white blood cells that the body sends to help protect against infection and help with the healing process," she explains. If the blister is small, your body will naturally re-absorb the fluid within a few days. (For additional advice on dealing with blisters properly, see page 62.)

Clean the burn. Gently cleanse the burn area at least twice a day with mild soap and cool water or with hydrogen peroxide, which kills germs, suggests Dr. Kleinsmith.

"Some burn centers recommend cleaning burns twice a day, especially if the wound seems infected or if the dressing becomes soiled be-

WHEN TO SEE A DOCTOR

When it comes to deciding whether or not to get medical attention for a burn, women doctors and other health care professionals offer these guidelines. See a physician if:

- The burn is larger than the palm of your hand, deep or severe—that is, characterized by deep ulcers and open sores.
- The burn is small but deep—that is, extremely tender, painful, swollen and blistered.
- The burn occurs on your face, hands, feet or genitals.
- The burn has pus, yellowish drainage or a yellowish crust.
- The area around the burn looks red or feels hot.
- You have signs of a fever.
- The burn causes unmanageable pain.

Electrical or chemical burns should always be treated by a doctor, because the burns may actually be much worse than they appear on the surface, says Candy Kuehn, R.N., nurse manager at the Burn Center at St. Paul–Ramsey Medical Center in Minnesota. And burns on children under the age of five or in elderly people (who may have weaker-than-usual immune systems) should generally be examined by a physician.

If in doubt, call a doctor or a burn center hot line for help in assessing burn severity. The St. Paul–Ramsey Burn Center, for example, provides a 24-hour toll-free information line, 1-800-922-BURN, which you can call from anywhere in the country for advice.

cause of your daily activity," says Kuehn.

Apply antibacterial ointments. These over-the-counter salves will help kill germs and prevent infection, says Dr. Kleinsmith. Avoid neomycin (an ingredient in some salves), though—it can cause a red, itchy allergic reaction in some people.

Bandage the burn. "For small burns an adhesive strip will suffice," says Dr. Kleinsmith. "For larger burns gauze dressings and tape work better."

Keep it mobile. Keep bandages loose and move the joint or burned area as much as possible, so that joints don't stiffen up and so that skin stays supple, says Kuehn. Movement also boosts circulation to the area, which helps with healing and clears out fluid buildup.

Moisturize skin. After the wound has healed over, thinly apply a moisturizing lotion. "A healing burn can have lots of itching and cracking, which interfere with the skin's ability to moisturize itself," says Kuehn. Moisturizers can help restore elasticity to the skin and reduce dryness and flakiness. Fragrance-free lotions are best.

Fill up on fluids. Water keeps skin hydrated and helps burns heal, says Michele M. Gottschlich, R.D., Ph.D., director of nutrition services at the Shriners Burns Institute in Cincinnati. Aim for eight eight-ounce glasses a day.

Eat plenty of protein. While your burn heals, beef up on high-protein foods such as skim milk, lean meats, nuts, beans, eggs, peanut butter and fat-free cheeses, says Dr. Gottschlich. "Protein helps speed burn healing by rebuilding collagen, a building block of skin tissue. So with any burn your protein needs will be higher—and the larger the burn, the more protein you need."

Eat C. To help your burns heal from the inside out, Dr. Gottschlich recommends eating a variety of foods, including fruits and vegetables. "Good nutrition is just as important to burn healing as is cleaning the wound." Vitamin C (found in foods such as oranges, grapefruit, broccoli, orange juice and tomatoes) helps rebuild collagen in tissue and speeds healing. "If it's difficult to change your eating habits on top of caring for a burn, consider taking a daily multivitamin supplement," she says.

Caffeine Withdrawal
Drink Less and Enjoy It More

The connection was painfully clear. Whenever she missed her daily dose of coffee, Jo-Ellyn Ryall, M.D., got a headache. An annoying one.

"If you're used to getting a certain amount of caffeine, and you don't get it, or you cut back abruptly, you can experience withdrawal symptoms, like headaches," notes Dr. Ryall, a psychiatrist in private practice in St. Louis.

Harmless as it might seem, the caffeine in coffee, tea, cola and chocolate can be quite addicting.

Cut off from caffeine or limited to considerably less than they're accustomed to, caffeine junkies complain of headaches, depression, difficulty concentrating and fatigue.

Given the consequences, why would anyone want to cut back?

"A fair amount of research suggests that moderately high doses of caffeine (more than a few cups of caffeine-containing beverages per day) can raise risks of miscarriage, fertility problems and, in some predisposed women, tachyarrhythmia (abnormally increased heart rhythm), high cholesterol and panic attacks," says Erica Frank, M.D., assistant professor in the Department of Family and Preventive Medicine at Emory University School of Medicine in Atlanta.

Some research indicates that high daily doses of caffeine may also boost a woman's risk of osteoporosis and aggravate fibrocystic breast disease, heart rhythm abnormalities, high blood pressure, ulcers and premenstrual tension, says Suzette Evans, Ph.D., assistant professor of psychiatry at Columbia University College of Physicians and Surgeons in New York City who has studied the physical effects of caffeine.

HOW (AND WHY) TO CUT CAFFEINE

If you're downing more than three or four 5-ounce cups of coffee, 8-ounce mugs of tea or 12-ounce cans of cola a day, you should cut back, Dr. Frank says.

The American College of Obstetricians and Gynecologists doesn't have a position on safe limits for caffeine consumption during pregnancy. But if you're pregnant or trying to conceive, you should cut back to less than two or three cups of caffeinated beverages, advises Elizabeth Livingston, M.D., assistant professor of obstetrics and gynecology at Duke University Medical Center in Durham, North Carolina.

You should also limit yourself to two cups of caffeinated coffee, tea or cola or less if you have fibrocystic disease, heart rhythm problems, high blood pressure, ulcers or premenstrual tension, says Dr. Ryall.

SURVIVING WITHDRAWAL

The worst symptoms of caffeine withdrawal—headaches, depression and poor concentration—usually let up after two days, and the rest dissipate within a week, notes Dr. Evans. After drinking less than your usual amount for a week or so, you won't miss it, since your body will adjust to the lower dose.

Better yet, women doctors say that there's actually a way to cut back, even give up, caffeine without experiencing withdrawal at all. If your doctor has advised you to cut back, here's how.

Have a little caffeine—for medicinal purposes. Are you in the throes of caffeine withdrawal right this very moment? Unfortunately, caffeine-free aspirin and other caffeine-free analgesics don't do a very good job combating the headaches that can accompany withdrawal, says Dr. Evans. And they don't offer any relief from the fatigue and depression.

The best remedy for the headaches and other withdrawal symptoms, says Dr. Ryall, is actually a moderate dose of caffeine—a pain reliever that contains caffeine (such as Excedrin Extra Strength) or a small cup of caffeinated tea, coffee or cola.

Rely on the 25 percent solution. Women experts say that by gradually cutting back, you can avoid headaches and other withdrawal symptoms in the first place.

"Each week, cut back on the amount of caffeine that you drink by 25 percent," says Kathleen Zelman, R.D., a nutritionist in Atlanta and a spokesperson for the American Dietetic Association. This method of gradually decreasing your caffeine intake will eventually allow you to eliminate it completely from your diet, while remaining withdrawal symptom–free.

Here is Zelman's formula: The first week, add decaffeinated coffee, tea or cola to your cup until it reaches the one-quarter mark. Then, fill to the top with regular. The following week, add decaf to the halfway mark

Grab a Nap

Elizabeth Livingston, M.D.

Craving caffeine?

Maybe you want caffeine, or maybe you think you need caffeine, when what your body really needs is a little more sleep, says Elizabeth Livingston, M.D., assistant professor of obstetrics and gynecology at Duke University Medical Center in Durham, North Carolina.

"Especially during pregnancy, women can feel more fatigued," says Dr. Livingston. "When I was pregnant, I used to come up to my office between clinics just so I could take a nap on the couch."

So if you find yourself reaching for caffeine to pull you out of a slump, Dr. Livingston suggests that you lie down for a 10- to 20-minute nap.

(For more practical advice on dealing with an afternoon slump or fatigue, see pages 5 and 214.)

and top off with regular. By week three your cup should contain three-quarters decaf to every one-quarter regular. If you started out with an eight-cup-o'-joe-a-day habit, you'll be drinking the equivalent of only two cups of coffee at this point. From here you can continue with this formula until you are drinking all decaf. If you are at home and don't want to make two pots of coffee to mix, you can blend caffeinated and decaffeinated coffee grinds following the same principles.

Reach for noncaffeinated beverages. An alternative strategy is to substitute a cup of decaf, herbal tea, skim milk, juice or water for a quarter, then half and, finally, three-quarters of the cups that you regularly drink, says Zelman.

Grab the biscotti, not the espresso. "You might also be experiencing a lull in energy because your blood sugar is low," Zelman explains. Rather than chug caffeine, have a little something to eat—half a bagel, an orange, a handful of raisins—to get your blood sugar back up there.

Take a hike. Cutting back on caffeine is particularly hard for women who rely on coffee or cola to propel them through tedious tasks or sluggish days. For a caffeine-free energy boost, Dr. Livingston suggests that you take a 20-minute walk.

Save caffeine for crises. If you're limited to just a cup or so of coffee, save it for when you most need a boost (like morning).

Calluses
Smooth and Soothe Hands

*A*ny woman who has ever raked leaves without wearing gloves, only to awaken the next morning with painful blisters on the palms of her hands, knows why the body produces calluses. In a word: protection. If you rake a few leaves a day for a week, your skin would toughen, forming a thick layer that we call a callus, which allows you to do many things that were at first painful on sensitive skin, says Loretta Davis, M.D., associate professor of dermatology at the Medical College of Georgia School of Medicine in Augusta. Without a callus, pressure and friction irritate your skin, and you end up with a blister.

"Calluses are functional and, ideally, should be left alone," says Dr. Davis. "Women shouldn't worry about how calluses look, but they do."

SOFTENING TACTICS

If a callus becomes annoying, overly large or too tough, it can be improved, says Dr. Davis. Here are some tips.

Look for lactic acid or urea. Dr. Davis suggests that women soften hard or rough calluses with a moisturizing cream with lactic acid or urea. "Moisturizers with alpha hydroxy acids, such as glycolic acid (from sugarcane) or lactic acid (from milk) are also effective and easy to find—every major cosmetic line has hand creams that contain them. Alpha hydroxy acids and urea are especially good for dry skin," she says.

Soak, then moisturize. Some women soak callused areas in water first and then apply the moisturizer, says Dr. Davis. "If you do this frequently, the callus begins to soften."

File gently. When you shower, carefully rub the callused area with a pumice stone marketed by hand-care product companies as nail stones, suggests Dr. Davis. "Never use these tools without water, or you could damage your skin." Make this part of your daily shower routine.

Don't forget your gloves. To prevent calluses in the first place, Dr. Davis recommends wearing an appropriate sports glove for sporting activities, putting moisturizer on under the gloves to minimize friction. It's also a good idea to wear cotton gloves when doing yard work or gardening.

(For practical ways to manage calluses on your feet, see page 145.)

Canker Sores
Wipe Out Pinpoints of Pain

*P*erhaps second only to unidentified vaginal discharges, canker sores are truly among the most vexing maladies known to women. Tiny as they may be to the eye, the crater-shaped sores inside your cheeks or along your gums or tongue can send you reeling with pain and make eating and talking difficult. Kissing, of course, is out of the question.

EXTERNAL AND INTERNAL TACTICS

Women doctors offer some surprising but effective tactics against vexing canker sores.

Apply an antihistamine. When canker sore pain gets too much to bear, duck into your local drugstore and buy a bottle of Benadryl liquid, an antihistamine commonly taken for allergies or colds, suggests Lenore S. Kakita, M.D., clinical assistant professor of dermatology at the University of California, Los Angeles, and an adviser to the American Academy of Dermatology. Pull apart a clean cotton ball and soak a canker sore–size wad in one-half to one teaspoon of Benadryl. Place the drenched cotton directly on your sore for five to ten minutes. "Apply the Benadryl three or four times a day, making sure that you don't swallow

WHEN TO SEE A DOCTOR

If your canker sores are severe, if you get them often or if they last for more than two weeks, women doctors say that you should call your doctor, dermatologist or dentist. Also, alert your doctor if you also develop a high fever or swollen glands, signaling an infection.

For canker sores that are beyond self-help, prescription corticosteroids recommended by your doctor or triamcinolone dental paste (Kenalog in Orabase) can help.

Saltwater Rinse Helps

Mahvash Navazesh, D.M.D.

Scientists aren't convinced that chocolate causes canker sores. But Mahvash Navazesh, D.M.D., associate professor and vice-chair in the Department of Dental Medicine and Public Health at the University of Southern California School of Dentistry in Los Angeles, thinks that it's more than a coincidence that when she indulges in the joys of chocolate, she pays a hefty price. Before long, a fiery, red-rimmed canker sore shows up inside her mouth. Here's what she does to relieve the pain.

"When I get a canker sore, I rinse my mouth often with salt and water," says Dr. Navazesh. "Or I make a mixture of half hydrogen peroxide and half water and rinse with that.

"If the sore really burns a lot, anything cool like ice has a soothing effect."

more than the precautions on the bottle advise. It tends to numb the area, so you can eat."

One caution: If you've applied a numbing agent, eat carefully, says Mahvash Navazesh, D.M.D., associate professor and vice-chair in the Department of Dental Medicine and Public Health at the University of Southern California School of Dentistry in Los Angeles. If you inadvertently bite your numbed mouth while chewing, the resulting injury can make your canker sore worse.

Apply canker sore salve. Over-the-counter products such as Zilactin or Orabase-B coat the canker sore with a sticky substance that acts as a protective shield, to help you talk and eat. Both are recommended by women doctors. Geraldine Morrow, D.M.D., past president of the American Dental Association, a member of a American Association of Women Dentists and a dentist in Anchorage, Alaska, also gives a thumbs-up to Kank-A, an over-the-counter medicine made by Blistex.

Eliminate acidic foods. Cutting down on acid fruits and vegetables and certain nuts, like walnuts, can help prevent canker sores, says Dr. Morrow.

(For practical ways to manage cold sores, which are caused by a virus and affect the lips only, see page 131.)

Cellulite

Practical Tactics against "Fem Fat"

Even when she was 8½ months pregnant and waddling like a duck, Colleen O'Callaghan, a former member of the American Ballet Theater in New York, had no cellulite.

Nor do any of the dancers she knows. They all have smooth, taut skin with not one hint of the dimpled, quilted or rippled effect that the cosmetic industry has dubbed "cellulite."

But why not? Why do dancers escape while so many others have to wrap themselves in beach towels every time they wear swimsuits?

"Cellulite is fat," answers Diana Bihova, M.D., a dermatologist in New York City and author of *Beauty from the Inside Out*. "And classical ballet dancers have very little or no fat. In either case, their thighs are so well-toned that the skin stays taut."

The difference between fat on your waist and cellulite is the way that it manifests itself, Dr. Bihova adds. You can develop it when you gain weight or when your skin gets a little lax from aging or lack of exercise. Then, the previously unobtrusive fat puffs out like the polyester fill in a comforter, and your skin looks as though it has been stuffed and stitched like a quilt.

WORK IT OFF

Although you probably won't have the cellulite-free thighs and buttocks of a dancer unless you're willing to put in whole days of leaps, twirls and twists *en pointe*, here's what women doctors say that you can do to improve the look of your cellulite-laced hips, thighs and backside.

Lose any extra fat. Weight loss frequently reduces the fat responsible for thigh and butt dimpling, says Allison Vidimos, M.D., a staff dermatologist at the Cleveland Clinic Foundation. So she advises women bothered by cellulite to drop any extra weight and exercise to tone muscles.

"People who lose weight through diet and exercise may note some improvement in the cellulite-prone areas," she says. Once the fat cells shrink, and muscle tone is improved, the contour of the skin may look more smooth.

Tone your lower body. Exercises that tone your thighs, hips and

105

lower buttocks will give dimpled areas a better look, says Dr. Bihova. And they're a great way to help you lose weight. In fact, exercise works better than dieting at improving the way your thighs and buttocks look.

Work your outer thighs. One of the best exercises to tone your outer thighs is the leg lift, says Janet Wallace, Ph.D., associate professor of kinesiology at Indiana University in Bloomington.

To begin, lie down on the floor on your side, with your legs straight, one above the other. Then bend the elbow that's on the floor and prop your head on your hand. Put your other hand flat on the floor in front of your waist. Now, keeping both your legs straight and your toes pointed straight ahead, lift your top leg from hip to toe as far as it will go, then lower it back to the floor. Repeat the lift 11 more times, then turn on your other side and do 12 more.

Try leg lifts three times a week, adding a couple more each time you do them, until you reach a maximum of 30 repetitions on each side, says Dr. Wallace. "Forget that 'go for the burn' stuff," adds Dr. Wallace. Your thighs will begin to look smooth and taut without it.

Add bands to your workout. When you get to the point that you're doing 30 leg lifts a day with no effort, get a resistance band from your local sporting goods store, says Dr. Wallace. It looks like a giant rubber band, and they come in various colors.

Loop the band around each of your ankles and do your regular set of leg lifts. The added resistance will make your legs work harder and help tone your muscles further.

Work your inner thighs. One of the best exercises to tone your inner thighs is to lie down on the floor just as you did for leg lifts, says Dr. Wallace. But this time, instead of raising your top leg, hold that leg still, move your bottom leg out in front a few inches until it clears your top leg, then try to lift your bottom leg up in front of your top leg. Lift it as far as you can, then lower your leg to the floor.

Repeat the lift 11 more times, then turn on your other side and do 12 more, says Dr. Wallace. Try the exercise three times a week, adding a couple of lifts to each workout until you're doing 30 lifts a session.

Build your butt. Lie facedown on the floor, with your arms out at your shoulders, your elbows bent and your palms flat on the floor, says Dr. Wallace. Now, keeping your right leg straight, try to lift it heel-first off the floor. Lift it as far as you can, then lower it to the floor.

Repeat the lift 11 more times, then repeat the exercise with your left leg. Try the lift three times a week, adding a couple of lifts every time until you reach a maximum of 30 lifts for each leg. By then your bottom may very well look as smooth as a baby's.

Cervical Dysplasia
Post-treatment Relief

*I*n the course of examining a woman's cervix—the opening to the uterus—a doctor may find that the cells are abnormal. Otherwise, with cervical dysplasia, there are no symptoms. It may go away on its own. Or it may not.

It's the "may not" that makes doctors most nervous. Cervical dysplasia can be the first step in the development of cervical cancer. Or it may not be cancer. As such, it's important to get prompt evaluation and treatment, says Diane Solomon, M.D., chief of the cytopathology section of the National Cancer Institute in Bethesda, Maryland.

EASING DISCOMFORT

If you've been diagnosed with cervical dysplasia, you and your doctor will have to decide on treatment—whether to adopt a wait-and-see approach or undergo laser surgery or another procedure to remove the abnormal cells.

Try rest, and an ice pack. If you're being treated for cervical dysplasia, your best bet is to follow your doctor's instructions and let nature heal, says Lila A. Wallis, M.D., clinical professor of medicine and director of "Update Your Medicine," a series of continuing medical education programs for physicians, at Cornell University Medical College in New York City. The wrong self remedies may cause more bleeding. "Sometimes rest and an ice pack to the lower abdomen will help," she adds.

Take an OTC painkiller. If you experience pain or discomfort after removal of the abnormal cells, acetaminophen can help relieve it, says Dr. Wallis. Follow the directions on the package. Avoid aspirin or ibuprofen, because they could interfere with the blood-clotting mechanism.

Skip sex for two weeks. You'll need a few weeks to fully recover from treatment, says Dr. Wallis. The time can't be too precise, because each woman's response varies. "The cervical tissue will be kind of like a cut on your knee. It will bleed until it's healed and makes scar tissue," she explains. Refraining from sex for at least two weeks will give your wounded tissue a better chance to stop bleeding and fully heal.

WHEN TO SEE A DOCTOR

Cervical dysplasia has no symptoms, so you have to count on your doctor to find it. "It is important for a woman to go for her regular Pap smear even if she is not having any problems," says Diane Solomon, M.D., chief of the cytopathology section of the National Cancer Institute in Bethesda, Maryland.

The National Cancer Institute recommends an annual Pap smear for three consecutive years. If all three tests are negative, the interval between screenings might be lengthened to every three years. However, Dr. Solomon notes, many professional medical societies still recommend an annual test. Furthermore, "It is important not to stop having your Pap smear just because you've become menopausal or are over the age of 60. In fact, about one-quarter of all invasive cervical cancers arise in women over the age of 60."

Do not douche or use vaginal creams or lubricants (except as advised by your doctor) for at least two days before a Pap smear, says Dr. Solomon. It can interfere with detection of dysplasia. Schedule your appointment for approximately two weeks after the start of your last period. A sample taken during your menstrual flow may not be adequate for laboratory evaluation, she explains.

PREVENTION ADVICE

Cervical dysplasia is one of the conditions that you'd rather not have to deal with in the first place. Here's what women doctors suggest.

Protect yourself. Studies have shown that certain strains of human papillomavirus (HPV), otherwise known as genital warts, increase a woman's risk of developing cervical dysplasia, says Dr. Solomon. Two proteins in HPV repress both the tumor suppressor gene P53 and the cancer-fighting retinoblastoma protein PRV. Other sexually transmitted diseases (STDs), such as AIDS, and immunologic factors may also be linked to cervical dysplasia.

To protect yourself against STDs when not in a mutually monogamous relationship, always use a condom during sex, says Dr. Wallis. She recommends the female condom, a device consisting of two plastic rings connected by a polyurethane sheath. "There's always stuff that leaks around the male condom," she says. "The female condom covers the whole vulva, so that you don't get exposed."

Take your vitamins. Women whose daily diets include insufficient intake of vitamin A, riboflavin and folate (B vitamins) and ascorbate (vitamin C) have a higher risk of cervical dysplasia, according to a study at the Comprehensive Cancer Center of the University of Alabama at Birmingham. Research has pointed to the importance of certain nutritional deficiencies in relation to cervical cancer, but the role of nutritional factors is still poorly understood. The study showed that about 75% of 257 women studied took less than the Daily Value of vitamin A, riboflavin, vitamin C and folate. That's 5,000 international units for vitamin A, 1.7 milligrams for riboflavin, 400 micrograms for folate and 60 milligrams for vitamin C.

Chafing
Friction You Shouldn't Ignore

Rub two sticks together and you'll make a fire. Rub two thighs together and you'll get the human equivalent: A patch of skin so red and inflamed that it looks as though it's been badly sunburned.

"Chafing occurs as a result of skin-to-skin rubbing," explains Mary Lupo, M.D., associate clinical professor of dermatology at Tulane University School of Medicine in New Orleans. Heat, humidity and sweat make chafing more likely occur, particularly in moist areas between the thighs, under the breasts and in the armpits of heavier people.

Chafing is more pronounced if you wear synthetic fabrics—polyester pants, lycra bike shorts, nylon panty hose and spandex tights, for example—that trap moisture and reduce airflow to vulnerable areas, says Deborah S. Sarnoff, M.D., assistant clinical professor of dermatology at New York University in New York City. And if you've recently been on antibiotics, chafing may make you more susceptible to a yeast infection in the affected area.

SOOTHING RILED SKIN

Women doctors say that, fortunately, chafed skin is easily soothed. Here's what they suggest.

Strip. Ideally, the best way to deal with chafing is to remove your clothes and walk around nude whenever you're at home, says Esta Kronberg, M.D., a dermatologist in private practice in Houston. If modesty or circumstances prevent you from taking that tack, pull on a peasant dress or caftan that allows air to circulate freely around your body. The air reduces excess moisture on the skin that interferes with healing.

Apply a medicated cream. If the chafed area feels really irritated, smooth on an over-the-counter cortisone cream such as Cortaid, says Dr. Kronberg. The cream will stop the inflammation and soothe your skin.

Try an antifungal cream. "If cortisone cream doesn't work, and the redness and tenderness get worse over the next 24 hours, you probably have a yeast infection," says Dr. Kronberg. Apply Lotrimin or Monistat to the area—yes, the same cream that's sold for vaginal yeast infections. Just follow dosage instructions on the package.

Rinse, then rinse again. After you bathe or shower, rinse your body thoroughly so that no soap remains on your skin, says Dr. Lupo. Soap residues can compound chafing by irritating the skin, and they can disrupt your body's natural moisture barriers that normally shield you from at least some of the friction generated by skin-to-skin rubbing.

Turn on your hair dryer. "Once you're out of the shower, put your hair dryer on a low setting and dry all areas prone to chafing and yeast," says Dr. Sarnoff.

"Be meticulous in drying," adds Dr. Lupo. "Lift your belly if it hangs down a bit and dry the skin underneath. Lift your breasts as well. And pay particular attention to your thighs."

Sprinkle on an absorbent powder. Sprinkle a light covering of Zeasorb powder in areas prone to chafing, says Dr. Lupo. The powder, which is available at your local drugstore, will actually absorb at least some excess moisture as you move through your day, and it will zap any errant yeast cells that might have plans for colonizing on your skin.

Use tampons, not pads. Since sanitary napkins prevent the free flow of air and cause a buildup of moisture where crotch and thigh meet, use tampons instead, suggests Dr. Sarnoff. If you can't use tampons, make sure that you change your sanitary napkin frequently and sprinkle a little Zeasorb-AF powder over fresh napkins.

Lose weight. If you're significantly overweight, the best way to prevent chafing is to lose excess pounds, says Dr. Sarnoff. Then you're much less likely to have sagging skin that can rub against the rest of your body.

Chapped Lips
From Parched to Pretty

*I*f your kisser more closely resembles the dry Sahara lake bed featured in *National Geographic* than the luscious smiles advertising makeup in *Glamour*, take heart.

Your lips are the first victims of the harsh environment around us, says Lenore S. Kakita, M.D., clinical assistant professor of dermatology at the University of California, Los Angeles, and an adviser to the American Academy of Dermatology. Lips contain none of the pigment imbued to your skin by melanin (which protects against sun damage to some degree), and therefore are ultrasensitive to the sun's damaging rays. They are also in an area that gets drier with the evaporation of water. Aggravating factors are drying winds, icy cold weather and moisture-sapping indoor heat.

HELPING NATURE

Most cracked, rough, reddened chapped lips can be softened up with just a few days of care and attention. If the cracking is severe, see your physician, says Dr. Kakita. You may need a prescription preparation to calm down the condition.

Quit licking and biting. Dr. Kakita says that it's natural—and automatic—to try and moisturize and relieve dry lips by licking. But all too soon, "air evaporates the moisture, making your lips even drier than before," she warns. If you tend to bite your lips—which can happen if they start to peel—you compound the problem. It tears away the protective top layer of skin from your already delicate lips. So concentrate on not licking or biting.

Drink up. Whether the furnace is cranked up at work on a wintry day, or you're hiking on a sun-baked trail over the Fourth of July weekend, you need to drink liquids, says Diana Bihova, M.D., a dermatologist in New York City author of *Beauty from the Inside Out.*

Humidify. Dry air sucks moisture out of your lips. So Dr. Bihova recommends using a humidifier at home and at the office.

Protect with lipstick. Years and years ago, lipstick tended to dry the lips. No more. Today's lipsticks are an asset—in more ways than

111

one: They moisturize and protect against the drying effects of the sun, says Dr. Kakita. For maximum effect, reapply often. Lip balms are also effective.

Build a barrier. Seriously chapped lips need strong protection in the form of a barrier ointment or cream. Dr. Kakita recommends Vaseline petroleum jelly, Aquaphor or Bag Balm applied often.

Think ahead. Planning on skiing, sailing or spending time outdoors in harsh conditions in any way? Boost your lip protection to a balm with sun protection factor, or SPF, of 30, Dr. Kakita advises. Look for extra-protective lip balms in sporting goods stores.

Say yes to yogurt. If the corners of your mouth have become red, chapped and cracked, your problem may be an overgrowth of yeast (a fungus organism), caused perhaps by antibiotics or stress, says Dr. Kakita. If you have a cold, or if saliva slips into the corners of your mouth when you're asleep, yeast can break down that sensitive skin. Head to the supermarket for liquid acidophilus yogurt, and swish it in your mouth several times a day, Dr. Kakita advises. Conditions such as diabetes may even be the culprit, so if the condition is consistent or severe, see your physician. An antifungus preparation or oral medication may be needed.

Chlamydia
Make This Episode Your Last

Chlamydia is sort of like the Stealth Bomber," says Judith N. Wasserheit, M.D., director of the Division of Sexually Transmitted Diseases Prevention of the National Center for HIV/STD and TB Prevention at the Centers for Disease Control and Prevention in Atlanta. "It comes along, and in most women, it has no symptoms. Many women don't know they have had the infection until they decide that they want to get pregnant and they can't—when they're diagnosed as infertile."

Chlamydia is the most common bacterial sexually transmitted disease (STD) in the United States, with some four million new cases of infection a year. It is caused by *chlamydia trachomatis*, a unique species of bacteria transmitted by sexual intercourse. Chlamydia infects cells along the endocervix, the center of the passageway between the uterus and the vagina. It doesn't affect cells in the vagina itself. It can, however, also infect cells in the urethra (leading to the bladder) or the rectum, says Kimberly A. Workowski, M.D., assistant professor of medicine in the Division of Infectious Diseases at Emory University in Atlanta.

Following its initial infection in the lower genital tract, chlamydia can advance to the upper reproductive tract if untreated. There it can lead to infertility when infection scars and blocks the fallopian tubes, where eggs and sperm are normally destined to mate. Ectopic pregnancies, or pregnancies outside the uterus—mostly in the fallopian tubes—can also result.

PERSONAL TACTICS TO SPEED HEALING

Fortunately, "it is possible to eradicate STDs like chlamydia," says Willa Brown, M.D., director of Personal Health Services at the Howard County Health Department in Columbia, Maryland. Early screening, prompt treatment of patient and partner with antibiotics and smart sex all play a part. Here's what she and other experts say that you can do to recover from chlamydia.

Take all your medication. Your physician may give you antibiotics—either a single dose of azithromycin (Zithromax) or a seven-day course of doxycycline (Vibramycin). Take doxycycline right after meals. This antibiotic can irritate your stomach, says Dr. Brown, so take it on a full stomach with a large glass of water.

It takes a few days for your body to absorb either drug. Antibiotics get your recovery rolling, but they don't knock out infection right away, says Dr. Wasserheit. "The medicine itself doesn't usually eradicate the infection. What it does is kill off enough of the bugs or slow them down enough so that your immune response can then do the rest of the work."

Protect yourself in the sun. "Doxycycline is a tetracycline drug that can increase sensitivity to the sun," says Barbara A. Majeroni, M.D., assistant professor and director of continuing medical education in the Department of Family Medicine at State University of New York at Buffalo. When you're heading outdoors, protect your skin with sunscreen with maximum sun protection factor (SPF), she advises. Shoot for an SPF of 15 or higher. Wear a hat and stay out of direct sunlight.

WHEN TO SEE A DOCTOR

More than 95 percent of patients will be cured with antibiotics, but early diagnosis of chlamydia is crucial to effective treatment. You may have symptoms such as abnormal vaginal discharge, frequent urination and burning in your urethra or vagina, dull pelvic pain, painful intercourse, bleeding between menstrual periods or heavier periods. But as many as 80 percent of women have no symptoms.

Your doctor may discover chlamydia during your annual gynecological exam, but testing for it is not part of the usual routine.

"A woman needs to prompt her health care provider to test for chlamydia," says Judith N. Wasserheit, M.D., director of the Division of Sexually Transmitted Diseases Prevention of the National Center for HIV/STD and TB Prevention at the Centers for Disease Control and Prevention in Atlanta. Be sure to ask for a test if you have had more than one sexual partner in the past three months, or if your partner has had more than one partner.

Women doctors say that some women are more comfortable going to a county health clinic or a Planned Parenthood center for testing instead of to their regular physicians.

Skip sex until a week after treatment. "We usually encourage people to wait until they are free of symptoms and they and their sex partners have completed medication before they have intercourse," says Dr. Wasserheit. If your partner starts treatment after you do, wait until after he completes treatment to be reasonably sure that he is no longer infected, either.

Absolutely don't douche. "There's no reason to douche at all, ever," says Dr. Workowski. Not only does douching have no effect on relieving or preventing chlamydia, but, she says, "it can also have the detrimental effect of pushing the infection up further into your urogenital tract," where it can do damage to your reproductive system.

Practice monogamy. Short of swearing off sex, cultivating a mutually monogamous lifetime relationship offers good protection against chlamydia and other STDs, says Dr. Majeroni, because you and your partner will not be bringing infections from others into your bedroom.

114

Chocoholism

Reign In the Sweetest Addiction

Can a woman actually be addicted to chocolate?

According to a study conducted in Scotland, self-described chocoholics do seem to have a few things in common with alcoholics and other bona fide addicts. Most say that their consumption is excessive and problematic.

On the other hand, self-professed chocoholics don't seem to go through withdrawal when they're denied chocolate. So other experts say that they aren't truly addicted.

"I don't think that you can be addicted to chocolate, though you certainly can experience frequent cravings," says Anne Kearney-Cooke, Ph.D., director of the Cincinnati Psychotherapy Institute, expressing a view held by many experts.

Addicted or not, many of us crave chocolate intensely. When it comes to chocolatey cravings, it seems, women take the (chocolate) cake. Studies show that while women crave chocolate more than any other food, men report more frequent yearnings for steak, hamburgers and other high-protein entrées.

According to Debra Waterhouse, R.D., a nutritionist in Orinda, California, and author of *Why Women Need Chocolate* and *Outsmarting the Female Fat Cell*, we women yearn for chocolate when certain feel-good neurochemicals (druglike substances released by our brains) are at low ebb in our bodies. As it turns out, levels of some of these neurochemicals wax and wane with levels of the female sex hormones estrogen and progesterone, Waterhouse notes. That may explain why we crave chocolate more than men do, and why our chocolate cravings vary over our menstrual cycles, peaking just before our menstrual periods. Eating chocolate, Waterhouse says, boosts levels of the necessary neurochemicals, improving our moods.

Besides, it tastes good. Even women doctors agree on that point. And substitutes don't cut it. In one study researchers at the University of Pennsylvania in Philadelphia found that chocolate cravers weren't satisfied by a tasteless capsule that contained chocolate's active ingredients—only by sweet, creamy, pleasing chocolate itself.

"Often, women who are obsessed with chocolate will tell me that it's the one thing they can count on to give them pleasure whenever they want it," Dr. Kearney-Cooke says. Amen to that.

CONTROL CRAVINGS (AND YOUR WAISTLINE)

As pleasant as chocolate may be to eat, too much can have an unpleasant effect on your health, notes Leah J. Dickstein, M.D., professor and associate chair for academic affairs in the Department of Psychiatry and Behavioral Sciences and associate dean for faculty and student advocacy at the University of Louisville School of Medicine and past president of the American Medical Women's Association. "If you eat a lot of it, you can gain weight, and the fat in chocolate can affect your heart," she explains. "If you have diabetes, or if it runs in your family, the sugar in chocolate can be a problem."

If you skip meals so that you can eat chocolate without gaining weight, your health still suffers. Though big on taste, chocolate is short on essential vitamins and minerals, notes Dr. Dickstein.

How to handle a chocolate craving? There's no single strategy that's right for everyone, the experts say, but one of the following should do the trick.

Wait a bit. Always try delay tactics first, Waterhouse advises. If a craving strikes, drink a glass of water and wait 15 minutes. Maybe it will pass. Occasionally, cravings go away of their own accord. And sometimes you need nothing more than to slake your thirst.

Substitute. If you're just plain hungry, you might try satisfying your craving with something more nutritious than chocolate—like a piece of fruit or a salad.

The more mature you are agewise, the more likely this advice is to work. "We found that people in their sixties and older were more likely to say that they could do this than younger people were," says Marcia Levin Pelchat, Ph.D., an experimental psychologist at the Monell Chemical Senses Center in Philadelphia who has studied cravings and addictions. "Some people said that they couldn't substitute anything for chocolate."

Eat a little. If you want to beat cravings now, not when you retire, or you know from experience that no substitute will suffice, Waterhouse suggests that you have a *small* piece of the real thing.

"A surprisingly small amount of chocolate will do it—the equivalent of half an ounce of chocolate," or three chocolate kisses. Calorie counters and fat-gram watchers note: Half an ounce of chocolate supplies about 75 calories and 4.6 grams of fat.

Scout out fat-free treats. If you're trying to eat less fat, you could also try to satisfy your craving with a few fat-free chocolate-flavored hard candies, a cup of fat-free hot cocoa, a low-fat fudge pop or one of the new low-fat candy bars, says Waterhouse.

Walk it off. If you crave chocolate, eat a small piece and then go for a walk, says Lisa Heaton-Brown, a chartered clinical psychologist in Huddersfield, England, who has studied chocolate cravings. Do that, or talk to a friend, head for a movie or dive into an engrossing book—anything to distract you from thoughts of going after another little bit.

Boost your daily pleasure quota. "If you rely on chocolate as a source of pleasure, you need to make sure that you have other sources of pleasure in your life, like good friends, sports that you love or hobbies that bring you joy," says Dr. Kearney-Cooke.

Chronic Fatigue Syndrome
Fight Endless Exhaustion

By itself, the name for what you have is enough to tire you out. Your doctor calls it chronic fatigue immune dysfunction syndrome, or CFIDS. Others call it chronic fatigue syndrome, or CFS, for brevity. You're not just tired, you're bone-achingly tired, and you've been feeling terrible for a long time. You may also feel feverish, forlorn or forgetful. You feel like you need an awful lot of sleep, but when you do sleep, you sleep fitfully.

What causes CFS? No one knows for sure. Some researchers theorize that the trigger is a viral infection, chronic stress or some other on-going trauma that continually activates the immune system. But studies have not been able to pinpoint a specific causes or causes, says Carol North, M.D., assistant professor of psychiatry at Washington University School of Medicine in St. Louis.

117

According to the Centers for Disease Control and Prevention in Atlanta, most people diagnosed with CFS are women—mostly Caucasian and mostly between the ages of 25 and 45.

SICK OR JUST PLAIN TIRED?

The hallmark of CFS is severe, unexplained fatigue that is not relieved by rest. Often women can recall exactly when they started to feel tired and could no longer go about their daily tasks.

If you've been diagnosed with CFS, you've probably been experiencing at least four of the following symptoms.
* Faulty memory or poor concentration
* Sore throat
* Tender lymph nodes (glands in the neck, armpits and elsewhere)
* Joint pain
* Muscle pain
* Headaches
* Exceptional fatigue after normal efforts
* Sleep that does not restore your energy

HELP YOURSELF FEEL BETTER

While the exact cause of CFS is a mystery, experts agree that you can take measures to help yourself feel better, and that feeling better can actually put you on the road to recovery.

Take the "morning test-walk." Symptoms of CFS differ from woman to woman—and from day to day in the same woman, says Jill Anderson, R.N., Ph.D., a clinical nurse specialist at the University of Illinois at Chicago Medical Center. "Test what kind of day that you're going to have by taking a short walk each morning." You'll know whether it's going to be a good day or a bad day by how you feel. Then measure your daily activities accordingly.

Use memory aids. Memory problems associated with CFS are most perturbing to women, says Dr. Anderson. "They feel terrible when they forget basics, like where they keep the coffee, for example. So organize your kitchen. Make lists. Write yourself notes and post them prominently. Label the drawers. And store necessities in visible places," she suggests.

Plan for some downtime. "If you have to attend an important but energy-draining function, like a wedding," says Dr. Anderson, "plan for the effort. Keep the day before the event free—and the day after—for rest."

Let wheels do the work. If you have to lug things around—like gro-

WHEN TO SEE A DOCTOR

"Those who seem to do best with chronic fatigue syndrome are those who start treatment within six months," says Dedra Buchwald, M.D., director of the Chronic Fatigue Syndrome Clinic and associate professor of medicine at Harborview Medical Center at the University of Washington in Seattle. "So I recommend that you see your doctor if you have unexplained fatigue that lasts for more than a month."

If you have chronic fatigue symptoms when you stand for a while, you may in fact have a blood pressure regulation disorder that causes the heart to pump less blood when it needs to pump more. Known as neurally mediated hypotension, it is treatable with diet and medication.

ceries—use a luggage carrier with wheels, says Dr. Anderson. "If your supermarket has a motorized riding shopping cart available, use it."

Sit down on the job. Keep a tall stool in the kitchen so that you can prepare meals or do the dishes sitting down. "And get a shower stool so that you can sit when you bathe," says Dr. Anderson.

Similarly, if you work in an office, the right chair, properly aligned with your desk or computer, can make you more comfortable, says Dedra Buchwald, M.D., director of the Chronic Fatigue Syndrome Clinic and associate professor of medicine at Harborview Medical Center at the University of Washington in Seattle. To find what works best, you may need to enlist the advice of an occupational therapist, says Dr. Buchwald.

Ask your spouse to help. "Among the women with chronic fatigue syndrome who do the best are those whose spouses are helpful, loving and supportive, but who still do as much as they can," says Dr. Buchwald.

Reach out and e-mail someone. "Online computer support groups help women with chronic fatigue syndrome keep their spirits up," says Dr. Anderson. "I know women with chronic fatigue syndrome who take fantasy cruises and plan dinner parties online."

Take a message. Dr. Anderson suggests that you arrange for caller identification service through your phone company so that you can screen calls and talk only when you feel up to it. "And keep your answering machine on," she urges. "That way, you can call people back when you feel like chatting."

Get your Zzzs. "Women with chronic fatigue syndrome need their sleep; it's a priority," says Dr. Anderson. (For tips on how get the most restful sleep that you can, see page 495.)

Chronic Lateness
You *Can* Get There on Time

When the *Toronto Star* asked 1,000 executives nationwide to recount the best excuses that they had heard from tardy employees, one told of a chronically late woman whose excuses grew increasingly incredible.

"One morning, more than two hours late, she called to explain that she'd awakened to discover two male window washers on scaffolding outside her bedroom window," he said. "Because she slept nude, she said, she was waiting for them to leave before she could get up and come to work."

CURES FOR TARDINESS

Her boss may have been somewhat amused by "Can you top that?" excuses, but yours may not. If you're chronically late and running out of excuses for your tardiness, you might try the following:

Apologize. If you're going to be late to your next meeting, plan to beg forgiveness. "If they don't know you well, apologize profusely and then get on with the business at hand," says Sandra Loucks, Ph.D., professor of psychology at the University of Tennessee in Knoxville and the University of Tennessee Medical Center. "If they know you, and this isn't the first time that you've been late, say, 'I have a problem with being on time, and I'm really working on it. Please forgive me, and know that I don't mean to be rude.'"

Analyze yourself. Try to figure out what's making you run late. While the supply of excuses for chronic lateness is infinite, the reasons are few.

120

Sometimes we miss deadlines because we underestimate how long projects will take, we get distracted and lose track of time, or we are unrealistic about our limitations and end up overbooking ourselves.

Draw a time line. If you underestimate how long things take, break down a task into its component parts and figure out how long each part actually takes you, says Camille Lloyd, Ph.D., professor in the Department of Psychiatry and Behavioral Sciences at the University of Texas Medical School at Houston. Be realistic—draw on past experience. Say that you need to be at work by 9:00 A.M. sharp. If you need a half-hour to read the paper, 20 minutes to shower and dress, 15 minutes to eat breakfast and 45 minutes for the commute, set your alarm for 7:00 A.M.

Time yourself. If you tend to lose track of time and forget to put the paper down after half an hour, set the alarm so that it goes off at again at 7:30 A.M., reminding you to hop in the shower, says Lenora Yuen, Ph.D., a psychologist in Palo Alto, California and co-author of *Procrastination.*

Set priorities. If you tend to try and accomplish too much in too little time—say, you start washing the dishes five minutes before you need to leave for the airport—chances are that you'll get a late start. "Recognize that you can't do everything," says Dr. Yuen. "Ask yourself what's really important and do that." The dishes will wait. The plane won't.

Watch the clock. Overbooking can easily make you late for appointments. On those occasions when you have no choice but to schedule appointments close together, be diligent about finishing each one on time. "When you arrive at each one, say, 'I wish I could spend more time today, but I absolutely have to leave at such-and-such time,'" says Dr. Loucks. "That way, when the time comes, everyone has been forewarned. You can leave early without feeling rude."

Just say no. If you always overbook, don't try to cram more obligations into an already tight schedule. "Women tend to be very responsive to other people's needs and have a harder time saying no when asked to do things," says Dr. Loucks. But saying yes to everything is self-defeating: Chronic lateness makes you look disorganized, inefficient and less competent, says Dr. Lloyd.

Kill time. If you habitually arrive late because you hate to be kept waiting yourself, imagine how you would feel if you were sitting there staring at your watch, says Dr. Yuen. Arrive on time and bring a book, magazine or stationery with you. That way, if you do end up waiting, you can use the time to read or catch up on correspondence.

Clutter

Restore Orderliness—And Your Sanity

*T*he backseat of your car looks like a dumpster. The clothes in your bedroom closet look as though they spent the night on "tumble." The top drawer of your bathroom vanity is a jumble of barrettes, brushes, tweezers, scissors, nail clippers, half-empty bottles of moisturizer—and about 2,000 pennies.

Pan to the living room: Two years' worth of magazines spill off the coffee table and onto the floor. Shoes and socks, doffed the night before, litter the area. The cat is fast asleep on a sweatshirt discarded after a session on the excercise bike.

This is clutter. And therapists say that it's one of the most insidious causes of stress in a woman's life today.

How does clutter cause stress?

"Women feel that clutter is a negative reflection on them," says Susan M. Satya, a psychotherapist, faculty member at the New School for Social Research in New York City and director of Catalysts for Change in Southampton, New York. Stress is an automatic reaction. "After countless messages from the culture, we feel that caretaking, pleasing and comforting others—which certainly includes creating a nurturing space—is a woman's responsibility," she says. So when we enter a room cluttered with the sneakers, books, bags and papers of our busy lives, we often unconsciously get uneasy or overwhelmed. Our stress levels go up, our self-esteem goes down and our general feeling of health and well-being hits the dirt. "The only hope for cleaning up this reaction is to take on only your share of the work, expect others to do their share and remind yourself that your worth is multifaceted and that clutter is a reflection of an involved and interesting life," says Satya.

Sometimes, though, clutter makes it more difficult for women to do the overwhelming numbers of things that they do on a day-to-day basis. "Life is easier if you know where everything is," says Marjorie Hansen Shaevitz, director of the Institute of Family and Work Relationships in La Jolla, California, and author of *The Superwoman Syndrome*. But clutter means that things are not where they should be and that you'll probably have to spend valuable time hunting for them.

FREE ADVICE

Clutter-control experts normally charge a hefty hourly rate to help the organizationally challenged. Here are some tips that you can use for free.

Tackle one problem area at a time. "Getting rid of clutter is like losing weight," says Stephanie Schur, founder of SpaceOrganizers in White Plains, New York, producer of the video *How to Organize Your Home* and founding member of the New York chapter of the National Association of Professional Organizers. "The 10 or 15 pounds that you need to lose seems impossible—until you divide that amount into smaller goals, like losing 2 pounds a week."

To conquer clutter, take a look at the whole house, decide what area bothers you the most and start there, says Schur. After you finish that area, work on the rest of your home on an area-by-area basis later.

Schedule a clutter clean-up day. Make an appointment in your personal planner or on your kitchen calendar to de-clutter, the same way that you would a doctor's appointment, says Schur. That way, it's harder to procrastinate.

Pick your best time to work. When do you have the most energy during the day? At 8:30 in the morning? Midnight? Work when you're fresh, says Schur. You're more likely to finish what you start.

Stick to the four-hour rule. Don't try to do major de-cluttering all at once, Schur says. Work up to four hours, tops. And make sure that you leave the last 30 minutes of that time to cart away stuff that you're recycling, giving away, throwing out or storing elsewhere.

Stock up on organizers. Car organizers, closet organizers, CD organizers, video organizers, desk organizers, shelf organizers, makeup organizers, bathroom organizers, drawer organizers, under-the-bed storage boxes—stroll through any hardware store or budget department store or flip through a catalog designed for organizing, and you can find a wide variety of products designed specifically to organize almost any kind of clutter that you would normally accumulate, says Schur.

Use baskets in clutter-prone areas. Baskets make great clutter collectors, because they are attractive and serve a purpose, says Schur. Put one beside the TV to hold the TV listings and remote controls; one beside the chair in which you do most of your reading so that you can toss magazines and newspapers that you plan to read, and so forth. Other key spots to target: the foot of any staircase (for fetching later), at the entrance to kids' bedrooms or playroom and on the kitchen counter.

Sort and pitch the mail. To sort the mail, stand over the trash can or recycling bin with letter opener in hand and sort as you go, suggests Schur. Keep the bills, bank statements and letters and put the catalogs and magazines that you want to look at later where you are most likely to read them.

Utilize door backs. Hang ties, scarfs, belts, and shoe bags on the backs of closet doors in your bedroom, says Schur. Hang measuring spoons, spice holders, lids, pot holders, even knife holders on the backs of kitchen cupboard doors.

Coffee Nerves
Soothe the Caffeine Jitters

While the occasional can of cola, cup of tea or mug of coffee can pick you up, too much of any caffeine-containing beverage can cause rapid or irregular heartbeat, jitters, anxiety, difficulty concentrating, gastrointestinal upset and headaches—the symptoms of what is commonly known as coffee nerves.

"Caffeine is a stimulant, and if you have too much—whether it's in coffee, tea or cola—you overstimulate your system," explains Kathleen Zelman, R.D., a nutritionist in Atlanta and a spokesperson for the American Dietetic Association.

How much caffeine is too much? That depends on your drinking habits. Since your body develops a tolerance to the amount of caffeine that you habitually guzzle, you won't get the jitters unless you swallow more than your usual amount, explains Suzette Evans, Ph.D., assistant professor of psychiatry at Columbia University College of Physicians and Surgeons in New York City who has studied caffeine's effect on the body.

"Someone who never drinks coffee can have an episode of coffee jitters after just one cup," adds Elizabeth Ward, R.D., a nutritionist in Boston. "But heavy users—people who habitually have at least three cups—would have to drink more." (If you're drinking that many cups, coffee nerves or no, many women experts say that you should try to cut back. To find out why—and how—see page 99.)

Taking oral contraceptives, for instance, makes your body metabolize caffeine more slowly, notes Dr. Evans. So cut back on your caffeine by approximately a third if you start taking the Pill, she says.

Ditto if you've just quit smoking. Studies find that male and female nonsmokers metabolize caffeine more slowly than smokers do, says Dr. Evans.

Jo-Ellyn Ryall, M.D., a psychiatrist in private practice in St. Louis, explains that nicotine stimulates the liver enzymes to metabolize caffeine and other substances more rapidly. Eliminating nicotine slows down the metabolism and results in a higher blood level of caffeine.

ANTIDOTES FOR CAFFEINE OVERLOAD

Fortunately, coffee nerves subside in time, usually within a couple of hours, says Erica Frank, M.D., assistant professor in the Department of Family and Preventive Medicine at Emory University School of Medi-

WHAT WOMEN DOCTORS DO

Knows Her Limits—Now

Erica Frank, M.D.

Running on empty after completing overnight duty in medical school, Erica Frank, M.D., downed three cans of Diet Coke in quick succession and learned firsthand that a caffeine overdose can be nasty indeed.

"My heart was racing at 160 beats a minute, and I had to get treated for an irregular heartbeat," says Dr. Frank, who survived the episode, graduated from medical school and is now assistant professor in the Department of Family and Preventive Medicine at Emory University School of Medicine in Atlanta.

Dr. Frank did the right thing: Physicians advise anyone whose heart rate exceeds 90 beats per minute from drinking caffeinated beverages (not from exercise or other exerting activities) to get it checked out. The problem could be something more serious than coffee nerves, like a heart or thyroid abnormality or anxiety.

For Dr. Frank the problem was a passing case of coffee nerves and nothing more lasting. Now she knows better than to chug so much caffeine in a short period of time.

cine in Atlanta. In the meantime, here's what you can do to ease the discomfort.

Take a break. If you feel jittery or anxious, or if you're having difficulty concentrating, take a breather, says Dr. Evans. Go for a walk, listen to soothing music, find a quiet spot and sit or lie back and relax. "Do something calming that takes your mind off the symptoms."

Doctor your digestive system. If OD'ing on coffee has given you diarrhea, try an over-the-counter remedy like Kaopectate, suggests Dr. Ryall.

Budget your caffeine. The best way to avoid a repeat occurrence of coffee nerves is to keep track of how much caffeine you swallow over the course of a day, notes Ward.

If you usually have two cups of coffee in the morning and a cola with dinner, but know that this particular afternoon you'll be having cappuccino with the gang over lunch, then make your dinnertime cola a decaf. That way, you'll stay within your daily caffeine budget.

Do your coffee arithmetic. To keep track of your caffeine intake, keep these figures in mind: A 5-ounce cup of coffee contains 70 to 115 milligrams of caffeine (and soup-bowl size mugs considerably more). A 5-ounce cup of regular black tea packs roughly 50 milligrams. A 12-ounce cola delivers 40 to 50 milligrams, and an ounce of dark chocolate contains 24 milligrams. For the record, over-the-counter stimulants like Vivarin and No Doz pack 100 to 200 milligrams of caffeine.

Colds
Old-Fashioned Remedies Work Best

Take two of these. Swallow a spoonful of this. Inhale some of that. Presto! Your aches, your stuffiness, your scratchy throat, your cough and all those other insufferably nasty cold symptoms are history.

Well, not really. You wouldn't know it from commercials for over-the-counter cold remedies, but no safe or effective cure for the common cold exists.

"Since no one has the time to just be sick for a day or two these days, the makers of cold remedies promise us instant relief," says Naomi Grobstein, M.D., a family physician in private practice in Montclair, New Jersey. More than 800 over-the-counter cold remedies compete for a slice of the multimillion dollar cold remedy industry. "But no matter what you take, cold symptoms won't vanish instantly."

"A cold is a collection of symptoms caused by any one of 200 or more different viruses," says Carole Heilman, Ph.D., chief of the respiratory diseases branch at the National Institute of Allergy and Infectious Diseases, part of the National Institutes of Health in Bethesda, Maryland. "To cure a cold, you'd have to find a remedy that was able to kill any one of the 200 different viruses that may be causing your particular cold. It's a real pain in the neck to find a substance that not only universally destroys viruses that don't behave in the same way but also doesn't-cause side effects. So far, no one has succeeded at finding the magic formula for a safe cold cure."

BETTER THAN STORE-BOUGHT

Busy women have come to expect instant relief from cold symptoms, says Dr. Grobstein. Yet taking over-the-counter cold remedies may actually prolong the misery. "I don't like over-the-counter cold preparations. I find that those who are sickest the longest are those who take over-the-counter remedies every four hours."

So what do women physicians and other women health professionals say that an achy, sniffly, sneezy woman should to do for the common cold? Their best advice follows.

Gargle for a sore throat. "A pinch of salt—a quarter-teaspoon—in a cup of warm water makes a good gargle for relieving throat pain," says Maureen C. Van Dinter, R.N., senior clinical nurse specialist at the University of Wisconsin Northeast Family Medical Center in Madison. "Warm liquids and salt can help shrink and dry mucous membranes."

Get steamed. "Turn on the shower full force with hot water, close your bathroom door, and sit on the closed toilet seat for 15 minutes," says Van Dinter. "Breathing the steam will shrink the swollen mucous membranes in your upper respiratory tract and promote drainage."

Slather on a metholated rub. "Rubbing your chest with an aromatic preparation like Vicks can make you feel better and less congested," says Van Dinter. "Research shows that it works."

Beef up your C intake. "Vitamin C can decrease the duration of a cold," says Carol S. Johnston, Ph.D., assistant professor of food and nutrition in the Department of Family Resources at Arizona State University in Tempe. "It's a natural antihistamine—and it may help counter congestion, runny nose and watery eyes triggered by substances known as histamines induced by the cold viruses."

Dr. Johnston recommends taking 500 milligrams of vitamin C a day—half in the morning and half at night—whether you're sick or well.

You'd have to eat lots of fruits and vegetables every day to get 500 milligrams, says Dr. Johnston. "Otherwise, I recommend taking a daily vitamin C supplement."

Once you actually have a cold, says Dr. Johnston, "The antihistamine effects that I've seen vitamin C provide are achieved at doses between 1,000 and 2,000 milligrams. I believe that people are better off taking vitamin C than antihistamine medications when they have colds, because antihistamines have side effects that include drowsiness. However, I don't recommend that people take more than 1,200 milligrams of vitamin C a day," she says.

Suck on a zinc lozenge. "Zinc is an important co-factor—a facilitator of sorts—for dozens of the body's metabolic reactions," says Katherine Sherif, M.D., instructor of medicine at Allegheny University of the Health Sciences and on staff at the Institute for Women's Health, both in Phildelphia. "It's likely that it helps the immune system." Zinc lozenges, used according to package directions, may help when you have a cold.

Water, yes; soda, no. Drinking plenty of fluids is especially important when you're fighting a cold, says Dr. Sherif. But drinks high in sugar are taboo.

"Women need eight glasses of fluid every day, and more when they have colds," explains Dr. Sherif. "Sweetened sodas and fruit juices act as diuretics—that is, they flush water out of your body—and will dehydrate you instead of replacing the fluids that your body loses in the virus-fighting metabolic process." Instead, she suggests, drink herbal tea (sans caffeine, also a diuretic), artificially sweetened soft drinks or water.

Choose the right herbal tea. Different herbal teas have different soothing properties, suggests Dr. Sherif. "Try mint tea if your cold comes with an upset stomach; anise tea is good for colds."

Have some chicken soup. Really. "Chicken soup is a wonderful symbol of nurturing," says Dr. Heilman. "And studies suggest that nurturing can promote healing."

And at least one study indicates that chicken soup itself might slow

Chicken Soup and Vitamin C

Physician Prescriptions

What do women physicians, pharmacists, nutritionists and medical researchers do when they come down with colds? Here's what they say.

"I throw some chicken and a bunch of vegetables into the slow cooker. Since the sense of smell is so closely connected to emotions, I feel better just smelling the soup as it cooks."
—*Janet Karlix, Pharm.D., assistant professor of pharmacology at the University of Florida College of Pharmacy in Gainesville*

"I don't get many colds, I think because I eat lots of fruit. When I do get one, though, I settle into bed, eat chicken soup, read trashy novels and watch old movies."
—*Judith Hallfrisch, Ph.D., research leader at the U.S. Department of Agriculture Metabolism and Nutrient Interactions Lab in Beltsville, Maryland*

"I drink plenty of water and juice. I try not to use decongestants, because they extend the period of stuffiness. If I'm really suffering, I use the daily allotment of acetaminophen. Then I lighten up and try to do the rest thing."
—*Michelle Lyndberg, Ph.D., an epidemiologist at the Centers for Disease Control and Prevention in Atlanta*

"I use zinc gluconate/glycine lozenges at the first sign of a cold."
—*Nancy Godfrey, Ph.D., a research scientist at Godfrey Science and Design in Huntingdon Valley, Pennsylvania*

"I take a couple of grams of vitamin C a day and nasal spray at night if I can't breathe." (One gram is 1,000 milligrams.)
—*Carol S. Johnston, Ph.D., assistant professor of food and nutrition in the Department of Family Resources at Arizona State University in Tempe*

"I come to work, keep my staff away from me, and when I get home, I make my kids feel guilty by acting like a martyr. Then they're really nice to me and bring me soup and toast until I start feeling better."
—*Carole Heilman, Ph.D., chief of the respiratory diseases branch at the National Institute of Allergy and Infectious Diseases, part of the National Institutes of Health in Bethesda, Maryland*

WHAT WOMEN DOCTORS DO

WHEN TO SEE A DOCTOR

"Colds don't typically produce much in the way of fever," says Anne L. Davis, M.D., associate professor of clinical medicine in the Division of Pulmonary and Critical Care Medicine at New York University Medical Center and attending physician and assistant to the director of Chest Service at Bellevue Medical Center, both in New York City. "But if you have a cold and run a fever above 101°F for more than a couple of days, see your doctor."

Dr. Davis suggests that you check with your doctor if:

• Your cold is accompanied by a new or worsening severe cough or a cough that produces green, yellow or bloody phlegm. Acute bronchitis, pneumonia, asthma and ear or nasal sinus infections can complicate the course of the common cold. If you develop sharp chest pain when coughing or deep breathing, wheezing or shortness of breath, earache or acute headache or facial pain and tenderness, you should call your doctor.

• You have a serious chronic medical condition of any kind (like chronic bronchitis or a heart condition). If you come down with a cold, avoid getting overtired. If your cold symptoms are worse than usual, be sure to let your doctor know right away.

Also, if you have a fever above 100°F and you are pregnant, consult your physician promptly, says Michelle Lyndberg, Ph.D., an epidemiologist at the Centers for Disease Control and Prevention in Atlanta.

down the inflammatory process of colds. In the study the researcher pitted his grandmother's chicken soup against neutrophils, the blood cells that rush into an infection site to combat the invading viruses and bacteria (which can lead to a cold's inflammation and discomfort). He found that the soup significantly decreased the neutrophil onslaught. Although the researcher admitted that certain commercial soups also had the same effect, grandma's homemade elixir won out on the basis of homemade taste appeal.

Make a hot toddy. "An old-fashioned honey, hot water and lemon toddy eases a cough and makes you feel better," says Anne L. Davis,

M.D., associate professor of clinical medicine in the Division of Pulmonary and Critical Care Medicine at New York University Medical Center and attending physician and assistant to the director of the Chest Service at Bellevue Medical Center, both in New York City. According to Dr. Davis, mix ingredients to taste.

Take to your bed. "That achy, tired-all-over feeling is your body telling you to get some rest," says Van Dinter. Taking it easy helps your body heal itself. "So staying home for a day or two might shorten the duration of your symptoms."

Quit smoking. "Having a cold is a great opportunity to quit smoking," says Dr. Grobstein. Smoking irritates membranes that are already irritated and will exacerbate your cold's symptoms, says Dr. Grobstein. Adds Dr. Sherif: "Avoid smoky rooms when you have a cold and don't let anyone smoke around you, either." Need further motivation? A study of more than 350 people showed that smokers got more colds than nonsmokers did, because smokers were more likely to get infections—and they were also more likely to develop illnesses following infections.

Cold Sores
Kiss Them Good-Bye

Any woman who has suffered the pain and embarrassment of one cold sore has probably been through the misery many times and knows the symptoms all too well: that slight, tingly, itchy, hot sensation at the edge of your lip. Maybe you feel feverish, like you have a touch of the flu.

Worse, cold sores seem to strike when they're least welcome—before a New Year's Eve party or some other special occasion. The usual herpes simplex I virus that causes cold sores is like annoying houseguests who just keep coming back, no matter how inconvenient you found their last visit.

131

Heavy-Duty Protection

Geraldine Morrow, D.M.D.

For Geraldine Morrow, D.M.D., past president of the American Dental Association, a member of the American Association of Women Dentists and a dentist in Anchorage, Alaska's beauty sometimes takes her breath away. She moved to Alaska from Boston and relishes the solitude, journeying 325 miles a week to deliver dental care to villagers in far-flung towns. Still, the state's climate can be harsh and the life rugged. When Dr. Morrow's resistance is down, or when she is exposed too long to the stark elements of cold, ice, wind and sun on snow, she sometimes feels a telltale tingle that means a cold sore is on its way. Here's what she does about it.

"If I keep the area covered with a heavy, greasy type ointment—either Carmex or DCT Blistex—it tends to almost prevent an imminent outbreak," she says. As a preventive tactic, Dr. Morrow smooths her lips with either one of those ointments every night. "I find it to be very valuable in keeping them away."

Cold sores spread through direct contact with someone who has them. Maybe you kissed someone who had an active cold sore, or you could have gotten the virus merely by touching the hand of someone who touched her own cold sore a few minutes before.

The first cold sore that you experience is probably the worst. Afterward, the virus lurks in your system forever, lying dormant among the nerve ganglia beneath your skin's surface, waiting to be reactivated, says Lenore S. Kakita, M.D., clinical assistant professor of dermatology at the University of California, Los Angeles, and an adviser to the American Academy of Dermatology. The good news, says Dr. Kakita, is that most women develop a slight immunity to them over the years, making outbreaks fewer and farther between.

In women stress is the biggest trigger for cold sores—although weather changes, especially excessive sunlight, can bring on outbreaks, says Dr. Kakita. When you get stressed, your resistance to disease drops, and that can awaken the dormant herpes virus within your nerve ganglia cells, prompting an outbreak.

Menstruation can also instigate cold sores in some women, but probably more as a result of stressful feelings at that time of the month rather than a direct result of hormone levels, adds Dr. Kakita.

BOLSTER YOUR DEFENSES

Left alone, a cold sore will normally last 10 to 14 days, says Dr. Kakita. Aside from taking the prescription drug acyclovir (Zovirax), here's what else you can do to minimize the discomfort on your own or shorten the duration of an attack. (For practical ways to manage canker sores, which affect the inside of your mouth and aren't caused by a virus, see page 103.)

Grab an ice cube. Applying ice directly to the sore can bring the swelling down and provide temporary relief, says Geraldine Morrow, D.M.D., past president of the American Dental Association, a member of the American Association of Women Dentists and a dentist in Anchorage, Alaska.

Dab on some lip balm with sun protection. If you have had an outbreak of cold sores in the past, you should wear a lip balm with a sun protection factor (SPF) of 30 at all times, but especially when you are outdoors in the sun, to prevent a cold sore, says Dr. Kakita. You can find lip balms with high SPFs in sporting goods stores and drugstores.

If you have an open cold sore, don't use the balm stick directly on your lips, or you'll spread the virus around, says Dr. Kakita. Instead, use a cotton swab to apply balm not only to your lips but also to the skin around the outside border.

Keep your hands off. People just don't realize how highly contagious cold sores are, says Dr. Morrow. "If you have a cold sore on your lip, don't pull it, don't stretch it, don't touch it." You could get "very, very painful" cold sores on your hands, especially if the fluids from the blister get under a hangnail, she says.

WHEN TO SEE A DOCTOR

Prescription medications such as acyclovir (Zovirax) are available to fight the herpes simplex I virus responsible for cold sores, and they can stop a cold sore in its tracks, says Lenore S. Kakita, M.D., clinical assistant professor of dermatology at the University of California, Los Angeles, and an adviser to the American Academy of Dermatology. If you're bothered by frequent, severe cold sores, it makes sense to see your doctor. Even if the cold sore develops, most women find that the outbreak will be milder, less painful and shorter if they're taking the medication.

Give lysine a try. Dr. Kakita recalls that before the advent of acyclovir, people swore by the preventive and healing properties of lysine, an amino acid that counteracts arginine, a substance in various foods that in some people seems to trigger cold sores. "Some people still take lysine tablets," she says. You can find it in health food stores or drugstores.

Sleep upright. If you have a cold sore, Dr. Kakita recommends propping a few pillows behind your head at bedtime, letting gravity help the blisters drain. Otherwise, fluid may settle in your lip during the night.

Reschedule your dental appointment. The last thing that you want to do when you have a cold sore is "open wide," says Dr. Morrow. The movement will stretch your lips, aggravating your tender cold sore, and it could cause it to break open and spread.

Colitis
Hope and Help
for Inflammatory Bowel Disease

If you have ulcerative colitis, you'll know it. Symptoms include diarrhea, bloody stools, cramps and abdominal pain, prompted by inflammation and sores in the large intestine.

If you have ulcerative colitis or Crohn's disease (forms of inflammatory bowel disease) medication is the primary treatment. But there are some ways that you can treat flare-ups at home.

WHAT TO DO DURING AN ATTACK

Ulcerative colitis or Crohn's disease attacks tend to come and go. During an attack you'll probably feel like crawling into bed. But if that's

WHEN TO SEE A DOCTOR

If you have frequent bouts of diarrhea, bloody stools, cramps and abdominal pain, see your doctor, so that she can confirm the diagnosis and prescribe the proper course of treatment. The symptoms of colitis can mimic other forms of inflammatory bowel disease, such as infectious colitis or other conditions, including irritable bowel syndrome. It's important that a clear initial diagnosis be made, says Sheila Crowe, M.D., gastroenterologist and assistant professor of medicine in the Department of Internal Medicine in the Division of Gastroenterology at the University of Texas Medical Branch at Galveston.

If you have known Crohn's disease or ulcerative colitis, and initial medication and dietary changes don't help during a flare-up, during which you have a fever, frequent stools or blood in your stool, you should see a doctor. Flare-ups may occasionally be caused by infections, which need to be treated differently than usual attacks.

not an option, here are some suggestions for keeping the discomfort to a minimum.

Drink deeply. If you have diarrhea (and you probably do), you may get dehydrated. To replace lost fluid, try to drink at least ten glasses of water or juice a day during an attack, says Sheila Crowe, M.D., gastroenterologist and assistant professor of medicine in the Department of Internal Medicine in the Division of Gastroenterology at the University of Texas Medical Branch at Galveston.

Eat sparingly. Diarrhea and cramps make it hard to tolerate any food at all when you're having an attack, says Dr. Crowe. To keep pain to a minimum, "eat very plain food, such as applesauce or boiled, skinless chicken or soft, cooked carrots—and not much of them," says Dr. Crowe.

For now, cut out the fiber. While your colitis is active, stick to bland, low-fiber, low-fat foods such as plain toast and gelatin, so that you won't irritate your colon, says Barbara Frank, M.D., gastroenterologist and clinical professor of medicine at Allegheny University of the Health Sciences MCP–Hahnemann School of Medicine in Philadelphia.

Pass up the popcorn. Seeds, nuts and popcorn irritate the bowel and, worse, impede its functioning during an attack, says Dr. Crowe.

If it hurts your stomach, stay away. There's no telling what might worsen the pain—for some it may be spicy foods, for someone else, acidic foods or a seemingly innocuous spoonful of cereal, or any food imaginable. "If you feel worse after eating any type of food at all, don't eat it during an attack," advises Dr. Crowe.

Congestion
Unplug Your Stuffy Nose

Whether caused by a cold, allergies or pollution, a stuffy nose is no fun. You can't breathe. You can't smell. You can't taste your food. And when you talk, you sound like a three-year-old.

SUFFER NO MORE

Whether you're trapped at home or trying to make it through the workday all stuffy and congested, women doctors offer these tips for relieving a stuffy nose. Try their recommendations, and see how quickly you'll be breathing easy again.

Use a decongestant only. The reality is, the fastest way to unclog your nose is with a decongestant. But what to buy? You can spend hours scanning cough-cold-flu-and-allergy products at your local drugstore trying to decide among decongestant/antihistamine combinations, decongestant/expectorants and myriad other over-the-counter remedies.

One woman doctor's shortcut: Buy a decongestant (such as Afrin nasal spray), not a combination product.

"If getting de-stuffed fast is essential, you can use Afrin nasal spray according to the package directions," says Karin Pacheco, M.D., staff physician in the Division of Allergy and Immunology at the National Jewish Center for Immunology and Respiratory Medicine in Denver. "But don't use it for more than three days, to prevent a rebound effect of a continually stuffy nose." In other words, your system gets used to it,

WHEN TO SEE A DOCTOR

"If you're frequently or chronically congested," says Karin Pacheco, M.D., staff physician in the Division of Allergy and Immunology at the National Jewish Center for Immunology and Respiratory Medicine in Denver, "then you should see a doctor, especially if your congestion is accompanied by itching or sneezing. You probably have an allergy."

Other signals that your congestion should be treated by a physician include:
- Greenish, yellowish or foul-smelling phleghm
- Severe headache or facial pain
- Fever
- Persistent cough

and when you stop using it, the congestion is worse than before.

Besides, there are plenty of nondrug options to try.

Mix yourself a homemade nasal spray. "Rinsing your nose with plain water can dry it out, because plain water is not the kind of fluid that the body normally produces," says Barbara P. Yawn, M.D., associate professor of clinical family medicine and community health at the University of Minnesota in Minneapolis and director of research at the Olmsted Medical Center in Rochester, Minnesota. "Spraying with a compatible saline solution can remove irritants like smoke, pollution, dust or pollen that cause your nose to swell and feel stuffy," says Dr. Yawn. Here's what to do.

"To one cup of lukewarm water, add a half-teaspoon of salt and a pinch of baking soda," says Dr. Pacheco. "Using a child-size bulb syringe, spritz the solution into your nose a few times, then blow your nose."

Pick up a drugstore saline spray. "Another option, of course, is plain saline nasal spray, such as Ocean, available over the counter," says Dr. Yawn. Follow the package directions.

Head for the showers. "If you're squeamish about nasal sprays," says Dr. Yawn, "taking a nice steamy shower will help relieve the congestion."

Add spice to your life. The fastest, no-fuss, no-muss remedy for your stuffy nose may be as close as your spice rack. "If your stomach can tolerate it, hot pepper will put an instant end to your congestion," says Carol Fleischman, M.D., staff physician at Allegheny University of the Health Sciences MCP–Hahnemann School of Medicine and at the Center for Women's Health, both in Philadelphia. "I recommend going to the nearest Indian restaurant and ordering a very hot curry dish." Or just sprinkle some red-pepper flakes into whatever you're having for dinner.

Constipation
Toilet Training for Adults

These days, there are no hard-and-fast rules on how often you need to move your bowels to be considered "regular."

Though most people average a bowel movement somewhere between once a day and three times a week, doctors say that you are not necessarily constipated if you move your stools less frequently. Constipation is defined as a decrease in your *usual* number of bowel movements.

So, let's say that you normally go once a day, and you suddenly only need to defecate once a week. That's constipation.

Doctors blame diets high in processed foods and low in fruits, vegetables, beans, grains and other sources of fiber. Fiber moves the bowels. Yet most Americans eat considerably less than the amount needed for a healthy colon. We should get 20 to 35 grams of fiber a day. Instead, we get as little as 5 grams a day.

Though opinions differ on whether women get more constipated than men, they definitely make more doctor visits. It is also known that hormonal changes during pregnancy and the pressure on the abdomen caused by childbirth often lead to constipation.

Women also often get constipated in the week or so before menstruation. This is because fluids that normally flow to the colon, softening and moving stools, are retained in other parts of the body, says Nicolette Francey, M.D., professor of medicine at New York Medical College in Valhalla and a medical consultant for primary care at the

Doctor's Consultants, a physicians' organization in New York City.

If you experience constipation, take heart. Women doctors say that retraining toilet habits, adding fiber to your diet and exercising regularly can get those sluggish stools on the go again.

GET MOVING NOW

"Except in rare cases, the last thing that you should take is a chemically based laxative like Ex-lax or Correctol," says Dr. Francey. That's because excessive laxative use is likely to make your bowel lazy, which means that you won't be able to go without help. Worse, laxatives often set up a vicious cycle, in which you are constantly alternating between constipation and diarrhea, and never have regular bowel movements.

But sometimes you just need something. Now.

Try hot broth (or other natural laxatives). "If you have mild discomfort from constipation because you're traveling and can't get to the gym or eat your fruits and vegetables, try a glycerine suppository, milk of magnesia or prune juice," says Joanne A. P. Wilson, M.D., a gastroenterologist and professor of medicine at Duke University Medical Center in Durham, North Carolina. "Sometimes even a warm cup of broth will help your bowels move more quickly."

Use a footstool. "If you're constipated, propping your feet up on a stool with your knees bent while you sit on the toilet will straighten the angle of your bowel and help you pass stool more quickly," says Jacqueline Wolf, M.D., a gastroenterologist, assistant professor of medicine at Harvard Medical School and co-director of the Inflammatory Bowel Disease Center at Brigham and Women's Hospital in Boston.

THE DIETARY FACTOR

What you eat and when has a significant bearing on regularity. Here's what women doctors advise.

Don't skip meals. Often women—especially dieting women—get constipated because they eat only one large meal a day, says Dr. Wilson. "Eating stimulates the reflex that causes stuff to move forward in the gut. Women who diet often eat fewer meals to cut calories. That decreases movement through the gut."

When nothing moves, you can't pass stool. Breakfast is particularly important, because that's what starts your digestive juices flowing every day.

139

Fill your meals with fruit. Fiber creates soft, mobile stools, says Elaine Feldman, M.D., professor emeritus of medicine at the Medical College of Georgia School of Medicine in Augusta. "You don't have to eat a pound of bran a day; just treat yourself to three servings of vegetables and two fruits a day and some whole-wheat bread."

Introduce fiber slowly. "Too much fiber too fast may solve your constipation, but replace it with gassiness, bloating and diarrhea," Dr. Feldman says.

Meanwhile, try a supplement. Some women complain that they can't digest that much fiber. If that describes you—or if you're working fiber into your diet—try a fiber supplement such as Metamucil, Citrucel or Fibercon, says Linda Lee, M.D., assistant professor of medicine in the Division of Gastroenterology at Johns Hopkins University School of Medicine in Baltimore.

Available in supermarkets and drugstores, supplements can be taken in granular form (mixed in water or juice) or wafer form, washed down with at least eight ounces of fluid. Fiber supplements soften and bulk up stool and nix constipation.

Drink a lot. Drink six to eight 8-ounce glasses of water daily to

WHAT WOMEN DOCTORS DO

Apples Do the Trick

Joanne A. P. Wilson, M.D.

Like many of her women patients, Joanne A. P. Wilson, M.D., a gastroenterologist and professor of medicine at Duke University Medical Center in Durham, North Carolina, has experienced the frustration and discomfort of constipation.

But what she recommends is apples.

"I tease my patients about an apple a day," she says. "I tell them that statement probably refers to constipation."

No surprise. Medically, eating apples makes sense—they're a good source of fiber.

Apples and other high-fiber fruits and vegetables are best for constipation, because the sugars in apples are harder for the body to digest. And what the body can't break down, it pushes out. So apples are a natural laxative.

Which is why you shouldn't go overboard. "Eat one apple a day, not four or five," says Dr. Wilson, so you don't get diarrhea.

WHEN TO SEE A DOCTOR

For some women, taking medications such as antidepressants or other prescription drugs can cause constipation. If you've recently started a new medication and you're suddenly constipated, see your doctor to see if she can address the problem. If you have irregular bowel movements, you could have a food allergy. Consult your physician for a blood test to see which foods could be upsetting you chronically.

Also, any of the following symptoms warrant medical attention.
• Blood accompanying a bowel movement
• A change in bowel movements, such as worsening constipation despite home remedies, or alternating constipation and diarrhea
• Fever
• Abdominal pain

soften the stool, says Robyn Karlstadt, M.D., a gastroenterologist at Graduate Hospital in Philadelphia. Fill an empty 64-ounce soda bottle with water and keep it at your desk, then help yourself until it's gone.

LEARNING NEW POTTY HABITS

To end constipation permanently, you'll also need to change some lifestyle habits, including the way you sit on the pot, says Dr. Wilson.

If you have chronic constipation, your bowel may have forgotten its job, because you've been ignoring its needs. You may need to relearn some good potty habits to refresh its memory.

Make a toilet date—and keep it. You wouldn't dream of leaving the house without doing your hair. So why not take the same care with your colon?

Eating, especially in the morning, is a wake-up call to the bowel, says Dr. Wilson. Yet what people do is get up, race out of the house, stop on the way for breakfast and head to the office. That doesn't give your bowel a chance to respond. And public bathrooms are not usually conducive to quiet time, and this causes further and further delays, says Dr. Francey.

The answer?

"Schedule time at home in the morning," says Dr. Francey.

"Usually, the bowel is ready to expel its contents about half an hour after the first meal."

Sit rather than strain. Trying to force out hard, dry, recalcitrant stool won't relieve your constipation; it may lead to hemorrhoids and a protrusion of rectal tissue through your anus, also known as prolapse of the rectum, says Dr. Wilson.

If you really can't go after 15 minutes, get off the pot and try again later.

Make a commitment to exercise. If nothing else, "just move around," Dr. Francey says. No one is sure why, but exercise stimulates bowel function. However, heavy exercise may cause dehydration, so remember to replenish water loss by drinking plenty of water, says Dr. Francey.

It doesn't take much. Walking, swimming or performing any other aerobic exercise for half an hour three times a week may be enough to cancel your constipation, says Dr. Francey.

Contact Lens Problems
Tips for Total Comfort

*D*isposable, extended-wear, soft, hard, gas-permeable. Whatever kind of contact lenses you wear, it's still a foreign object in your eye. So it only makes sense that to avoid problems—like redness, irritation and infection—your eyes need special attention. You already know that. But what you may not know is that being female can create a unique set of problems.

Hormonal changes that occur as a result of pregnancy and menopause can make your perfect-wear lenses suddenly less than perfect. And some ingredients found in makeup and hair spray can stray into your lens-covered eyes and cause infections, leading to impaired vision, says Anne Sumers, M.D., an ophthalmologist in Ridgewood, New Jersey, and a spokeswoman for the American Academy of Ophthalmology.

"The chemicals in hair spray coat your lenses as they coat your hair," says Sumers. "If you sprayed hair spray on your car windshield, it would be hard to see through."

And then there are universal problems. Almost everyone who wears lenses has experienced dryness, redness or irritation from a piece of grit trapped under a lens.

WHAT TO DO RIGHT AWAY

When your contacts find you literally crying for help, here's what to do.

Remove the lens. If you try to tough it out and leave an uncomfortable lens in your eye, it will increase the irritation and may lead to infection, says Dr. Sumers. If a lens feels uncomfortable, remove it.

Rinse, clean and (maybe) reinsert. If you pop a dirty lens back in your eye, you may not get rid of the irritant, and you could end up with an infection, says Dr. Sumers. So make sure that you clean it with a sterile saline solution. "Remember, bacteria live in 'clean' water, and distilled water is not sterile water."

Make sure your lenses are in correctly. An inverted soft lens (inserted with the convex curve against your eye) will feel uncomfortable. "It may sound obvious, but it's quite common to do this. Especially if you're in a rush or are a first-time contact lens wearer," says Gerri Goodman, M.D., an ophthalmologist and an instructor at Johns Hopkins Hospital in Baltimore. Soft contact lenses are made to feel very comfortable on the eye. You know that you have it in wrong if your eye feels really uncomfortable. Take it out and check it.

Right lens, right eye? If your lenses feel okay but your vision is blurry, "check that the left lens is in the left eye and the right lens is in the right eye," says Dr. Goodman.

If your vision is still blurry, take out your lenses. Protein deposits can film up your lenses, making it seem like you're looking through a smeary windshield. Once protein deposits settle on your lenses, cleaning won't help. You'll need a new pair. This process of accumulation may take months or years, depending on how meticulous you are, among other factors. "Those who are allergic will build up deposits more quickly. It also happens to those who aren't as meticulous with their lens-cleaning," says Dr. Goodman.

WHEN TO SEE A DOCTOR

The following are signs of possible infection; they also can cause an infection that jeopardizes vision. See a doctor if you wear contacts and experience any of these symptoms.
- Persistent redness or irritation in the eye
- Eye pain
- Blurry vision
- Vision loss
- Eye discharge

Look for specks. Eyelashes, bits of makeup, grit, sand and, yes, even bugs can get in your eyes, causing contact lens discomfort, says Dr. Sumers. To get them out, remove your lens, rinse your eye and lens with a sterile saline solution and reinsert the lens.

Refresh with artificial tears. They'll remoisten your eye and help flush out debris that you can't see, says Dr. Sumers.

If it still hurts, take it out again. If you continue to wear a lens that hurts, you might scratch your cornea, the eye's front window. Cuts and scratches are painful. And they can develop into a secondary infection, causing scarring and resulting in a very hazy window, says Penny Asbell, M.D., associate professor at Mount Sinai Medical Center in New York City and president of the Contact Lens Association of Ophthalmologists. "The eye should feel comfortable without the lens," says Dr. Asbell. "If it doesn't, don't reinsert the lens."

If the pain or discomfort doesn't subside within 30 minutes, make an appointment right away so that you can rule out serious conditions like corneal infections, says Dr. Asbell. It's a good idea to always carry a pair of glasses and your lens case for just these types of situations.

FINDING A "LOST" LENS

Lenses can't really get lost in your eye, Dr. Sumers says. A thick membrane called the conjunctiva keeps the lens from going behind your eye to your brain. But a lens can slip off your cornea and under your upper lid, where it seems to disappear.

You may have to try more than one tactic to retrieve the prodigal lens. Here's what to do—in this order.

Rewet your eye. One or two drops of artificial tears can help unstick a lens, says Dr. Sumers, especially if your eyeball is dry.

Or exert gentle pressure. If your lens has slipped off your cornea and onto the flatter part of your eyeball, don't put your finger in your eye. "Close your eye, press lightly on the lens underneath your eyelid and guide the lens back onto your cornea, which is more curved to keep your lens in place," says Dr. Sumers.

Corns and Calluses
A Tender Touch for Tough Feet

Rub your feet the wrong way with the wrong shoes long enough, and they'll respond by growing corns or calluses—extra layers of hard, dry skin that help protect pressure points on the foot. Some women, for example, develop cone-shaped corns between their toes, where bones rub together. Others, especially women with high arches, develop a sheet of calluses that may cover a part, or the whole ball, of the foot. And calluses or corns are common where shoes rub against bony prominences.

If a corn or callus grows thick enough to press on nerves, it can hurt. "A large corn can be as irritating as a pebble in your shoe," says Kathleen Stone, D.P.M., a podiatrist in private practice in Glendale, Arizona.

LESS PAIN IN MINUTES

Here's what women doctors advise to help stop the pain.

Soak, then rub. Soften corns or calluses by soaking your feet in plain lukewarm water for five or ten minutes. Then use a pumice stone or a synthetic abrasive pad, available at drugstores, to rub off dead skin a little at a time. "I recommend the new synthetic spongelike pumice pads, which contain abrasive material and can be wetted with water and liquid soap and used in the bath or shower," says Dr. Stone.

WHEN TO SEE A DOCTOR

If your corn or callus pain persists despite self-care, see a podiatrist. She can trim the corn or callus and perhaps prescribe orthotics (shoe inserts) that take the pressure off that area of your foot. If you have diabetes, or if you have diminished sensation or decreased circulation in your feet, it's wise to see a podiatrist for any foot problem.

Note: If you have diabetes, decreased sensitivity or decreased circulation, check with a podiatrist before you attempt this, says Cheryl Weiner, D.P.M., a podiatrist in Columbus, Ohio, and president of the American Association for Women Podiatrists.

Oil 'em up. After soaking and rubbing, use a moisturizing cream to help keep your feet soft, says Dr. Stone. "I like vitamin E cream or vitamin E oil (not vegetable oil), which penetrates the skin very nicely."

Cushion the worst offenders. To lessen pain from soft corns between your toes, work a tuft of lamb's wool between your toes, suggests Dr. Stone. Lamb's wool is available at drugstores.

Pad 'em. Traditionally, adhesive-backed felt, called moleskin, was used as a doughnut-type pad around corns and calluses to take pressure off them. The women whom Dr. Stone treats seem to prefer a new synthetic material, Cushlin, available at most drugstores in Dr. Scholl's products. The material is thin, soft, resilient and rubbery. It doesn't flatten out and holds up well. Cut sheets of the material to pad around, not over, your corn or callus.

Buy shoes that fit. Narrow shoes can contribute to corns and calluses; shoes with room for the toes are less likely to do so. To size up prospective shoes, says Nancy Elftman, a certified orthotist/pedorthist (a professional shoe fitter) in La Verne, California, trace your foot on a sheet of paper and take the paper with you when you go shopping for shoes. Then place the shoes you like on top of the tracing. If any of your foot tracing shows, the shoe is too short or narrow for your foot.

Lace up to save your toes. If you have corns on top of your toes, Elftman suggests lacing your sports shoes so that one lace goes from one bottom eyelet to the top eyelet on the opposite side. The other lace is alternated through the lace holes. Then, by pulling on the single lace, you can lift the toe box and give your toes more room. (This also helps if you have a long second toe.)

Coughing
Quiet the Hacking and Quacking

Coughing is such a nuisance, interrupting your sleep (or another's sleep), disturbing your work, drawing unwanted attention in class and meetings. In a way, coughing is worse than sneezing. And when your simple sniffle evolves into an infuriating, roof-rattling, throat-tickling, phlegm-producing cough, you want relief, and fast.

Coughing occurs for a reason: It's your body's reflex, designed to rid your lungs or airways of foreign material or mucus.

BE STILL, MY THROAT

Provided that your doctor has ruled out asthma, a lung infection or other serious condition, here are some tips for quieting your cough.

Put on the kettle. A cough with a tickle needs hot tea to settle it down, says Penelope Shar, M.D., an internist in private practice in chilly Bangor, Maine. To coat your throat, sweeten your cup with some honey and breathe in some steam while it's brewing, she advises. (To avoid a steam burn, don't get too close.)

Create a steamy situation. Another way to give your airways the humidity that they crave is to use a vaporizer, says Sally Wenzel, M.D., associate professor at the University of Colorado School of Medicine and a pulmonary specialist at the National Jewish Center for Immunology and Respiratory Medicine, both in Denver. Or luxuriate in a warm shower to ease congestion that prompts coughing.

Have a piece of candy. Suck on sugarless hard candy or licorice. Women doctors say that they will probably quiet your cough just as well as most lozenges.

Know when to leave well enough alone. If your cough is bringing up phlegm, doctors would call it a productive cough. Dr. Wenzel advises against taking anything to suppress such a cough, since it is clearing out your congested airways. "If you can't sleep, take cough medicine just before bed," she says. And don't swallow phlegm—your body is trying to get rid of it.

Look for the "D" word. For simple, dry coughs Dr. Wenzel recom-

WHEN TO SEE A DOCTOR

Coughs can be serious business, so women doctors say that it's wise to see a doctor if your coughing:

- Is persistent
- Awakens you at night
- Gets worse or changes
- Interferes with your daily activities

"It's especially important to get medical attention if your cough isn't getting better and if you have other symptoms, such as fever, chills, chest pain, ear pain or swollen glands," says Penelope Shar, M.D., an internist in private practice in Bangor, Maine. "If you're feeling rotten and your mucus is greenish, don't delay: Antibiotics will help." Or you may simply need a stronger cough medicine.

mends syrups containing dextromethorphan. But like many doctors, she discourages overuse of any type of cough medicine. Many of them are filled with ingredients (guaifenesin, terpin hydrate, phenothiazine promethazine) that you don't need, since they haven't been proven to do anything beneficial for your cough.

Keep the liquids flowing. Even if your cough is the last remnant of a cold, drink plenty of water, juice and broth, recommends Dr. Wenzel. Drinking plenty of fluids—including chicken soup—will thin the mucus in your airways and lungs.

Consider taking an antacid. If your cough comes on suddenly at night, it may be caused by gastroesophageal reflux, or a backing up of juices from your stomach. Taking an antacid before bed might help. Also try raising the head of your bed and cutting out food and alcohol for a few hours before you retire for the night.

(For practical ways to deal with colds, influenza, sore throat and postnasal drip, see pages 126, 306, 505, and 437.)

Crow's-Feet
Delay Fine Wrinkles Indefinitely

*I*f you take twin sisters, and one becomes a lifeguard while the other takes a desk job, chances are that on their thirtieth birthday, the lifeguard will have more crow's-feet—tiny lines radiating from the corners of her eyes—than the office worker. And if the lifeguard smokes, the difference will be even more marked.

"Crow's-feet are usually the earliest wrinkles to appear on a woman's face," says dermatologist Debra Price, M.D., clinical assistant professor of dermatology at the University of Miami School of Medicine and a dermatologist in South Miami. But they're not necessarily a sign that you're aging. "Crow's-feet are caused primarily by exposure to the sun—what we call photoaging."

Squinting into the sun contributes to the process as well, explaining why outdoor enthusiasts may be more susceptible to crow's-feet than less-exposed women, says Margaret A. Weiss, M.D., assistant professor of dermatology at the Johns Hopkins Medical Institutions in Baltimore. Once the skin has been exposed to sunlight over the years, it loses its elasticity. Squint long enough and often enough, and temporary wrinkle patterns formed at the corners of your eyes eventually become permanent.

Women smokers may develop crow's-feet earlier than women who don't smoke. According to Dr. Weiss, smoking makes you unconsciously squint as your eyes try to avoid the smoke's irritating and drying effects.

TAKE STEPS TO PREVENT CROW'S-FEET

Women dermatologists agree: If you never smoke, squint or tan your face, you'll get fewer crow's-feet. So the sooner you take steps to prevent crow's-feet, the younger the skin around your eyes will look. If the damage is already done, there are ways to minimize their appearance.

Here's what women doctors suggest for preventing crow's-feet in the first place—or preventing existing lines from getting worse.

Go glycolic. You can minimize the appearance of existing crow's-feet by moisturizing the area with an eye cream that contains glycolic acid—one of a group of alpha hydroxy acids—originally derived from sugarcane, says Dr. Weiss.

Glycolic acid encourages wrinkled cells to slough off and newer ones to emerge. The moisturizing agents in the cream will prevent any wrinkling from dryness.

Not many over-the-counter eye creams contain glycolic acid, says Dr. Weiss. One is Murasome Eye Complex 10 by Murad (developed by a dermatologist at the University of California, Los Angeles). To find a store near you that carries Murad products, call 1-800-33MURAD.

Whatever you do, *never* use higher strength skin lotions with glycolic acid (10 percent strength formulated for use on the face and neck) around your eyes without the supervision of a dermatologist. You could get a nasty burn. Around your eyes stick with 5 percent strength.

Turn back the sun. Since crow's-feet appear only after sunlight has begun to destroy the skin's elastin and collagen fibers over time, the best way to prevent crow's-feet is to use a sunscreen around the eyes, says Dr. Price.

Use a broad-spectrum sunscreen made especially for the eye area. Dot it gently around your eyes, including your upper and lower eyelids. Reapply every few hours. Dr. Price suggests using only fragrance-free sunscreens in the eye area, since some people might find fragrances irritating to delicate eye tissue.

Wear sunglasses and hats. In addition to applying sunscreen, wear dark sunglasses and wide-brimmed hats that shield as much of your eye area as possible, says Dr. Price.

Avoid smoke. Chalk up another reason for giving up cigarettes: Smoking, or spending a lot of time in a smoke-filled environment, makes you squint, so avoiding tobacco smoke helps prevent crow's-feet, adds Dr. Weiss.

Cuticle Problems

Patch Rips, Nicks and Tears

Cuticle means "little skin" and refers to that tiny rim of near-transparent tissue that peaks out from underneath your skin, covering part of your nails.

Unlike your appendix or other body parts that you can live without, cuticles are there for a reason. They serve as barriers to protect nails from infection, says Loretta Davis, M.D., associate professor of dermatology at the Medical College of Georgia School of Medicine in Augusta.

NO SELF-SURGERY

Many women insist on trimming the cuticle away from the curve of the nail. But performing self-surgery on cuticles is not advised. "That can lead to trouble, including bleeding and swelling," says Dr. Davis.

Here is women doctors' advice for keeping your cuticles problem-free.

Soak up some suds. Soften cuticles in warm, sudsy water for several minutes. This prevents drying and cracking, says Marianne O'Donoghue, M.D., associate professor of dermatology at Rush-Presbyterian–St. Luke's Medical Center in Chicago.

Follow with petroleum jelly. Keeping cuticles soft is the key to keeping them healthy, according to Dr. O'Donoghue. "I push mine back with a washcloth or an orange stick and then cover them with petroleum jelly. It helps hold in the moisture." Moisturizing your cuticles nightly will help keep them from drying out, especially in winter.

Push them back—gently. "Your nails will look wonderful with the natural cuticle right where it should be," says Trisha Webster, a hand model with the well-known Wilhelmina Modeling Agency in New York City. "My hands are photographed all the time, and I know that they look perfect with the cuticle simply pushed back."

Webster pushes back her cuticles with an orange stick wrapped in cotton gauze.

151

Cuts and Scrapes
How to Mend Broken Skin

*W*omen are no less prone to cuts and scrapes than their kids are. It's easy to accidentally slice your thumb while cutting a bagel or gash your hand on a piece of broken glass while doing dishes. Or perhaps you've slipped on loose gravel, scraping your knee or elbow.

Your skin is designed to repair itself—provided that you take steps to prevent infection and promote healing, say women doctors.

"Researchers have microscopically videotaped cells in action, and they found that cells in the top layers of skin actually do little cartwheels over each other as they find the spots that they need to fill in to heal a wound," says Sheryl Clark, M.D., assistant clinical professor of dermatology at Cornell Medical Center and an assistant attending physician in medicine at the New York Hospital, both in New York City.

SPEED UP THE REPAIR PROCESS

If your cut doesn't warrant stitches or other medical attention, here's what women doctors say that you can and should do.

Apply pressure. Gently press a clean, damp towel against a cut or scrape for up to 20 minutes, until the bleeding stops, says Dr. Clark.

Wash the wound. It is vital that you clean dirt out of a cut or scrape so that it doesn't cause infection, says dermatologist Karen E. Burke, M.D., Ph.D., an attending physician at Cabrini Medical Center in New York City and at Greensboro Specialty Surgical Center in North Carolina. "Gently rinse a scrape under running water until it is totally clean."

"For a minor cut or scrape all you need is plain old soap and water," says Wilma Bergfeld, M.D., head of clinical research in the Department of Dermatology at the Cleveland Clinic Foundation. "Try Hibclens, a brand-name soap available in drugstores. It's a superior cleanser, not irritating to tender skin."

Don't use hydrogen peroxide—some women doctors say that it's too strong. "Along with killing bacteria in the cut or scrape, it also kills the healthy skin cells that are trying to heal the wound," says Dr. Clark.

Repeat three times a day. Sizable cuts or scrapes should be cleaned three times a day, says Dr. Bergfeld.

WHEN TO SEE A DOCTOR

If a cut is deep or large (more than a half-inch long), you definitely need stitches, says dermatologist Karen E. Burke, M.D., Ph.D., an attending physician at Cabrini Medical Center in New York City and at Greensboro Specialty Surgical Center in North Carolina.

"Stitches help the cut heal faster and reduce the chance of scarring. And a cut is less apt to get infected if it is stitched closed," explains Dr. Burke.

But how can you tell if you need stitches?

If a cut shows white or flesh color, then it's not deep enough to require stitches. But any cut that is deep enough to reveal a rich yellow color has cut into the layer of fat underneath skin, and it must be stitched closed to heal properly. See a doctor, even if you're in doubt, say women doctors. To keep swelling down apply pressure and ice (with a bandage and ice pack), then make an appointment for some time within the next 24 hours.

Other times when you may need a physician's care:

• The cut area is red, tender, inflamed, oozing or discharging pus.
• You also have a fever or swollen lymph nodes.
• You have multiple cuts and scrapes.

You may need an antibiotic, says Wilma Bergfeld, M.D., head of clinical research in the Department of Dermatology at the Cleveland Clinic Foundation.

You should also see a doctor if:

• Cinders, gravel or other foreign material is imbedded in the cut. "Your doctor may need to anesthetize (numb) the wound and remove the debris," says Dr. Bergfeld.
• You get a cut on your face or other prominent area.
• You have mitral valve prolapse, an artificial heart valve or a hip replacement and you get a deep cut. You may need to take an oral antibiotic, says Dr. Burke.

Top it off with ointment. For years doctors thought that cuts and scrapes heal better when they are dry. Research shows, however, that the opposite is true: "If you keep wounds moist, they heal more quickly and with a nicer cosmetic result," says Dr. Clark. "They need a moist environment so that they can maneuver around and form nice, flat, beautiful layers of skin."

So after cleansing, apply an antimicrobial ointment such as Bacitracin or Polysporin to keep the wound moist and bacteria-free and to speed healing, suggests Dr. Bergfeld.

Seal it to heal it. Women doctors recommend a new type of over-the-counter product called a colloidal dressing. "It's a porous, gelatin-like material that sticks on your skin like contact paper," says Dr. Bergfeld. It also contains an antimicrobial medication to fight bacteria.

These membranes form a "breathable" membrane over the wound, which is like a second skin. "They allow oxygen to pass back and forth across them, but they don't allow water to pass. So they keep the wound moist, and fluid stays in," says Dr. Clark. She recommends Tegasorb (by 3M) and Spenco Second Skin.

"These dressings can cut healing time in half," says Dr. Bergfeld. "They're especially good on scrapes or cuts on your legs, where healing time is prolonged."

Leave it alone. Leave the dressing on for two to five days. "It will naturally loosen and come off on its own—or it will wash off in the shower. Then you can replace it if necessary," says Dr. Bergfeld.

Tape it shut. If you don't have any colloidal dressing available, traditional bandaging will do. To keep both edges of a small cut together and help it mend, pull the cut closed and stick the edges together with a small strip of surgical tape. "Or try one of those little narrow strips that you find in a Band-Aid box," says Dr. Bergfeld.

Put on the covers. Protect the wound with a gauze bandage and tape, if necessary, or with just an adhesive bandage if the cut or scrape is small, says Dr. Clark.

Apply the bandage loosely so that the wound can air out without being constricted, says Dr. Burke.

Dress and undress. Change the dressing two or three times a day—whenever you wash the injury, says Dr. Clark.

Give it some support. If you have a large cut or scrape on your leg or a lower extremity, support the surrounding tissue and reduce swelling by putting on an elastic bandage or pulling on an elastic knee-high stocking or some support hose, says Dr. Bergfeld. "You don't want it to be tight—just supportive," she says.

Dandruff

Fight Feisty Flakes

Compared with earthquakes, floods and other natural disasters, dandruff is a minor problem. But walking around with white flakes on your head and shoulders is embarrassing—doubly so if your dandruff flares up just before an important job interview or romantic encounter.

A short lesson in the biology of dandruff can help you select the remedy that works best for you.

"Dandruff can be associated with oily hair," says Diana Bihova, M.D., a dermatologist in New York City and author of *Beauty from the Inside Out*.

Another cause is yeast infection of the scalp, adds Yohini Appa, Ph.D., director of product efficacy at the Neutrogena Corporation in Los Angeles. And while they don't cause dandruff, hormonal and seasonal changes can also exacerbate the problem, she says.

Dandruff is characterized by accelerated cell turnover—in other words, the cells on the surface of your skin build up like crazy.

"Typically, it takes 21 days for new cells to migrate to the surface of your scalp, where they are shed," Dr. Appa says. "Ideally, it's an invisible process. But with dandruff, the cell reaches the surface in half the time." As a result, cells build up on your scalp in clumps before they're shed. And when they do shed, they look like tiny white flakes.

ANTI-DANDRUFF STRATEGIES

Fortunately, dandruff can be conquered with these tips from experts.

Use a dandruff shampoo. Choose an anti-dandruff shampoo that contains coal tar, salicylic acid, pyrithione zinc, sulfur or selenium sulfide, says Patricia Farris Walters, M.D., clinical assistant professor of dermatology at Tulane University School of Medicine in New Orleans and a spokesperson for the American Academy of Dermatology.

Each ingredient reduces dandruff in a different way, explains Dr. Appa. The tar-based shampoos slow cell production, while salicylic

WHEN TO SEE A DOCTOR

If tiny white flakes appear on your shoulders, use a hand mirror to help you check your scalp carefully in a wall mirror, says Patricia Farris Walters, M.D., clinical assistant professor of dermatology at Tulane University School of Medicine in New Orleans and a spokesperson for the American Academy of Dermatology. Persistent scaling that's accompanied by redness and itching could be seborrheic dermatitis, an inflammation of the oil glands.

You should also consult your doctor anytime that dandruff is severe or is accompanied by redness or itching, says Dr. Walters. Your doctor will probably prescribe a medicated shampoo containing the antifungal agent ketoconazole, or a cortisone preparation.

acid–based shampoos slough off dead cells before they clump. And both shampoos have antifungal properties and help fight invading yeast microbes, which is one of dandruff's most persistent triggers. Pyrithione zinc and selenium sulfide reduce cell turnover, while sulfur is believed to cause slight skin irritation—just enough to lead to the shedding of flakes.

Some shampoos on the market contain more than one ingredient, adds Dr. Walters. Trial and error is the only way to sort out which one will work for you. (It doesn't matter which one you pick first, says Dr. Walters.)

Rub vigorously. Regardless of which dandruff shampoo you're using, a little elbow grease can enhance its effectiveness. When you wash your hair, lather once, rinse, lather a second time and really rub your scalp as you shampoo, says Dr. Appa. Your fingers will help dislodge excess cells.

Let it sit and soak. After you lather a second time, let the shampoo sit on your head for at least five minutes, suggests Dr. Bihova. That way, you give the anti-dandruff ingredients time to work.

Rinse well. Now that you've loosened all those little cells, rinse and rinse again, says Dr. Appa. If you don't rinse them all out, they'll end up on your clothes as dandruff.

Shampoo daily. "The more frequently you shampoo, the better," says Dr. Walters. It prevents your scalp from accumulating dead cells that will precipitate a major outbreak.

Rotate your shampoo. "If you've been using one shampoo successfully for several months, and your dandruff suddenly returns, just switch shampoos," says Dr. Walters. No one knows why a perfectly good dandruff shampoo suddenly stops working, but they sometimes do.

Alternate dandruff shampoos with regular ones. Shampoo every other day with a regular nondandruff shampoo suited to your particular natural hair type—dry, oily or normal, says Dr. Walters. This will protect your hair from the harsh chemicals in dandruff shampoos, which, over time, have a tendency to dry your hair.

Condition with tar. If your hair starts to feel dry after you've been using a dandruff shampoo for a while, don't reach for a heavy after-shampoo conditioner. Instead, switch to a tar-based shampoo like T-Gel, suggests Dr. Walters.

"Tar softens and conditions," says Dr. Walters. "So you can use it to get soft, tangle-free hair without having to use the heavier conditioners that can exacerbate dandruff."

Spray on sun protection. Since sunburn can cause dandruff by drying out your scalp, it makes sense to spray a sunscreen—one made especially for hair—on your hair and scalp before you hit the beach or jump in the pool, says Dr. Bihova. A light spray will protect your hair and scalp from both sunburn and the nasty, drying effects of chlorine. Just spray it on, comb it through and go. Reapply according to package directions.

Dark Circles under the Eyes
No More Tired-Looking Shadows

*C*osmeticians worked hard to make Sally Field look old enough to play Tom Hanks's mother in the Oscar-winning movie *Forrest Gump*. They put dark circles under her eyes. But if you have under-eye shadows, the only kind of recognition that you'll hear is concerned remarks like, "Are you feeling tired?"

157

Dark circles can be aggravated by fatigue, allergies, overexposure to the sun, menstruation or pregnancy. But they're usually hereditary; if your parents have them, chances are that you do, too, says Marianne O'Donoghue, M.D., associate professor of dermatology at Rush-Presbyterian–St. Luke's Medical Center in Chicago.

Sometimes what you're seeing isn't really darkened skin, but engorged blood vessels under your eyes. Because the skin under your eyes is thinner than skin anywhere else on your body, blood vessels there are more noticeable, especially if you're fair-skinned, says Monica L. Monica, M.D., Ph.D., an ophthalmologist in New Orleans and spokesperson for the American Academy of Ophthalmology.

Usually, dark circles are caused by hyperpigmentation—higher-than-average amounts of melanin, the substance that gives your skin its pigment. They tend to show up in people of Mediterranan descent and can run in families.

FROM DARKNESS TO LIGHT

Medically speaking, dark circles are harmless, say doctors. Still, if you'd prefer to blot them out, here are a few lightening tips.

Try a cold compress. Close your eyes and cover them with a cold washcloth for about five minutes, says Dr. Monica. Repeat several times throughout the day. That will help constrict your blood vessels, minimizing darkness, and it may help minimize tissue swelling and eliminate some of the darkness.

Hide 'em. More opaque than foundation makeup, cream concealer is made to order for under-eye darkness. Select a cream concealer that's a little lighter than your skin when wearing it under foundation (or the same shade as your skin when wearing the concealer alone), says Fatima Olive, product developer for Aveda Corporation, a cosmetics and health products manufacturer in Blaine, Minnesota. "Paint" the concealer with a small brush into the dark areas. Then take your pinky finger and very lightly pat the edges to blend it in. Finally, powder lightly to help the concealer stay put.

Spread on the sunscreen. Use a sunscreen especially made for the face with a sun protection factor (SPF) of at least 15, but preferably 20, "all day every day," to keep the sun's rays from darkening the skin under your eyes, says Dr. O'Donoghue.

Supplement your foundation. Some foundation makeups contain SPFs of 6 or 8, says Dr. O'Donoghue. For full protection you'll still need either a moisturizer or a sunscreen lotion with an SPF of 15.

Eye cream: The newest option. If your circles persist, try an opaque eye cream such as Lancome's Expressive, says Dr. O'Donoghue.

Alpha hydroxy acids, used in many newer eye creams "decrease wrinkles and lighten and smooth the skin," says Wilma Bergfeld, M.D., head of clinical research in the Department of Dermatology at the Cleveland Clinic Foundation. The most common alpha hydroxy acids are glycolic acids (extracts derived from fruit and other plants). Other new eye creams that look promising include Renova and the cosmetic Cellex-C eye contour cream or gel (a topical vitamin C).

Depression
Treat an Illness, Not a Weakness

If you're depressed to the point that you can't sleep, can't concentrate and don't want to get out of bed, you're not alone. More than twice as many women as men have severe depression that can linger for several months, even years, if not treated. Sometimes depression can lift only for symptoms to recur, says Ellen McGrath, Ph.D., a clinical psychologist in Laguna Beach, California, and New York City, chairperson of the American Psychological Association's National Task Force on Women and Depression and author of *When Feeling Bad is Good.*

Women are also more likely than men to experience mild depression—to feel overwhelmed, powerless, discouraged, ineffective or sorrowful and possibly angry or guilty. These feelings last longer than the blues but typically lift after several hours or days, says Dr. McGrath.

WHY SO SAD?

Research suggests that our genes and biochemistry, our circumstances and our personal history can all—independently or in combination—contribute to depression. It's an illness, not a character flaw, and experts say that it runs in families. People with severe depression seem to

159

have a brain chemistry that predisposes them to bouts. Hormonal changes that precede menstruation and follow pregnancy also appear to play some role. Losses, disappointments, difficult relationships, stress and past trauma can all contribute. So can other illnesses or certain prescription drugs, including oral contraceptives.

"We don't know why depression is more common in women, but a number of theories exist," says Leah J. Dickstein, M.D., professor and associate chair for academic affairs in the Department of Psychiatry and Behavioral Sciences and associate dean for faculty and student advocacy at the University of Louisville School of Medicine and past president of the American Medical Women's Association. "In addition to hormonal and biochemical differences, it may be caused by the added stress in a society where women don't get the same opportunities and respect that men do. Differences in the ways that boys and girls are socialized may also leave women more vulnerable."

Then there are relationships: Unhappily married women run 25 times the risk of depression that happily married ones do, says Carol Landau, Ph.D., clinical professor of psychiatry and human behavior at Brown University School of Medicine in Providence, Rhode Island. No big surprise. But it doesn't end there: Dissatisfaction with other roles—as mother or as employee—can have a similar effect. A study comparing stay-at-home moms and working mothers found that the mothers who were most depressed were those who were unhappy with their roles—whatever they were.

WHAT YOU CAN DO FOR MILD DEPRESSION

Studies suggest that depression takes a toll on the immune system, leaving us more susceptible to illness, and may increase our risk of heart disease. If severe, it can lead to thoughts of suicide, so severe depression warrants professional treatment. Mild depression can respond to some tender self-care, says Dr. McGrath. Here's what she and other experts suggest.

Get some exercise. Studies show that exercise alleviates depression by reducing stress and raising levels of feel-good substances in the brain, notes June Pimm, Ph.D., a clinical psychologist and associate professor of pediatrics and psychology at the University of Miami School of Medicine.

So get up and walk, even if it's the last thing that you feel like doing, says Dr. McGrath. "Remind yourself, 'I can do this. It'll be worth it; I only have to take a few steps,'" she says. Set a goal of exercising 20 minutes a day, three times a week.

WHEN TO SEE A DOCTOR

If you have five or more of the following symptoms for more than two weeks, experts recommend that you consult a physician or counselor.

- Persistent sad, anxious or empty feelings
- Loss of interest or pleasure in activities
- Feelings of hopelessness and pessimism, guilt, worthlessness or helplessness
- Insomnia or oversleeping
- Appetite loss or overeating
- Fatigue
- Restlessness
- Irritability
- Difficulty concentrating or remembering
- Persistent headaches, digestive trouble or chronic pain that won't respond to treatment

Even if you have none of the above symptoms but have thoughts of death or suicide, you should seek help, stresses Leah J. Dickstein, M.D., professor and associate chair for academic affairs in the Department of Psychiatry and Behavioral Sciences and associate dean for faculty and student advocacy at the University of Louisville School of Medicine and past president of the American Medical Women's Association.

You should also seek help if:

- Depression interferes with your work or relationships.
- You experience periods of depression alternating with periods of extreme euphoria, or mania.

Your doctor should first attempt to identify or rule out physical illnesses—like thyroid disorder—that can cause symptoms similar to those of depression, says Dr. Dickstein. If your physician diagnoses depression, she may prescribe antidepressant medication to correct brain chemical imbalances that can perpetuate it, along with talk therapy or cognitive or behavioral therapy.

Explore your feelings on paper. "If you don't feel like yourself, it may not be enough to sit down and ask yourself, 'Why am I feeling different? Am I depressed?'" (Although it's a start, suggests Dr. Pimm.)

It can help to write about or illustrate your feelings in a journal,

161

says Dr. McGrath. Note the time, place and situations in which you feel out of sorts. Eventually, patterns may emerge. You may find that you're likely to get depressed in certain circumstances. "The writing stops you from obsessing and ruminating so much, so the issues become clearer," Dr. McGrath says.

If you can determine what is contributing to your depression, the next step is to figure out how to address it, says Dr. McGrath.

Confide in friends. When you're depressed, bed may seem the safest place. It isn't. Social isolation contributes to depression, says Dr. Landau. If you're down, make a particular point of seeking out and confiding in supportive friends, even if only by phone.

While it's important to get out there and be with people, avoid taking on too many responsibilities, since stress feeds depression, warns Dr. Pimm. "The conventional wisdom is that a large social network is a buffer against depression, but that isn't necessarily true for women," she says. "For many women a large social network means a lot of responsibility—for children who can create anxiety, for parents who need to be taken care of, and so on."

Steer clear of whiners and complainers. Try to avoid relationships that are all work and no gain. By all means, don't let guilt or a sense of obligation keep you in a relationship that you don't enjoy, says Dr. Landau. They'll make you feel worse, not better.

Diabetes
Easy Ways to Control Blood Sugar

*W*hat do actress Mary Tyler Moore and *Empty Nest* TV actress Park Overall have in common? They both have diabetes, and they both live full, rich lives.

Diabetes is a metabolic problem that affects your body's ability to make or respond to insulin, a hormone. Insulin regulates the delivery of blood glucose (blood sugar) to your body's organs and tissues, where it's used for energy. Type I, or insulin-dependent, diabetes, is an inherited disease that affects the pancreas, destroying that organ's ability to make insulin. Type I diabetes usually occurs during childhood or adolescence.

Nine out of ten people with diabetes have Type II, or non-insulin-dependent, diabetes. For them, the body can't use insulin that's manufactured. Type II diabetes usually occurs after age 30.

SMART SELF-CARE

Women doctors say that if you have been diagnosed with diabetes of either type, you should be under medical supervision (usually a physician, and often a registered dietitian, a nurse practitioner/educator and an ophthalmologist, all working as a team). Changes in diet, exercise and other self-care strategies that follow are important, but should be checked with your doctor or other health care professionals, especially if you plan to have children. With proper blood sugar management, women with diabetes can get pregnant and deliver healthy children, says Kathleen Wishner, M.D., Ph.D., medical director of the Endocrine Global Business Unit of Eli Lilly and Company in Indianapolis and past president of the American Diabetes Association.

"Make sure that your blood sugar is meticulously controlled before you get pregnant," says Marie Gelato, M.D., Ph.D., associate professor of medicine at State University of New York at Stony Brook Health Sciences Center School of Medicine.

Here's what women doctors say you can do to control diabetes.

Lose fat, lose weight. Four out of five women with Type II diabetes are overweight, and they may even control their diabetes or reduce their medication if they lose weight, says Dr. Wishner. Calorically, fat is denser than protein or carbohydrates, so if you reduce the grams of fat that you eat, you automatically reduce calories. "To lose weight, aim for a diet with fat grams comprising 20 to 30 percent of your total calories," she says.

Start with cereal. "Foods high in fiber may help people with diabetes control their blood sugar," says Dr. Wishner. "Fiber slows the absorption of carbohydrates that you ingest. And after eating a high-fiber meal, you feel full. This can also help with weight loss."

Eating a big bowl of high-fiber cereal (like All-Bran) for breakfast and a big bowl of chili for lunch, for example, could help keep your blood sugar levels stable. According to one study, people with Type II diabetes who ate meals with 20 grams of fiber had significantly lower post-meal blood sugar than others who ate meals with only 10 grams of fiber.

Reach for some cornstarch. "We use uncooked cornstarch from the grocery store in people being treated for diabetes who experience

163

WHEN TO SEE A DOCTOR

According to the American Diabetes Association, nearly 8.4 million women in the United States have diabetes, but only half know it. See your doctor if you have any of the following symptoms for more than a week.

- Increased thirst, urination or appetite
- Dry mouth
- Vomiting
- Diarrhea
- Blurred vision
- Rapid or irregular heartbeat
- Dizziness
- Unintentional weight loss
- Recurrent yeast or urinary tract infections

Also, see your doctor if you have diabetes and you're pregnant or thinking of starting a family. Women with poorly controlled diabetes have higher risk of complicated pregnancies that could affect mother and baby.

Women with diabetes are also prone to problems with circulation or loss of feeling in their feet. So inspect your feet for red, dry, cracked skin; infections; calluses or blisters. And see your doctor if you see signs of infection. Untreated, even minor cuts or infections can lead to serious medical problems.

episodes of hypoglycemia, or low blood sugar," says Francine Ratner Kaufman, M.D., associate professor of pediatrics at the University of Southern California School of Medicine in Los Angeles, director of the Comprehensive Diabetes Program at Children's Hospital of Los Angeles, and a member of the American Diabetes Association Board of Directors. "Uncooked cornstarch is a very slow release type of sugar—it takes up to six hours for your body to break it down and absorb it.

"Stir one or two teaspoons of uncooked cornstarch into a glass of milk or sprinkle it into pudding," says Dr. Kaufman. She suggests consuming cornstarch with an evening snack to prevent low blood sugar during the night, or before exercise, which affects blood sugar levels.

Consider a chromium supplement. Tests show that people with diabetes may have lower blood levels of chromium than people without diabetes. "Chromium may help people with Type II diabetes, because the body needs chromium to be able to respond to insulin," says Dr. Kaufman. "It is sometimes difficult to get beneficial amounts of chromium from food, so look for a multivitamin that supplies the recommended amount for chromium—50 to 200 micrograms daily."

Eat just one. In the past, people with diabetes were told that they could not eat certain foods—namely, refined carbohydrates like cookies or sweets, says Davida F. Kruger, R.N., a nurse practitioner at Henry Ford Hospital in Detroit and senior vice president of the American Diabetes Association. "But research shows that all carbohydrates will elevate blood sugar the same way; a cookie is equal to a piece of bread, which is equal to a piece of fruit.

"If there's a food that you really like, make sure to include it in your diet," says Kruger. "If your favorite snack food is cookies, but you never eat them, it's easy to feel deprived and frustrated, and that can lead to bingeing. Have one cookie and enjoy it. The key here is to treat yourself in moderation—don't eat the entire bag."

Walk, swim, cycle, dance. Exercise burns fat and calories and can help you lose excess pounds. For women with diabetes, exercise offers added bonuses: Exercised muscles are more sensitive to insulin, improving the way your body metabolizes sugar. Plus, studies show that regular exercise lowers the risk of heart disease, a special concern for people with diabetes.

"The current recommendation is to exercise at least three times a week for about 30 to 40 minutes," says Dr. Gelato. "Start out slowly, then work your way up. Walk, swim, cycle, dance—do whatever you enjoy." This should be done under a doctor's supervision, she adds, as your medication and diet may need adjustment to accommodate your increased activity.

Diarrhea
On-the-Spot Relief for the Runs

Everybody has had diarrhea at least once—those loose, watery stools that have you on the toilet seat eight or ten or more times a day. Diarrhea is the body's way of saying, "Out with the bad"—a quick fix that will put your digestion back in balance.

A sudden attack of the runs can originate from a number of sources, most commonly bacteria in food or water, a virus or, more rarely, a parasite picked up while traveling.

TAMING LOOSE BOWELS A.S.A.P.

If you have a sudden sharp attack of diarrhea, it probably won't last longer than three days, even if you do nothing. But while you're going-going-going, diarrhea is all-consuming. And if you suffer from the chronic diarrhea usually associated with irritable bowel syndrome (IBS), as many women do, you know all too well what a crimp it can put in your day-to-day life. Either way, diarrhea can leave you feeling limp and lousy.

But don't worry. Easing the pain and getting your bowel function back to normal is simple.

Avoid milk. When you have diarrhea, you temporarily lose the ability to digest lactose, a milk sugar, says Sheila Crowe, M.D., gastroenterologist and assistant professor of medicine in the Department of Internal Medicine in the Division of Gastroenterology at the University of Texas Medical Branch at Galveston. So while you have the runs, dairy products won't be absorbed. In fact, they make diarrhea even worse.

Eat lightly. "The less food that your system has to process, the fewer symptoms of cramping and diarrhea you will experience," says Dr. Crowe. If you're hungry, eat bland, light foods such as toast, cooked rice or bananas.

Try the pink stuff. If you can't stay home and ride it out, over-the-counter antidiarrheal remedies such as Imodium A-D, Kaopectate and Pepto-Bismol all will help stop the runs, says Dr. Crowe.

Pepto-Bismol binds toxins produced by bacteria in the bowel, says Barbara Frank, M.D., gastroenterologist and clinical professor of medi-

Hot Tea Works Wonders

Elaine Feldman, M.D.

Like most women, Elaine Feldman, M.D., professor emeritus of medicine at the Medical College of Georgia School of Medicine in Augusta, has had bouts of diarrhea.

Her home remedies:

"Strong hot tea without too much sugar is binding. I can't say whether it's temperature that makes a difference or something in the tea."

Boiled rice, plenty of fluids and sometimes warm, flat ginger ale also do wonders, she says.

If all else fails, she tries strawberries when they're in season. Yep, strawberries, a remedy from one of her former professors. "They're very good for controlling diarrhea," says Dr. Feldman.

cine at Allegheny University of the Health Sciences MCP–Hahnemann School of Medicine in Philadelphia.

"I generally don't take medicines," says Dr. Frank. "But when my husband and I went to South America, we took Pepto-Bismol from the minute we got on the airplane." Result: No diarrhea.

Drink as much as you can. When you have diarrhea, your body loses water every time you use the toilet, so you can easily become dehydrated very quickly. "Try to drink at least ten glasses of clear liquid a day," says Dr. Crowe.

Try chicken bouillon. Fluids that contain salt and small amounts of sugar, such as chicken bouillon or sports drinks like Gatorade, are also good, because they help the body replace not only fluids but also minerals and nutrients lost during an episode of diarrhea, Dr Crowe says.

DEALING WITH CHRONIC DIARRHEA

You may not be able to say an eternal adieu to diarrhea if you have a chronic condition such as IBS, but if you follow these steps, you may be stopped up by the runs a lot less often.

Eat a lot of fiber. If you have diarrhea because of IBS, a high-fiber diet is the number one tool for a calmer, happier colon.

If your stool is normally watery and moves out of your bowel too

WHEN TO SEE A DOCTOR

Simple diarrhea usually disappears within 72 hours; other symptoms may be signs of a more serious condition. See your doctor immediately if you notice blood in your stool, you have worsening pain or fever, you're vomiting or you have severe cramps. You should also see your doctor immediately if the diarrhea is severe enough to make you dehydrated (dizzy or lightheaded when you stand up). Other reasons to see a physician about diarrhea that lasts include:

- You wake up at night with diarrhea.
- You have severe diarrhea.
- You have diarrhea for longer than three days.
- You have recently camped out or traveled. You may have the parasite *giardia*, which can be treated with antibiotics.
- You have recently added or changed a medication. (They can cause diarrhea.)

quickly, fiber will bulk it up and slow it down.

For optimal bowel function, we need at least 20 to 35 grams of fiber daily, says Ann Ouyang, M.B., B.S. (the British equivalent of an M.D.), professor of medicine and chief of the Division of Gastroenterology at the Milton S. Hershey Medical Center of the Pennsylvania State University College of Medicine in Hershey.

Eat cereal every morning. High-fiber foods include fruits, vegetables, beans, whole-grain bread and bran-based cereals, says Dr. Ouyang. Examples: A serving of Kellogg's All-Bran with Extra Fiber contains 15 grams of fiber per half-cup serving; Fiber One contains 13 grams and Bran Buds, 11. A half-cup of cooked baked beans—another good source of fiber—has 7 grams.

Try a fiber cocktail. If you're not used to eating high-fiber foods like vegetables and bran, your diarrhea may even get worse—at first. That's where fiber cocktails—supplements mixed with water or juice—can be helpful.

"It takes months for the gastrointestinal tract to adjust to eating more fiber," says Dr. Crowe.

So while you slowly up your fiber count—perhaps by one vegetable or fruit a week—"try fiber in tiny little doses, like a quarter dose of Citrucel" or other natural supplement, says Dr. Crowe. You can buy fiber supplements in supermarkets and drugstores. The granular form is mixed with water or juice. If you find the taste too grainy, try fiber in wafer form and wash it down with water or juice.

Cut back on meat. "Fatty foods are hard to digest and may often lead to diarrhea," says Dr. Frank. So avoid high-fat snacks, and eat lean meat and nonfat dairy products, not full-fat versions.

Stay away from artificial sweeteners. Sorbitol, found in sugarless gums and mints and many diet sodas, often leads to the runs, because it's not easily digested, says Dr. Ouyang.

(For practical ways to manage lactose intolerance, which can trigger diarrhea, see page 336.)

Difficulty Getting Out of Bed
An A.M. Jump-Start for Mind and Body

*T*here's 50 times more information written about an exotic virus that most of us probably won't contract than there is about a problem that's likely to affect every single woman at least once in her lifetime: the ubiquitous, but seldom fatal, disorder unofficially known as "difficulty getting out of bed in the morning."

WHY ARE YOU STUCK?

No self-help group, no 12-step program, no not-for-profit support organization, no newsletter exists to aid those in need of a little push in the morning. But happily, there are some medical experts familiar with the problem. Here's what they advise.

Think like Scarlett O'Hara. "Women sometimes have trouble getting out of bed because they exhaust themselves ruminating over their

169

The Rosemary Alarm Clock

Jeanne Rose

As president of the National Association for Holistic Aromatherapy and author of The Aromatherapy Book, *Jeanne Rose knows the link between pleasant scents and well-being—and uses selected scents to help her start the day fresh.*

"In my bedroom I have two scent diffusers set on timers. In the morning I wake to the reviving, refreshing aroma of rosemary; at bedtime, I go to sleep with the relaxing scent of ylang-ylang. I always wake refreshed and raring to go."

You can buy essential oils of rosemary and ylang-ylang, among other relaxing or refreshing scents, at aromatherapy shops. Look for true essential oils, not synthetics.

Scent diffusers can be purchased at aromatherapy shops or by mail order from Amrita Aromatherapy (call 1-800-410-9651). They cost about as much as a good toaster.

problems in the middle of the night," says Margaret Jensvold, M.D., director of the Institute for Research on Women's Health in Rockville, Maryland. "Then they feel too tired to move in the morning. So when they go to bed at night, I urge them to put aside their worries until the next day."

Make plans. "Having difficulty getting going in the morning can be linked to depression," says Dr. Jensvold. "Though you may feel like withdrawing, you must make an action plan to carry you through the day. Account for every hour to give your day structure and to help you feel less anxious."

Think of a mental carrot and stick. "Plan your day while you're still in bed. Be sure to include some things that you really want to do," says Dr. Jensvold. "Maybe it's lunch with a dear friend, a manicure or an uninterrupted bubble bath. Make sure that you have spots of pleasure worked into every day's plan."

Take a wake-up bath, not a shower. "Showers are for cleansing; baths are for the mind," says Jeanne Rose, president of the National Association for Holistic Aromatherapy and author of *The Aromatherapy Book*. Rose recommends scenting a morning bath with essential oils like stimulating peppermint, rosemary or grapefruit. Spikenard oil, she says, is especially euphoric.

170

Take baby steps. Borrowing a technique that she uses when treating women for depression, Gillian Kaplin Adams, M.D., a family physician in private practice in Bel Air, Maryland, suggests taking one step at a time—literally. "Set very short term goals for getting out of bed." Tell yourself to first put your feet on the floor. Plan your path to the bathroom. Concentrate on how you'll literally walk through each step—then do it.

Get a life. "Sometimes women who have the most trouble getting out of bed each morning are those who have the least to do," says Carol North, M.D., assistant professor of psychiatry at Washington University School of Medicine in St. Louis. "Having nothing to do is an energy sapper. If no one needs you or wants you, you may feel as if you have no reason to rise each morning. Volunteer your services, offer your assistance to an overburdened friend, join a club or take some classes."

Diverticulosis
Best Advice for Colon Cramps

A few years ago, the comedy writers for *Saturday Night Live* came up with a satirical ad for a fictional high-fiber cereal called Colon Blow, touted as a way to keep the colon free and clear of nasty digestive obstructions. In creating the ad the writers must have done some medical research: Trying to pass hard, dry stools puts a lot of pressure on your colon, sometimes causing pea-size pouches known as diverticula to form on the colon walls. The problem is called diverticulosis.

Lots of people have these pouches—about 10 percent of people over age 40 and about half the population that's over age 60.

Most of the time, you won't even know that you have diverticulosis; there will be no symptoms. Occasionally, you may experience dull cramps and the constipation that often causes diverticulosis.

About 20 percent of the time, the pouches become infected and inflamed—that's diverticu*litis*, a more serious condition that, in a small number of cases, must be treated surgically.

WHEN TO SEE A DOCTOR

Severe pain in the lower left part of your abdomen, with or without a fever, warrants a visit to your doctor. You might have a burst diverticular sac or an infection (or both), and you may need antibiotics or other medical treatment.

THE ROAD TO RELIEF

If you are troubled by diverticulosis, the key to a comfortable life is in making a few dietary changes.

Make every meal a high-fiber meal. Constipation—characterized by hard, dry stools that are difficult to pass—often leads to diverticulosis. The main way to a softer, bulkier, faster-moving stool? "A high-fiber diet and water," says Robyn Karlstadt, M.D., a gastroenterologist at Graduate Hospital in Philadelphia.

Doctors recommend 20 to 35 grams of fiber a day, but most Americans eat far less. To up your fiber count, "try to eat at least one serving of fruits, vegetables or grains at every meal," says Elaine Feldman, M.D., professor emeritus of medicine at the Medical College of Georgia School of Medicine in Augusta.

Or try a supplement. Sometimes women with diverticulosis find that high-fiber foods make them feel even more crampy. If fruits, beans and vegetables are a problem for you, try a fiber supplement such as Metamucil or Fibercon, says Linda Lee, M.D., assistant professor of medicine in the Division of Gastroenterology at Johns Hopkins University School of Medicine in Baltimore.

Available in supermarkets and drugstores, supplements can be taken in granular form (mixed in water or juice) or wafer form (washed down with at least eight ounces of water). Supplements soften and bulk up your stool, which should keep pouches from forming.

Sprinkle on the bran. Wheat bran or oat bran, found in health food stores, are also good sources of fiber. But if you think that bran tastes like sawdust, "disguise it by sprinkling it on top of a tossed salad or add it to a meat loaf or casserole," says Dr. Karlstadt.

Load up on water. Drink six to eight eight-ounce glasses of water or other low-calorie beverages a day, Dr. Karlstadt says. That will also help soften and bulk up your stool and prevent the pressure that causes pouches.

Cut out the java. Sometimes people drink a lot of coffee to try and get their stools to pass. That's the wrong approach, says Dr. Karlstadt.

Steady high doses of coffee will harm, not help, your diverticulosis. Caffeine is a diuretic, and stools without water get hard, which is what causes pouches to form. Lots of caffeine can also cause the muscles in the colon to contract more, which prevents the stool from passing along. So if you have diverticulosis, switch to decaf—or at least cut down on the leaded stuff.

Double Chin
Lose It or Hide It

Who would have guessed that back in your twenties, when you and your girlfriends wrapped aluminum foil over record album covers to help tan your necks, what you were doing—inadvertently—was contributing to double chin?

Sunlight breaks down the elastin and collagen fibers in your skin that keep your neck smooth and taut, explains Alison Vidimos, M.D., a staff dermatologist at the Cleveland Clinic Foundation. And that encourages skin to sag.

But sunlight isn't the primary cause, says Dr. Vidimos.

"Double chins are caused by excess fat, or by a combination of excess fat and a loss of muscle tone as you age," says Dr. Vidimos. And like other facial features, double chins sometimes run in families. Add sun-damaged, sagging skin to even a little extra fat, and you have a double chin.

NONSURGICAL OPTIONS

Here's what you can do to help ditch double chin.

Peel pounds. You're not likely to have a double chin unless you are carrying at least a little extra fat, says Debra Price, M.D., clinical assistant professor of dermatology at the University of Miami School of Medicine and a dermatologist in South Miami. Her advice: "Try to get back to a healthy weight."

Eat less, exercise more. Use your double chin as motivation to cut calories and increase the amount of physical activity in your life, says Maria Simonson, Sc.D., Ph.D., director of the Health, Weight and Stress Clinic at the Johns Hopkins Medical Institutions in Baltimore.

Cut the amount of food that you put on your plate in half, for example. Or drink a glass of water before meals to fill you up. Learn to savor the taste and texture of your food. This will slow you down.

Apply sunscreen. To keep the sun from damaging your skin any further and making the problem worse, smooth on a broad-spectrum sunscreen that reflects both ultraviolet rays A and B, says Dr. Price. She recommends sunscreen products that contain titanium dioxide, microscopic particles that reflect ultraviolet light. Apply the sunscreen to your neck every day. (And don't forget to apply it to your face as well.)

Dry Eyes
More Moisture—In Seconds

When it comes to dry eyes, the causes vary. Overheated rooms. Air-conditioned rooms. Air-conditioned cars. Pollution. Working at a computer for hours. A bit of grit in your eye. Allergies. Allergy medicines. Other medicines.

And let's not forget aging. As we get older we may still cry at romantic movies, but we produce fewer moistening tears. And more women than men experience dry eyes, because of hormonal changes— specifically, a drop in estrogen production that accompanies menopause.

"Most women over age 40 have dry eyes," says Anne Sumers, M.D., an ophtalmologist in Ridgewood, New Jersey, and a spokeswoman for the American Academy of Ophthalmology.

If you wear contact lenses, dry eyes may become a problem

sooner—around age 35, says Monica L. Monica, M.D., Ph.D., an ophthalmologist in New Orleans and spokesperson for the American Academy of Ophthalmology. Contact lenses are uncomfortable when eyes are dry, so dryness is more noticeable in lens wearers.

Ironically, crying or excessive tearing can still leave your eyes dry. Normally, every time you blink, your eyes create tears that keep them moist and dewy. But when you cry or get a piece of grit in your eyes, your eyes shed more diluted "fighter reflex" tears that run out of your eyes too quickly to wet them.

One thing is for sure—dry eyes hurt.

"Dry eyes look red and they burn, tear excessively or feel irritated and scratchy," says Dr. Monica.

H$_2$O TO THE RESCUE

Regardless of the cause, relief is just seconds away.

Splash a little water in your eye. If closing your eyes for a few minutes doesn't relubricate them, step into the nearest washroom and splash water in your eyes, says Dr. Monica. (If you wear contact lenses, skip this remedy. Otherwise, bacteria routinely present in water could interfere with your wetting solution or lodge under your lens and lead to infection.)

Apply a cold compress. If you have the time, wet a towel or washcloth and apply to your eye for a few minutes two or three times, says Dr. Monica.

Buy artificial tears. If you wear contact lenses, use rewetting drops, or if tap water and cold compresses aren't convenient, go to the drugstore and buy over-the-counter artificial tears such as Moisture Drops, Hypotears or Tears Naturale. Apply immediately and repeat as often as necessary, says Dr. Monica.

DAY-TO-DAY STRATEGIES

Once you have found immediate relief, follow these tips for lasting comfort.

Use tears liberally. Use artificial tears as often as you like—doctors say that most people underuse artificial tears. "You can use them as often as needed—from once or twice a day to every 20 minutes," says Dr. Monica. These over-the-counter drops will cleanse your eyes and restore the right kind of tears.

Go preservative-free. If you wear contacts or use artificial tears more than once or twice a day, choose a preservative-free brand such as

When to See a Doctor

Many medications—decongestants, antihistamines and sleep aids or sedatives—can dry your eyes. Artificial tears can help. If they don't, talk to your doctor—she may be able to suggest an alternative.

When accompanied by other symptoms, dry eyes can be a sign of infection that, untreated, can cause vision loss. See a doctor if:

- Your eye remains pinkish-red, despite frequent use of artificial tears.
- Your eye hurts.
- Your vision changes.
- You notice pus or discharge from your eye.
- You have dry eyes, dry mouth and arthritis (these symptoms may be a sign of Sjögren's syndrome, a rare but treatable condition that sometimes affects women at midlife).

Hypotears PF or Celluvise. Otherwise, your eyes may sting or your contacts may react adversely to the preservatives, says Dr. Monica.

Don't use medicated eyedrops such as Murine or Visine. They are decongestants and shrink the eye's blood vessels, treating redness, not dryness, says Silvia Orengo-Nania, M.D., assistant clinical professor of ophthalmology at Baylor College of Medicine in Houston.

Moisten your eyes before blow-drying your hair. Do you use a hair dryer every morning? To keep from drying your eyes along with your tresses, use artificial tears before and after you blow-dry, says Dr. Monica. For extra measure, moisten your eyes halfway through, too.

Humidify your work space. If you suspect that a bone-dry work space is contributing to your problem, put a humidifier near your desk, or if possible, open a window, says Dr. Sumers.

Skip the alcohol. Drinking alcohol can leave your mouth parched. It can dry out your eyes, too. If you go out for a social drink, keeping alcohol to a minimum (or choosing a nonalcoholic beverage) is kinder to your eyes, says Dr. Monica.

Stay smoke-free. "Smoking is notorious" for causing dry eyes, says Dr. Monica. If you smoke, or if you live with someone who does, using artificial tears will keep your eyes moistened. Quitting, of course, solves the underlying problem.

Wear your lenses part-time. To ease the strain of dry eyes, "Remove your lenses at the end of the workday, just like you kick off your shoes," says Dr. Monica. If you have dry eyes, this might be a good idea whether you have daily-wear or extended-wear lenses.

Pretreat at bedtime. If you wake up with scratchy, burning eyes, use tear ointment such as Lacri-Lube before you go to bed, says Dr. Monica. It's thicker than artificial tears and available over the counter at your drugstore. It will help keep your eyes lubricated, but it's only for overnight use, because it blurs your vision.

(For more solutions to contact lens problems, see page 142.)

Dry Hair
Moisturize That Mane

Dry hair is the pits. It sticks out straight and dry like the bristles on a broom. It won't curl, it won't wave, it won't shine. All it does is make you feel grouchy every time you look in the mirror.

"Dry hair is a tough problem," sympathizes Patricia Farris Walters, M.D., clinical assistant professor of dermatology at Tulane University School of Medicine in New Orleans and a spokesperson for the American Academy of Dermatology. "Generally, dry hair is caused by overprocessing—bleaching, coloring, straightening and perming—further aggravated by use of heat-intensive devices like blow-dryers and curling irons."

Normally, the cells in each strand of hair line up in straight rows like the shingles on a roof, explains Yohini Appa, Ph.D., director of product efficacy at the Neutrogena Corporation in Los Angeles. But if tiny sections of your hair's outer cell layer have been chipped or stripped away by harsh chemicals or intense heat, exposing the inner layers of the hair shaft, the hair loses moisture. Also, damaged hair doesn't reflect light the way that healthy, smooth hair does, so dry hair looks dull and lifeless.

HELP FOR THE FRIED AND DRIED

Fortunately, say women doctors, you can repair the damage that causes dry hair with a few simple changes in your hair-care routine.

Shampoo, then condition. Proper shampooing is the first step to a healthy scalp and manageable hair, but don't use a conditioning shampoo, says Dr. Appa. Two-in-one products that combine shampoo and conditioner really can't do a good job of either cleansing or conditioning. After all, how can a product effectively remove and add substances at the same time?

Instead, use a gentle shampoo to cleanse, then follow with a conditioner specifically geared for dry hair every time you shampoo. Don't worry about shampooing too often. Today's gentle shampoos are designed for frequent use.

Deep-condition regularly. To fill nicks and chips in the hair's damaged outer layer and restore shine, Elizabeth Whitmore, M.D., assistant professor of dermatology at Johns Hopkins University School of Medicine in Baltimore, recommends that you deep-condition. Depending on the condition of your hair, once a week or once every few weeks is all that is needed. Consisting of various combinations of natural and synthetic ingredients (including proteins, polymers or other additives), deep conditioners don't "feed" your hair; they just fill in defects and coat the hair shaft, resulting in a smooth, flat surface that will reflect light and restore shine to your hair.

For maximum effectiveness Dr. Whitmore suggests that you apply a deep conditioner before you shampoo. Gently work the conditioner into your hair with your fingertips and allow it to be absorbed for a few minutes. Then shampoo and follow with your regular conditioner.

Pat your hair dry. Hair dryers and blowers—and even vigorous towel-drying—can rough up the outer layer of hair cells. So whenever possible, pat or gently squeeze your hair dry with a towel and avoid rough handling, suggests Dr. Appa.

Use thermal styling conditioners. If you must blow-dry your hair, says Dr. Appa, spray it with a thermal conditioner such as HeatSafe before you plug in your dryer. HeatSafe combines four different types of moisturizers designed to both treat and prevent dry hair.

Protect your tresses. To prevent the sun from drying your hair or exacerbating hair that's already dry, mist your hair with a sunscreen made for hair before you hit the beach or head for the pool, says Dr. Whitmore. Or wear a hat whenever you're out in the sun.

Dry Hands

From Sandpaper to Satin

hey crack, burn and itch. They snag on your panty hose. And they look like the appendages of a crustacean, not a human being. They're dry, chapped hands—the scourge of women who spend time with their hands in and out of water or working in the super-dry air of office buildings.

"Even here in Oregon, where the air is moist year-round, dry skin can be a real problem for hands, because once we turn on the heat, it dries out the skin," observes Phoebe Rich, M.D., clinical assistant professor of dermatology at Oregon Health Sciences Center in Portland.

SOAK, SEAL AND PROTECT

Women doctors say that there is plenty you can do to relieve dry hands. "How we care for our skin can make a major difference in how our hands look," says Loretta Davis, M.D., associate professor of dermatology at the Medical College of Georgia School of Medicine in Augusta. Here's what to do.

Wash with a superfatted soap. "Soaps in general strip oil from your skin, so look for less irritating products," says Dr. Davis. Look for soaps that contain emollients—such as Dove and Oil of Olay.

Replace lost oils. At first, dunking your parched hands in water soothes the itching and discomfort. But repeated exposure only exacerbates dry skin, say women doctors.

"Water is the biggest culprit to hands, especially in combination with soaps and detergents," says Dr. Rich. She advises that women moisturize their hands immediately after washing them, to seal in the water that the skin has absorbed, helping prevent drying and chapping.

Skin-care specialist Lia Schorr, owner of Lia Schorr Skin Care Salon in New York City, suggests looking for hand lotions and creams that contain mineral oil or glycerin. Others recommend mild lotions such as Cetaphil, Moisturel, Aveeno, Eucerin or Purpose.

Wear protective gloves. "Hairdressers, who come in constant contact with chemicals, experience dry hands more than anyone else," says Dr. Rich.

179

For everyone else household cleaning products are a problem. Bathroom cleaner, ammonia and bleach tend to be especially drying to the hands, says Dr. Davis.

To protect your hands, Dr. Rich advises wearing rubber gloves with cotton liners. "The liners keep your hands from sweating. Otherwise, the sweat, just like water, dries out your skin."

(For practical ways to manage eczema, a skin condition that resembles dry skin, see page 193.)

Dry Mouth
Wet Your Whistle

*I*f your mouth is chronically dry and you've seen your doctor, she has probably probed possible causes, including medication or disease. In women, a disorder called Sjögren's syndrome is a possible cause of dry mouth as well as dry eyes. It tends to hit women after menopause.

Women with diabetes are at increased risk for dry mouth, says Heidi K. Hausauer, D.D.S., instructor of operative dentistry at the University of the Pacific Dental School in San Francisco and a spokesperson for the Academy of General Dentistry, as are women who have have had radiation for head and neck cancer, which can damage the salivary glands.

And some women find that their mouths simply get drier as they get older, for no medical reason, Geraldine Morrow, D.M.D., past president of the American Dental Association, a member of the American Association of Women Dentists and a dentist in Anchorage, Alaska.

BRUSH, FLOSS, CHEW, SIP

Whatever the cause, solving dry mouth is important—and not just for comfort, say women doctors.

"Bacteria forms in plaque, and it eats the same sugars that we eat, creating acid as a by-product," says Dr. Hausauer. "Acid causes tooth

WHEN TO SEE A DOCTOR

Saliva helps your teeth resist decay and gum disease. So if your mouth becomes uncomfortably dry for more than a few days, or if it recurs often, you should make an appointment to see your doctor or dentist, says Geraldine Morrow, D.M.D., past president of the American Dental Association, a member of the American Association of Women Dentists and a dentist in Anchorage, Alaska. The cause might be medication you're taking.

Dry mouth is a possible common side effect for more than 400 drugs, from antihistamines to high blood pressure medications, among others. If medications are to blame, perhaps your prescription can be changed.

In the event that your doctor concludes that dry mouth is caused by some underlying health condition, she'll probably prescribe an artificial saliva rinse and a prescription fluoride rinse or gel to be used daily to protect your teeth against decay.

decay, but in a normal mouth, saliva buffers that acid." Here's what you can do.

Floss and brush with fluoride toothpaste—religiously. Above all, a woman with dry mouth needs an intensive brushing and flossing program with a fluoride toothpaste, notes Dr. Morrow. "The healthier you keep your mouth, the less chance you give bacteria to set up shop."

Drink water, not soda. Dr. Hausauer tells women with dry mouth to carry around a bottle of water, sipping all day, to keep their mouths fresh and moist. Water is a better choice than soft drinks or fruit juices, since you want to avoid sugar and you lack the saliva necessary to neutralize the acids formed by plaque.

Tote some saliva spray. Both Dr. Morrow and Dr. Hausauer recommend artificial saliva rinses or sprays, available over the counter.

Chew away. If your mouth is dry, chew sugarless gum—it will encourage your natural saliva production and moisten your mouth, says Diane Schoen, dental hygienist and clinical assistant professor and coordinator of the Preventive Dentistry Program at the University of Medicine and Dentistry of New Jersey in Newark. Studies have found that saliva flow improves significantly when people chew gum for ten minutes an hour.

Change your rinse. Some mouth rinses and denture cleaners can dry out your mouth, says Dr. Morrow. So try changing these products to see if this will bring some relief.

Dry Skin
Stop the Itch-Scratch Cycle

*Y*ou don't need an expert to tell you if your skin is dry. Look for rough, scaly patches on your legs, back, arms or waist. They're the areas that you forget about in your concentration on moisturizing your face and hands, and they can itch. You might scratch. "I often see scratch lines on people," says Dee Anna Glaser, M.D., assistant professor of dermatology at St. Louis University School of Medicine. A few even draw blood. Scratch too much, and an itchy patch can get infected or result in a permanent scar.

AHHH, RELIEF!

No need for things to get that dire, says Mary Lupo, M.D., associate clinical professor of dermatology at Tulane University School of Medicine in New Orleans. "There's so much that women can do for dry skin—more so than for oily skin. A whole new generation of moisturizers and skin products are available to help dry skin, so it really needn't be a problem anymore."

Some golden oldies still work, too. Here's what women doctors advise.

Milk it down. If your itchy winter skin is driving you nuts, "go to the refrigerator and get a quart of milk. Pour it into a bowel or basin. Dip a washcloth or a piece of gauze in the cold milk and apply it to your skin for five minutes," says Susan C. Taylor, M.D., assistant clinical professor of medicine in the Department of Dermatology at the University of Pennsylvania School of Medicine in Philadelphia. "Milk has anti-inflammatory properties that often take the itch away. It stops the vicious itch-scratch cycle."

"Milk is very soothing to the skin," says Karen S. Harkaway, M.D., clinical instructor of dermatology at the University of Pennsylvania School of Medicine and a dermatologist at Pennsylvania Hospital, both in Philadelphia. "Some milk contains lactic acid, which is beneficial to skin."

Grease up. For dry, itchy skin the best moisturizer is one that's thick and heavy. "Watery, scented lotions are next to useless for dry skin," says Diane L. Kallgren, M.D., a dermatologist in private practice in Boulder, Colorado. "I recommend pretty strong, thick creams or emollients. The least expensive is petroleum jelly."

Petroleum jelly may be too thick and greasy for some women. "If so, warm it up in your hands first—then it will spread easier," says Dr. Taylor. If you find petroleum jelly messy, use it at night when you're in bed.

Moisturize while damp. The best time of all to oil or cream your face and body is after a bath or shower, while you're still damp and your skin is plump with moisture, says Dr. Glaser. Moisturizing lotions are formulated to lock in moisture so that it doesn't evaporate.

Take the overnight cure. This overnight treatment from Dr. Glaser "will make your dry skin feel markedly different when you wake up the next morning," she says.

"First, soak in a lukewarm tub almost to the point where your fingers shrivel up like prunes—your skin will be fully hydrated. Get out of the tub and pat yourself semidry, then apply a layer of oil. It doesn't have to be an elegant, expensive oil—Crisco shortening is one of the very best, because it is solid, and you can slather on a thick layer. Then put on your pajamas and get into bed."

It's a little messy, so use old pajamas and sheets. "Do this when your skin is very dry," she says. "You'll feel a difference."

Grease and seal super-dry spots. Often the very driest of dry skin occurs on your heels, hands and elbows. But you can seal them with grease, too, says Dr. Glaser. Wear gloves to bed over greased-up raw, sore hands. Wear socks over your cracked heels. And wear a long-sleeved pajama top or T-shirt with snugly fitting sleeves over chapped elbows.

SKIN STRATEGIES TO TRY

Once you've salved your scratchy skin, keep it soft with these techniques.

Forming a Habit

Susan C. Taylor, M.D.

Philadelphia isn't Fairbanks, Alaska, but its winters are mighty harsh on skin, nonetheless. Susan C. Taylor, M.D., assistant clinical professor of medicine in the Department of Dermatology at the University of Pennsylvania School of Medicine in Philadelphia takes these steps to protect her skin.

"As a mainstay, I apply moisturizer twice daily: in the morning after a shower and at night when I take my clothes off at the end of the day. That's when you feel most itchy, so it's a good time to reapply moisturizer.

"There's not a day in my life when I don't apply moisturizer after a shower. It's the optimum time to apply lotion, because it locks in the moisture from the shower, and it can make a big difference.

"Make moisturizing a habit, like applying deodorants," she says. The improvement motivates her to stick with her post-shower routine. "I also use a heavier moisturizer in the middle of winter, when the air is so dry."

Aim for an AHA. When it comes to preventing dry skin, women doctors rave about moisturizers with alpha hydroxy acids (AHAs), originally derived from milk, fruit or sugarcane. AHA moisturizers do double duty. "They remove dry, dead, crusty, scaly skin and they trap moisture in your skin," says Dr. Taylor.

"Some over-the-counter AHA products are better than others," says Dr. Harkaway. "In general, the thicker the moisturizer, the better."

Bathe or shower with tepid water and mild soap. The water temperature should be lukewarm, says Dr. Harkaway. "Use a very mild soap—like Dove, Lever 2000, Tone or Caress. If your skin is dry, stay away from strong antibacterial soaps," she says.

Earaches and Ear Infections

Turn Down the Pain

*W*omen doctors agree: The term *earache* is a commonly used yet unscientific term for a whole range of problems that run the gamut from minor annoyances to serious infections.

At the minor end is simple ear discomfort, says Jo Shapiro, M.D., instructor of otology and laryngology at Harvard Medical School and associate surgeon of otolaryngology at Beth Israel Deaconess Medical Center and Brigham and Women's Hospital, both in Boston.

"Annoying but uncomplicated achy ears are usually the result of a cold. The eustachian tube (the pencil-size canal that leads from the back of your nasal passages to your ear) becomes congested. Since there is less air in the middle ear, it creates a negative pressure, sometimes associated with fluid accumulation," says Dr. Shapiro. "Because of this, you won't feel sharp pain, but you will feel discomfort or pressure or have muffled hearing."

Ear pain can also occur when the eustachian tube becomes inflamed or congested from a cold, allergy or sore throat.

HELP FOR SIMPLE EARACHES

If you have an earache, you want relief, and you want it fast. Here's what to do.

Warm 'em up. "Heat is excellent for earaches," says Jennifer Derebery, M.D., assistant clinical professor of otolaryngology at the University of Southern California in Los Angeles. "Heat promotes blood flow and marshals infection-fighting white blood cells in the area." She recommends using a hot-water bottle, a hot towel or a heating pad, warmed to a comfortably hot level and wrapped in a towel. Keep the heat on your ear for 20 minutes or until the pain goes away, whichever comes first.

Reach for the hot sauce. "Food that is so spicy that it makes your

No More Ear Pain

Donna Jean Millay, M.D.

In the hills of Vermont, below-zero winter temperatures can cause painful earaches. But that doesn't stop Vermonters from venturing out. When Donna Jean Millay, M.D., assistant professor of otolaryngology at the University of Vermont and staff physician at Fletcher Allen Medical Center, both in Burlington, goes outdoors, here's what she does to keep her ears warm and pain-free.

"I'm a runner," says Dr. Millay. "But I avoid hats when I run, because they make me too hot.

"So when it's chilly, I roll up a cotton bandana and tie it around my head, covering my ears. When it's really freezing, I wear a fleece headband to cover my ears."

Once home, Dr. Millay says, she rubs her hands together, then places one on each ear to warm them up after her run.

nose run can ease earaches associated with congestion," says Evelyn Kluka, M.D., director of pediatric otolaryngology at Children's Hospital in New Orleans. "Try a good hot-and-sour soup or, better yet, an authentic New Orleans gumbo loaded with hot peppers."

Humidify your nose. "Use a plain saline nasal spray, available over the counter, several times a day when your nose is congested. It will reduce the congestion caused by a cold or allergies, thereby reducing your ear discomfort," says Dr. Kluka.

Breathe away an ache. According to Effie Chow, R.N., Ph.D., a certified acupuncturist and Qigong master who teaches the Chinese healing discipline Qigong at the East/West Academy of Healing Arts in San Francisco, Qigong's deep-breathing techniques are effective for earaches and other pain, because they oxygenate the body, strengthen the immune system and open blockages.

"Breathe in deeply from your diaphragm, not your chest, bringing air in through your nose," says Dr. Chow. "Imagine the area right behind your naval to your upper chest area as an accordion, and fill it with air through your nose. Keeping your lips closed, expand the accordion. Then exhale, collapsing the accordion, and allow the air to escape through your lips. Continue this exercise until you feel relaxed and the pain eases." Dr. Chow suggests that this breathing be done from time to time over a 24-hour period.

TIPS FOR AIRBORNE ACHES

When your eustachian tubes are congested, changes in air pressure—during aircraft landings, scuba dives or even rapid trips in high-rise elevators—can hurt your ears. Excess mucus prevents your middle ear from equalizing the pressure. A vacuum forms, sucking the eardrum inward and stretching the eardrum. Sounds are muffled or blocked, and you feel discomfort. If you have a cold and must fly, try these tips.

Try the Frenzel maneuver. Pinch your nose and push your tongue against the back part of the roof of your mouth, says Laura Orvidas, M.D., senior associate consultant and instructor in the Department of Otorhinolaryngology at the Mayo Clinic in Rochester, Minnesota. That will work a little air through your eustachian tubes without damage.

Yawn or chew (or both). To clear that full-ear feeling during take-off or landing, force yourself to yawn, says Dr. Orvidas. Or quietly chew on a stick of gum.

WHEN TO SEE A DOCTOR

See your doctor as soon as possible if your ear pain is:
- Severe
- Accompanied by drainage or discharge from your ear
- Accompanied by a fever of 102°F or higher
- Not accompanied by a cold
- Not caused by water in your ear

Symptoms that may require emergency treatment include:
- Sudden change in hearing
- Sudden onset of dizziness
- Inability to concentrate
- Muscle weakness on the same side of your face as the affected ear

"Any one of these four symptoms could mean that your infection has spread and is more aggressive than usual," says Donna Jean Millay, M.D., assistant professor of otolaryngology at the University of Vermont and staff physician at Fletcher Allen Medical Center, both in Burlington. "See your doctor—or visit an emergency room—immediately."

Also, people with diabetes need immediate attention when their ears ache.

Pretreat with a decongestant. One hour before flight time, take a decongestant like Sudafed, says Dr. Orvidas. Follow package instructions.

Or, use a decongestant spray. "A spray or two in each nostril of Afrin or Neo-Synephrine reaches the exact area that you want to decongest," says Dr. Orvidas.

Dr. Kluka advises using nasal spray when you're in the terminal, about 20 minutes before boarding the plane, then again once you board your flight.

EARACHE OR EAR INFECTION?

Most ear infections start with an earache, says Dr. Shapiro, but not all earaches are ear infections. If you have an infection, it's time to see Ye Olde Family Physician. "She will prescribe antibiotics. Many people ask if antibiotics are really necessary. I tell them that the ear is close to many delicate structures, including the brain. An untreated infection can spread and cause problems, including mastoiditis—an infection of the bone tissue surrounding the ears. Antibiotics eliminate ear infections—and potentially serious problems—safely and rapidly," says Dr. Shapiro.

To ease discomfort until you see the doctor, here's what you can do.

Try an OTC painkiller. To ease severe ear pain and reduce fever, take ibuprofen or acetaminophen according to package instructions, says Donna Jean Millay, M.D., assistant professor of otolaryngology at the University of Vermont and staff physician at Fletcher Allen Medical Center, both in Burlington.

Decongest. A decongestant like Sudafed, taken according to package instructions, relieves congestion and discomfort, says Dr. Millay.

Earlobe Problems
First-Aid for Rashes and Gashes

*A*s body parts go, earlobes are low-maintenance, trouble-free equipment. So you probably don't give your earlobes much thought—until one accidentally tears or develops a crusty, itchy rash.

"Earrings can get caught on clothing, tangled in long hair, pulled out by hairbrushes or even, rarely, ripped through earlobes on extremely windy days," says Hilary E. Baldwin, M.D., assistant professor of dermatology and director of dermatologic surgery at the State University of New York Health Science Center at Brooklyn.

FAST ACTION FOR A TORN LOBE

If you tear your earlobe, it may bleed quite profusely. But don't panic, says Dr. Baldwin. Here's what to do.

Put the pressure on. First, pinch the lobe with a clean tissue, towel or cloth and press firmly for a full five minutes. "No peeking. If you remove the pressure and the tissue too soon, you won't give the blood a chance to clot," explains Dr. Baldwin.

Repeat as needed. If, after five full minutes, you remove the tissue and your earlobe is still bleeding, try again, this time for ten minutes. Again, no peeking.

Cream the germs. Once the bleeding has stopped, keep the wound moist with an antibacterial ointment such as Polysporin.

SOOTHE THE IRRITATION

If your earlobes redden, itch or weep, the problem could be your earrings or an allergy to the antibacterial ointment that you used on your earlobes. Here's what to do.

Say no to nickel. "Earrings containing nickel can cause allergic reactions in many women," says Dr. Baldwin. "And most jewelry contains nickel. Some women even have trouble with 14 karat gold, because it may contain trace amounts of nickel. So it's best to stick with sterling silver or hypoallergenic stainless-steel posts. In fact," she adds, "if your skin is sensitive, any part of the earring that touches your ear should be nickel-free."

Swab your earrings. To prevent infections, Dr. Baldwin advises women to keep earrings as clean as possible: Swab the posts or fasteners with a cotton ball soaked with rubbing alcohol before each wear.

PROBLEM-FREE PIERCING

To minimize problems associated with newly pierced ears, follow these tips from Dr. Baldwin.

Reduce germs. To prevent infection, swab newly pierced earlobes with rubbing alcohol and apply an over-the-counter antibiotic ointment such as Polysporin at least once a day.

Avoid chunky or "chandelier" earrings. Freshly pierced lobes need time to toughen, so don't wear heavy earrings for at least two months after you've had your ears pierced, says Dr. Baldwin.

F.Y.I. to African-American Women: Stick to Clip-Ons

Researchers don't know why, but melanin—a pigment-producing substance in the skin—seems to leave African-American women more prone to large, irregularly shaped scarlike skin growths known as keloids, says Hilary E. Baldwin, M.D., assistant professor of dermatology and director of dermatologic surgery at the State University of New York Health Science Center at Brooklyn. In her study Dr. Baldwin found that African-American women are 25 percent more likely to develop keloids than the general population.

Since the female hormone estrogen seems to play a role in the production of keloids, Dr. Baldwin advises African-American women against having their ears pierced if they are:
- Pregnant
- Taking birth control pills
- On estrogen replacement therapy

Dr. Baldwin also advises African-American women who have had keloids in the past to avoid future piercings. "If you already have a keloid, there is a 50 percent chance that you'll develop another one," she says.

WHEN TO SEE A DOCTOR

If you tear an earlobe and let it heal on its own, the hole will close. So if you want to wear pierced earrings again, see a doctor within 24 hours. Stitches can keep the hole open while it heals, says Hilary E. Baldwin, M.D., assistant professor of dermatology and director of dermatologic surgery at the State University of New York Health Science Center at Brooklyn. If the hole has closed, don't repierce it yourself—have a doctor do it.

You should also see a doctor for a torn earlobe if:

- Your earlobe feels hot to the touch.
- Your earlobe is red or swollen.
- You see pus.

It may be infected. Also, Dr. Baldwin warns women who have developed elongated holes in their earlobes against wearing heavy earrings. "Those holes are more likely to tear," she says. "They're unsightly but relatively easy to fix. So get them fixed before they tear completely."

Just the lobe, please. "I advise women to pierce their lobes only, not the cartilage on the outer or upper ear," says Dr. Baldwin. "The cartilage is more likely to get infected; it has a limited blood supply, so fewer infection-fighting white blood cells reach the cartilage than reach the fleshier lobe. And if it does get infected, cartilage is more difficult to treat. Also, infected cartilage can easily become deformed—that is, floppy or misshapen."

Earwax
Too Much of a Good Thing?

*T*hink of earwax as the gatekeeper to your very delicate inner ear structures, and you're likely to be a lot more respectful about how you go about removing the stuff.

Before you reach for that cotton swab, bobby pin or paper clip, listen to Donna Jean Millay, M.D., assistant professor of otolaryngology at the University of Vermont and staff physician at Fletcher Allen Medical Center, both in Burlington: "Never, ever poke around in your ear with *anything*, for any reason whatsoever! You could easily puncture your eardrum."

You might not even need to remove earwax, says Evelyn Kluka, M.D., director of pediatric otolaryngology at Children's Hospital in New Orleans. "Earwax usually acts as a lubricant and as a protective cleanser. A certain amount of earwax enables debris to slide from the inner to the outer part of the ear canal, where it can be wiped away with a cloth."

TIDIER EARS, WITHOUT PROBING

Here's what women doctors say about earwax removal.

De-wax your outer ear. "Remember hearing Mom remind you to wash your ears when you took a bath?" asks Barbara Hopson, R.N., a certified nurse practitioner at the Veteran's Administration Medical Center Occupational Health Unit in Dallas. "Well, Mom was right. When you don't cleanse away excess earwax, it can build up, harden and plug up your ears, which results in hearing loss." To remove excess wax in your outer ear easily and safely, she recommends using a washcloth that's just slightly damp, not soaked, to gently wipe out the outer portion of your ear, without poking the towel in your ear canal.

Oil away excess wax. If you can see wax on the cloth, says Dr. Kluka, you have too much wax in your ear. To soften and liquefy hardened earwax, she recommends warming baby oil or olive oil to body temperature and placing a few drops in your ear. "Hold your head to one side, put the drops in, rub your ear, then tilt your head over to let the drops run out. The drops should carry the excess wax out with them."

Use a baby syringe. "I like the over-the-counter wax removal products like Debrox or Cerumenex," says Hopson. She recommends removing excess wax monthly. For easy-does-it removal, she suggests that you "use a baby-size car syringe instead of the bulb syringe that comes with the kit to flush the wax away after using the drops. The adult version uses too much pressure. Or, instead of a syringe, stand under the shower and let warm water flow gently over your ear."

"If you have a reaction, like itching or irritation, discontinue using the product," adds Dr. Millay.

Eczema

Help for Overly Sensitive Skin

*I*f you have allergies, hay fever, hives or dry, overly sensitive skin, you may also have bouts of eczema, typified by a red and dry rash that itches like crazy.

There are about ten types of eczema, but atopic dermatitis—allergic inflammation of the skin—is among the more common kinds.

"The eczema rash typically appears as red, swollen patches or blotches on the face and neck and the folds of the elbows and knees, but it can also affect the hands and feet—or the whole body," says Kristin Leiferman, M.D., professor of dermatology at the Mayo Medical School in Rochester, Minnesota. And no one knows what causes it, but it's not contagious.

Less Wool, More Moisture

Karen K. Deasey, M.D.

Dermatologists aren't immune to the dry, itchy skin that typifies eczema, says Karen K. Deasey, M.D., chief of dermatology at Bryn Mawr Hospital in Pennsylvania. Here's what she does to soothe her itching skin.

"I make sure to moisturize my skin at least once a day, and sometimes twice," she says. "And I know that stress plays a role in my skin condition, so I try to keep the stress under control.

"Plus, I'm really beginning to believe in the benefits of aromatherapy. I bought a pretty, scented 'stress relief' candle at a Bath and Body Works store at a nearby mall. I burn it while I'm eating dinner, or in my bedroom while I'm reading or getting ready for bed."

Dr. Deasey also makes it a point to wear cotton or soft, natural-fiber clothing, and she avoids wool and heavy, scratchy materials that would aggravate her skin.

A CYCLIC PHENOMENON?

Eczema symptoms come and go. One day your skin may be fine, and the next, you may experience a flare-up of redness and itchiness. Triggers include exposure to harsh soaps or household cleaning products, a skin-drying environment like when the furnace comes on in the fall and early winter, coarse or scratchy clothes and possibly even stress.

Many women also report that they experience eczema flare-ups at the same time during their menstrual cycles each month—either premenstrually or during their periods, says Dr. Leiferman.

ANTI-ITCH SUGGESTIONS

Women doctors say that while there is no cure for eczema, there are things that you can do to keep your skin smooth and clear and keep outbreaks under control. Here's what they recommend. (For other practical ways to deal with dry hands and dry skin, see pages 179 and 182.)

Baths help. Doctors used to tell eczema patients not to bathe frequently. Now many believe that one or two baths or showers a day can be very helpful, says Dr. Leiferman.

Turn down the temp. "Bathe in lukewarm water—it's less drying than hot water," says D'Anne Kleinsmith, M.D., a staff dermatologist at William Beaumont Hospital in Royal Oak, Michigan.

Take 10. "It's important to stay in the water for at least 10 to 20 minutes—long enough for your skin to soak up water," says Dr. Leiferman. "You'll know that you've been in long enough when your skin starts to pucker and crinkle," she says. "Your skin cells actually absorb water through their membranes and become hydrated."

Go easy on the soap. "To avoid drying out your skin, use soap only on those body parts where you think you need it," recommends Karen K. Deasey, M.D., chief of dermatology at Bryn Mawr Hospital in Pennsylvania. And stick with mild, nonirritating soaps. She recommends Dove or Oil of Olay Beauty Bar.

Other good choices are superfatted soaps such as Basis or Aveeno, according to Dr. Kleinsmith.

Glycerinated (see-through) soaps are also a good bet, Dr. Leiferman says. But avoid deodorant soaps, which tend to be harsh and irritating.

Seal in water with moisturizer. The best time to slather on moisturizer is immediately after you step out of the bath or shower. "Just blot off excess water with a towel and liberally apply moisturizer while your skin is still damp," says Dr. Kleinsmith. This after-bath treatment helps trap the moisture that has gotten into your skin while bathing.

Go fragrance-free. "I advise patients to look for bland moisturizers that don't have a lot of fragrance, color or additives that could irritate skin," says Dr. Leiferman.

"Read the labels and pick one that is right for you," agrees Dr. Deasey, who recommends Cetaphil moisturizing cream, Aveeno cream or lotion, and Lubriderm products. Sometimes she suggests a specialized lotion called Lac-Hydrin Five for extremely dry skin.

Keep moisturizers handy. "Stock up on small travel-size tubes of moisturizer and carry them around in your purse or pocket," says Dr. Kleinsmith. "That way, every time you wash your hands, you can reapply a coat of moisturizer."

Wash that itch right out of your clothes. Use mild laundry detergents, such as Tide and Ivory, and rinse your clothes twice when washing to clear away all traces of detergent, advises Dr. Deasey. "I stay away from those newer, blue liquid detergents, because I find that they leave residues on clothes that make people itch. I also avoid fabric softeners, because the fragrances in them can make your skin itch."

Protect your hands. Wear gloves whenever you do dishes or housework, because soap and water, cleaning products and even dust can irri-

WHEN TO SEE A DOCTOR

If you have eczema, you can probably handle most flare-ups on your own. You should see a doctor if:

- The itch is so severe that you can't sleep, or you can't get relief from over-the-counter products such as hydrocortisone cream. "A doctor can prescribe itch-relieving medication, such as antihistamines or hydroxyzine (like Atarax) or doxepin (like Zonalon Cream)," says Karen K. Deasey, M.D., chief of dermatology at Bryn Mawr Hospital in Pennsylvania.

- The eczema is open and oozing, because your skin may be infected. Your doctor may prescribe an antibiotic, which can also help reduce itching and redness.

tate your skin, advises Dr. Kleinsmith. "However, rubber gloves tend to get hot and make your hands sweaty, so wear cotton glove liners inside the rubber gloves to absorb perspiration," she says. "You can get cotton gloves in drugstores or in medical supply stores."

Heal with hydrocortisone cream. If your skin is really inflamed and itchy, over-the-counter hydrocortisone creams can help soothe the itch. They may also diminish some of the redness, says Dr. Kleinsmith.

Emphysema
Boost Your Lung Power

Most of us know what it feels like to struggle to catch our breath when we're running, biking or trying to keep up with the latest aerobics video.

"People with emphysema experience shortness of breath when performing very simple daily activities such as brushing their teeth, taking a shower and even eating," says Lisa Schulz, a respiratory therapist at the National Jewish Center for Immunology and Respiratory Medicine in Denver.

As the disease progresses, however, a stroll through a garden, or just walking from the house to a car may leave you gulping for air like a goldfish.

Emphysema is bad news. It involves irreversible damage to the air sacs inside the lungs where the vital exchange of oxygen and carbon dioxide takes place. The air sacs lose their elasticity, making it hard to exhale fully. So the lungs remain filled with stale, oxygen-poor air, and fresh air can't get in.

This lung damage doesn't happen overnight, says Sally Wenzel, M.D., associate professor at the University of Colorado School of Medicine and a pulmonary specialist at the National Jewish Center for Immunology and Respiratory Medicine, both in Denver. "Most people with emphysema are long-term smokers or former smokers who develop this condition in their fifties and sixties," Dr. Wenzel says. "And these days, almost as many women as men get the disease, as more long-term female smokers hit middle age and beyond."

HELP YOURSELF BREATHE BETTER

People with severe emphysema use pressurized oxygen to get around. A new surgical procedure called lung reduction surgery also helps people with emphysema to better use the remaining good parts of their lungs.

These additional tactics can help damaged lungs work their best.

Pucker up and blow. An exercise called pursed-lip breathing helps people with emphysema move more stale air out of their lungs with each exhalation, says Dr. Wenzel.

To do this exercise, inhale fully through your nose, purse your lips as though you are going to blow out a candle and then, after holding your breath for a second or two, exhale slowly and fully for a count of at least six. "I tell people to hold the back of their hand three to five inches away, facing their mouth," says Betty Booker, a respiratory therapist and pulmonary rehabilitation coordinator at University Hospital in Denver. "If they can feel their breath on the back of their hand, they are exhaling really well."

Pursed lips provide a little resistance that maintains air pressure in airways. "That keeps the airways from collapsing before air has left the lungs, which can happen in people with emphysema," says Dr.

WHEN TO SEE A DOCTOR

If you have emphysema, you should be seeing your doctor regularly for checkups. That's because labored breathing can put a big strain on your heart. If your symptoms seem to be worsening, if you have congestion in your lungs or have swelling in your legs, see your doctor as soon as possible, says Sally Wenzel, M.D., associate professor at the University of Colorado School of Medicine and pulmonary specialist at the National Jewish Center for Immunology and Respiratory Medicine, both in Denver.

And be sure to line up early for flu shots. Add an acute infection to a chronic disease, and you have the potential for deadly trouble. "I tell my patients to get flu shots every year as soon as the shots are available, usually in October," says Dr. Wenzel.

If you feel like you're getting a cold or the flu or if you have fever, chills or severe coughing, you should also get to a doctor quickly for antibiotics or other treatment. Don't wait, Dr. Wenzel says.

Wenzel. "That's what traps stale air in the lungs and makes it even harder to breathe."

Most people do pursed-lip breathing during exertion if they feel short of breath, Schulz says. "It can require a little practice initially, especially to exhale slowly and fully, but it is very relaxing. We also encourage people to do it whenever they feel short of breath or anxious."

Breathe from your belly. To take deep breaths that fill your lungs with air from the bottom up, you need to properly use your diaphragm, the sheet of powerful muscles that create the vacuum that makes your lungs fill.

"You can learn to do this while lying down, sitting up straight in a hard chair or standing," says Schulz.

Place your hand on your belly, relax your belly and then inhale slowly through your nose, concentrating on relaxing your abdomen so that your diaphragm drops down and your belly expands. When exhaling, pull the abdomen in and the diaphragm up, to slowly push the air out of the lungs through pursed lips. "People can learn to focus their energy on certain muscles or on certain areas of their lungs to breathe more efficiently," Schulz says. "It takes concentration and practice, but it works."

Position yourself for better breathing. "Some people with emphysema can actually get in more air if they lean forward and place their forearms on a table or shopping cart," says Karen Conyers, a respiratory therapist at the University of Kansas Medical Center in Kansas City. Most other times you'll want to sit or stand up straight, keeping your belly relaxed. "This allows your diaphragm maximum movement," she says.

Shake a leg. It's a vicious cycle. People with emphysema tend to become more and more sedentary—a nice word for doing nothing. "The gradual reduction in activity is barely perceptible to most people, but the less they do, the less they are able to do," Conyers says.

Although exercise won't improve your lungs' function, it does improve endurance, Dr. Wenzel says. "It helps the heart and other muscles to use available oxygen more efficiently, so people can do more."

Most people with emphysema can walk, on a treadmill or outdoors, or use a stationary bicycle. It's best to check with your doctor first if you haven't been active, says Dr. Wenzel. You can be tested to see if you do better getting supplemental oxygen while you're exercising.

Some people may begin with as little as two minutes of walking before they need to rest. "But once they get past two weeks or so, they see their endurance begin to pick up and they are willing to extend the time more," Booker says. "Some really get into it." Their goal isn't marathons, but to be able to do simple activities without hauling an oxygen tank.

Don't be passive about smoke. Chances are it's cigarette smoke that damaged your lungs in the first place. So you want to avoid it—even secondhand smoke. "This can be really hard for people whose friends still smoke," Schulz admits. (If you have emphysema and still smoke, see the chapter on nicotine addiction on page 397.)

In the air, get extra oxygen. Cabin pressures on airplanes can lower blood oxygen levels enough to cause problems for people with lung disease, Dr. Wenzel says. You won't be allowed to bring your own oxygen tank onto the plane, but many airlines can arrange for supplemental oxygen during a flight if they have advance notice.

Drink enough water. Aim for at least eight glasses of water, juice or the equivalent a day, says Dr. Wenzel. "Being well-hydrated thins out mucus in the lungs, making it easier to remove."

Dress loosely. Clothes that pinch you around the waist make it hard to breathe properly, Dr. Wenzel says.

Eat like a bird, not a boa constrictor. In other words, don't eat so much that you become uncomfortably full, Dr. Wenzel says. "The size of meals is very important. If you eat too big a meal, your stomach pushes up on your diaphragm and you can't breath properly."

Guard against girth. Just as a full belly can cramp your diaphragm, so can weight around the middle, Dr. Wenzel says. "If you can keep your weight normal, you'll have fewer problems."

Endometriosis
Take the Edge off Pelvic Pain

*A*s disorders go, endometriosis is as mysterious as it sounds. Normally, the endometrial tissue—soft tissue that lines your uterus—alternately thickens and sheds each month with your period. But in some women the endometrial tissue migrates outside the uterus and starts to grow on and around other pelvic organs, such as the ovaries, colon and bladder or the fallopian tubes, which carry eggs from the ovaries to the uterus.

Just like uterine tissues, errant endometrial tissue thickens monthly in response to release of the female hormone estrogen, and it may cause painful cramps and heavier-than-usual monthly bleeding. Worse, the renegade tissue may exert pressure on the organs and result in pain. Endometriosis may also lead to painful sexual intercourse, infertility or both.

A TAKE-CHARGE APPROACH

No one knows why otherwise well-behaved uterine tissue suddenly decides to creep beyond its bounds and cause trouble. If you've been diagnosed with endometriosis, your doctor will work with you to find the best medical treatment. "Meanwhile, dealing with the chronic nature of the discomfort is an ongoing, day-to-day challenge," says Mary Lou Ballweg, president of the Endometriosis Association. "The women who take the bull by the horns and do everything they can do to improve their overall health do the best."

Women doctors offer these tips on dealing with the day-to-day and long-term challenges of endometriosis.

Eat a low animal fat diet. Meat, fatty fish and poultry, dairy products and eggs contain dioxins—chemical residues that may be linked to both the onset and severity of endometriosis, says Linda Birnbaum, Ph.D., director of the Experimental Toxicology Division of the U.S. Environmental Protection Agency. By-products of industrial processes such as incineration, dioxins are released into the environment and are consumed by animals, then stored in fat tissues. When we eat animal products, we also consume dioxins, which our bodies store for long periods of time.

Studies have shown that laboratory animals that are fed dioxins exhibit an increase in the incidence and severity of endometriosis, says Dr. Birnbaum. Researchers in her own lab have found that when laboratory mice and rats are treated with dioxin, endometriotic sites grow bigger. The chemicals appear to do their dirty work by short-circuiting the body's complex hormone system. They also cause problems with the immune system, affecting antibodies and other important disease-fighting immune cells called lymphocytes.

"The Public Health Service recommends a diet with less animal fat and more green and leafy vegetables and complex carbohydrates like pasta. This will lead to a slightly lower level of these compounds in your body. And it's also good for your heart," says Dr. Birnbaum.

Counter constipation. "If you're constipated and bloated, you're going to feel a lot worse," says Deborah A. Metzger, M.D., Ph.D., director of the Reproductive Medicine Institute of Connecticut in Hartford, especially if the endometrial tissue has encroached into your bowel area. So be sure to eat plenty of vegetables and other high-fiber foods and drink lots of water to keep your bowels moving.

Change sexual positions. Painful sexual intercourse may be remedied by choosing a position in which the woman has greater control over penetration, says Dr. Metzger. "The missionary position is not the best for control. The female on top is better. The best thing to do is experiment to find the most comfortable position."

Exercise if at all possible. A program of regular exercise, three times a week for at least 30 minutes, can help relieve pain and menstrual cramps, says Sue Ellen Carpenter, M.D., an obstetrician and gynecologist with the Emory Clinic in Atlanta.

Exercise reduces menstrual flow and, therefore, the endometrial irritation and inflammation. It also increases your body's production of endorphins, natural pain-blocking substances released by the brain, says Dr. Metzger.

Walking is a good basic exercise, says Dr. Metzger, though some women with endometriosis may find it too jarring. In that case, swimming or doing a routine of stretches are good ways to keep the juices flowing.

Take a painkiller. The pain of endometriosis can be severe, especially during menstruation, says Dr. Carpenter. Tiny endometrial growths called petechiae are very active in producing prostaglandins, substances linked to the symptoms. Over-the-counter nonsteroidal anti-inflammatory drugs such as ibuprofen can help by interfering with prostaglandin production. Just follow the package directions.

Relax progressively. Chronic pain causes a release of stress hormones, which in turn increases pain sensitivity by reducing the produc-

WHEN TO SEE A DOCTOR

These symptoms may suggest endometriosis and warrant medical attention.
- Painful menstrual periods with heavy, irregular flow
- Pain before and after your period, often accompanied by lower-back pain
- Pain in your pelvis
- Diarrhea
- Painful bowel movements during periods
- Painful intercourse
- Inability to conceive

You may also experience fatigue, exhaustion and low energy.

Medical treatment for endometriosis ranges from hormone therapy to surgery.

tion of endorphins, says Alison Milburn, Ph.D., a health psychologist who specializes in chronic pain and former co-director of the Chronic Pelvic Pain Clinic at the University of Iowa Hospitals and Clinics in Iowa City. "The added complication is that people with chronic pain tend to position their bodies to try and compensate." They might sit differently or walk differently, and this sets up patterns of chronic muscular tension that can cause muscle spasms and such.

A technique called progressive muscle relaxation can help by systematically tensing and relaxing individual muscle groups in your body, Dr. Milburn says. Close your eyes, take a few deep breaths and tense the muscles in your face. Hold for a few seconds, then take a deep breath and release. Repeat this in your neck, shoulders, arms and down through your body. The whole process should take about ten minutes. "Try to do it regularly, daily or even three or four times a day," Dr. Milburn says. "You don't want to do it only when the pain is bad. It's a skill that you need to practice regularly."

Enlarged Pores
Concealment Tactics to Minimize Flaws

*Y*ou have great skin, great hair and a great body. In fact, the only thing standing between you and a cover girl's perfection may very well be the enlarged pores around your nose that deflect attention from your sweet nose and sparkling eyes.

Just about everyone gets enlarged pores, says Deborah S. Sarnoff, M.D., assistant clinical professor of dermatology at New York University in New York City. That's because pores are actually tiny openings in your skin that provide a way for the oil glands underneath to lubricate and protect the surface of your skin.

Pores enlarge during puberty, when oil glands in your skin begin to increase the amount of oil that they pump through your pores. The pores get bigger so that they can handle the increased output. And they stay enlarged until somewhere around menopause, when they shrink into the perfect, totally unnoticeable size that you've always wanted.

SHRINK, FILL, COVER

You're most likely to notice enlarged pores around your nose, because that area has more oil glands per square inch than any other part of your body, says Dr. Sarnoff. But it's still possible to shrink your pores and minimize their appearance. "Even models have enlarged pores; they just know how to hide them."

Here's what experts suggest.

Reach for the right skin cream. After washing your face, smooth a lotion containing alpha hydroxy acids (AHAs) over your skin to peel away old skin cells that build up around your pores, says Mary Stone, M.D., associate professor of dermatology at the University of Iowa in Iowa City. The AHAs are fruit and milk acids that encourage older cells to peel off, leaving younger, smoother skin underneath. You can buy an AHA-containing lotion in most drugstores.

Use an alpha hydroxy acid product that is 10 percent glycolic acid and follow package directions. "You can improve the appearance of your pores by removing dead skin cells," says Dr. Stone.

Smooth on a pore-minimizing lotion. "Use a foundation that suspends powder in liquid and apply it like a putty," says Carole Walderman, national education director for Matrix Skin Care Products in Solon, Ohio.

Make sure that the base you use is noncomedogenic and oil-free, says Dr. Stone.

"Clinique has one called a pore minimizer," says Walderman. After you smudge it over your enlarged pores, the liquid evaporates, leaving your pores full of powder, like applying putty to a hole in the wall.

Apply a water-based foundation. Let the pore minimizer dry for three to five minutes, then apply a water-based foundation over top, says Walderman. "Your face—including the enlarged pore area—will look as smooth as silk."

Episiotomy Pain
Heal Tender Tissues

Sometimes, under the force of expelling a full-term baby, the tissues between the vulva and anus tear or the pelvic muscles weaken and lead to a bulge in the bladder or rectum. To prevent tearing the tender area (called the perineum), physicians and midwives sometimes take preemptive action and make a neat, clean cut (an episiotomy) to enlarge the birth opening. Then it is stitched up after delivery.

PATIENCE AND PAMPERING

If you've had an episiotomy or tear, healing will take a while, says Mindy Smith, M.D., associate professor in family practice at the University of Michigan in Ann Arbor. In fact, you may feel uncomfortable for as long as three to six months.

Here are some things that you can do to help yourself, right from day one.

Cool it. To reduce swelling, apply ice packs, wrapped in a towel, to the incision for the first 12 hours after delivery, suggests Martha Barry,

R.N., adjunct clinical faculty member of the University of Illinois School of Nursing and a certified nurse midwife with Illinois Masonic Hospital, both in Chicago. "Look for cold packs that are about the size of sanitary pads and contain dry ice, sold in drugstores and medical supply stores. You crack the pack, and it becomes cold."

Sitz it. Relaxing in a tub of water, either a shallow sitz bath or a deep regular bath, provides relief, says Barry. Make sure that your bathtub is clean so you don't invite bacteria in.

"One study compared cold sitz baths with warm ones," says Barry. "The researcher found that the women who took the cold ones had less pain afterward. Cold acts as an analgesic. But if warm water feels better to you, that's fine, too. Warmth increases circulation to the area and aids healing."

Use an herbal wash. To soothe tenderness, relieve inflammation, aid cell repair, protect against bacteria and improve circulation, try this herbal combination as recommended by Mary Bove, a naturopathic physician with the Brattleboro Naturopathic Clinic in Vermont and a licensed midwife. Into a pint of boiling water put one handful each of calendula flowers, comfrey root, yarrow flowers and rosemary leaves. Remove from the heat, cover and steep for several minutes. Strain the liquid and transfer into a plastic squirt bottle. Then use it to wash your vaginal area after you urinate. Or make a large batch and use it as a sitz bath. You can store the solution in the refrigerator for two to three days. Allow it to warm to a comfortable temperature before using.

Apply vitamin E. Vitamin E has skin-healing properties and is often prescribed to patients who have undergone surgery, says Barry. If you have had an episiotomy, wait a couple of weeks for the laceration to heal a little. Then open a liquid vitamin E capsule and apply it to the area.

WHEN TO SEE A DOCTOR

If you have had an episiotomy—a surgical incision to enlarge the birth opening—the pain will gradually improve after the first few days, but call your doctor if:

- Pain does not subside after two weeks.
- Pain worsens.
- Bleeding suddenly occurs.

These symptoms may signal an infection that needs treatment.

Eyebrow Problems
Tricks for More Flattering Brows

*W*hether you want Madonna's strong, defined brows or Drew Barrymore's pencil-thin curves, great eyebrows can be as flattering as a great manicure. The trick is knowing where to begin, what to do—and when to stop.

"All you generally need to do is remove a few strays or add a line here and there," says Natasha Salman, a face treatment and waxing specialist at Elizabeth Arden's Red Door Salon in New York City.

TAMING TOO-FURRY BROWS

If your problem is too many hairs, here's the easy way to remove them.

Give them ten days. If your eyebrows seem too furry, and you're not satisfied with the results of your current plucking strategy, let them grow in for at least ten days before you try to shape them, says Salman. That way, you'll make sure that you have enough hair in the right places before you try to artfully shape them.

Tweeze with the grain. Unless you have your brows waxed at a salon, tweezing is the most practical way to shape your brows. For best results Salman says that you should tweeze in the same direction as hair growth. To better enable your tweezers to grip brow hairs (which can be slippery because of natural hair and skin oil), apply powder lightly before tweezing.

Shape naturally, with finesse. When shaping your brows, the arch of each brow should peak over the outer edge of your pupil, says Marcia Turnier, a makeup artist and eyebrow specialist at Elizabeth Arden's Red Door Salon. If your face is very long, flatten the arch by taking a little off the top. If your face is too round, tweeze from below to accentuate the arch. If your eyes seem as though they're too close, shape the brows to widen the distance between them.

Dull the pain. Some women let their brows grow au naturel because they hate the pain of tweezing. To relieve pain, apply pressure with your fingers to the eyebrow area for 10 to 15 seconds after each hair is removed, says Salman. Then, if the area still feels a little tingly, apply a cold compress for 5 minutes to soothe the area.

OVERTWEEZED OR SPARSE BROWS

If you've overtweezed your brows, the only real solution is to let them grow in for four to five weeks. If your natural brow line is sparse, experts offer these tips for making your brows look fuller.

Pick up a pencil. If your brows are permanently or temporarily sparse and need further help, fill in the "missing" hairs with a sharp eyebrow pencil that's a shade darker than your eyebrow, suggests Turnier. If your eyebrows are black, use black. To further keep the pencil's work from becoming too obvious, use short, feathery strokes and brush with an eyebrow brush.

Extend-a-brow. If your eyes are wide-set, use an eyebrow pencil to extend your eyebrow closer to the bridge of your nose, says Turnier. If your brows stop short of the line above the outer corner of your eyes, extend them outward.

Take control. If individual hairs tend to stray out of place during the day, trim the long unruly ones with a cuticle scissor and brush them down with an old toothbrush coated lightly with hair spray, says Turnier.

Eye Irritations
Stop the Misery—Right Away

Unless you wear protective goggles 24 hours a day, sooner or later, you're going to get something in your eye—a speck of dust, grit or makeup, for instance. The misery is intense.

Even if your eyes are fortunate enough to escape invasion by a foreign object, they're subject to dryness and allergies, both of which are highly irritating.

WHEN TO SEE A DOCTOR

If you get something in your eye and manage to remove it, but it still feels like something is in there, you may have scratched your cornea, the eye's protective cover.

Keep your eyes shut for half an hour. Then see your doctor if, when you open your eyes:

- Your eye hurts.
- Your eye is red.
- You have vision loss.

OUT WITH IT

Fortunately, simple solutions are at hand.

Blink. Blinking stimulates your eyes to generate tears—tears that help your body flush out foreign invaders, like grit, dust and dirt, says Silvia Orengo-Nania, M.D., assistant clinical professor of ophthalmology at Baylor College of Medicine in Houston.

Work it down—and out. If blinking doesn't work, you can use your eyelids to gently push the speck down and out, says Kathleen Lamping, M.D., associate clinical professor of ophthalmology at Case Western Reserve University in Cleveland. Grasp the eyelashes of your upper lid between your fingers, then pull your upper lid over your lower lid. This allows your lower eyelashes to brush the speck off the inside of your upper lid. Then blink a few times.

Sometimes this maneuver moves the offending particle to the corner of your eye, says Dr. Lamping. If that happens, use the corner of a cloth handkerchief or moist tissue to draw it out. If you don't have a handkerchief or tissue, use your fingertip—gently.

Flush it out. Ordinary tap water can flush a speck out of your eye. "Go to the faucet and splash in as much water as it takes to remove the speck," says Dr. Lamping.

Try artificial tears. Artificial tears—available over the counter—not only flush out foreign objects, but help soothe and remoisten your eye, says Dr. Orengo-Nania. If you have some handy, use them.

Wearing contact lenses? Take them out. Once your eyes are irritated, contact lenses aggravate the situation. "The irritating item may be on your contact, not in your eye," says Dr. Lamping. "Remove your lens right away."

Standard tactic: A cold compress. Allergies—to ragweed, makeup, pet dander or just about anything—can make your eyes itch. A cool compress will cut down the itch and soothe your eyes. Wet a washcloth or towel and place it on your closed eyes whenever they itch—for at least 2 minutes or as long as 20, says Dr. Orengo-Nania.

Wear protective goggles for chores. As a regular form of exercise, mowing and weed whacking can keep you and your lawn in great shape. But stir up grass and dirt, and you're apt to get some in your eyes. Protective goggles or safety glasses will eliminate that problem, says Dickie McMullan, M.D., an ophthalmologist in private practice in Atlanta. They're a good idea when using or cleaning paint brushes and rollers, too.

Put on watertight goggles before the plunge. Chlorine in pool water will sting and irritate eyes. So protect your eyes with watertight goggles, says Anne-Marie Cavallero, O.D., an optometrist in private practice in Houston.

Eyelid Problems
Anti-itch Strategies That Work

The thin skin of your eyelids is all that protects your eyes from the wind, grit and goldenrod of the world. As such, eyelids are prime targets for irritation or infection, says Monica Dweck, M.D., an ophthalmologist in Allentown, Pennsylvania, who specializes in eyelid problems. Sometimes, adds Dr. Dweck, leaving eye makeup on overnight leaves your eyelids irritated instead of beautified.

The most common eyelids problems, say ophthalmologists, include:
- Itching (caused by allergic or nonallergic reactions to makeup, nail polish—when you rub your eyes—or pets, or from hay fever)
- Eyelid dermatitis (dry, scaly lids usually caused by nonallergic reactions to makeup, makeup remover, nail polish, perfume, skin lotion or skin cream)
- Blepharitis (an inflammation of the oil glands marked by scaly,

crusty lids). This resembles greasy dandruff in the eyelids, says Charlotte Saxby, M.D., an ophthalmologist with the Group Health Cooperative of Puget Sound, in Seattle.

Each eyelid has between 20 and 30 oil glands. Makeup that is left on overnight or not completely removed can seep into the glands and clog them up, says Dr. Dweck. Stress and estrogen fluctuations during menstruation and pregnancy also can cause blepharitis.

- Conjunctivitis (bacterial infection of the inner lid called the conjunctiva) Commonly known as pinkeye, it's a highly contagious infection. This requires medical attention, because it can easily lead to long-term problems that need to be monitored. (For practical ways to manage pinkeye, see page 428.)
- Sties (inflammation of the eyelash follicles, similar to a pimple. See page 515 for more on sties.)

EASING THE IRRITATION, RIGHT NOW

Whether your eyelids are simply dry and irritated, allergic or inflamed, soothing the irritation is the first order of business. Here's what to do.

Find something else to do with your hands. Try to resist rubbing your eyes or scratching an itch, says Dr. Dweck. If you claw at your eyelids, you'll only irritate them further. You may even scratch your cornea, which can lead to scarring or vision loss.

Make a cold compress. Wet a four-inch by four-inch gauze pad or a clean washcloth with cold water and apply to your eyes, says Monica L. Monica, M.D., Ph.D., an ophthalmologist in New Orleans and a spokesperson for the American Academy of Ophthalmology. Compresses work best if they conform to the shape of your eye. "Use compresses as frequently as possible for as long as possible," says Dr. Monica. Ballpark: A minimum of 2 minutes, a maximum of 20.

Apply cold, wet tea bags. "The tannic acid in tea bags (another form of cold compress) will soothe and cool down the itch," says Wilma Bergfeld, M.D., head of clinical research in the Department of Dermatology at the Cleveland Clinic Foundation. Wrap the tea bags with paper towels to avoid any staining of the eyelid.

Drop in artificial tears. The surface of the eye is covered with a thin film of watery fluid created by tears. Tears lubricate the eye so that the lid can move over it smoothly and wash away foreign bodies. When you don't produce enough tears, your eyelids can't blink away irritants.

Artificial tears, such as Moisture Drops, Hypotears or Tears

WHEN TO SEE A DOCTOR

Stubborn itching, scaling and other eyelid discomfort may call for medical attention. You should see your doctor if:

- After using artificial tears or tear ointment for two days, your eyelids still hurt.
- You have a bump on your eyelid that is painful, changes shape or color, doesn't go away or keeps coming back.

Naturale—available over the counter—moisten and soothe the eye and make it possible for the eyelid to move smoothly over it, says Dr. Dweck.

Use artificial tears whenever your eyes feel irritated or dry—once a day or as often as every 20 minutes, says Dr. Dweck.

If you wear contact lenses, use preservative-free tears, says Anne Sumers, M.D., an ophthalmologist in Ridgewood, New Jersey, and a spokeswoman for the American Academy of Ophthalmology. Otherwise, the preservatives can make your eyes itch. If your doctor has prescribed rewetting drops, those can work just as well, says Dr. Sumers.

Use a tear ointment at bedtime. If your eyes still feel irritated, an over-the-counter tear ointment, such as Lacrilube, will help ease the scratchiness while you sleep, says Dr. Dweck. The ointments differ from artificial tears, because they last longer, lubricating your eyes. But they blur your vision and should only be used overnight.

Eyestrain
Relief for Overworked Eyes

*Y*our eyes worked overtime again last night. You were reading the latest Judith Krantz romance novel. As you sighed over "The End" in the wee hours, your heart sang—but your eyes hurt.

Spending hours with your eyes locked on a romance novel or other close work strains your eye-focusing muscles.

"Any muscle held in one position too long will strain," says Charlotte Saxby, M.D., an ophthalmologist with the Group Health Cooperative of Puget Sound in Seattle. It's much like the sort of muscle strain that occurs if you, say, repeatedly practice skating on one leg while learning to figure skate (on a much smaller scale, of course).

As you normally go about your day, switching from task to task, your inner eye muscles flex and contract to focus and refocus on numerous and varied items—near, far and in between. When you concentrate on a task—reading, working at the computer or watching television—for any length of time, your inner eye muscles tighten up, and you forget to blink. "So your eyes get irritated, dry and uncomfortable," says Dr. Saxby.

If you're out in the sun, you may strain the facial muscles around your eyes by squinting, adds Dr. Saxby.

WINK, BLINK AND NOD

If you're over age 40, eyestrain may also be a sign that you need reading glasses or have chronically dry eyes for some reason. Generally, though, eyestrain stems from overuse. So the solutions are simple.

Here's what women doctors suggest.

Close your eyes. Shutting your eyes for a few minutes—or even several seconds—will refocus them and ease the strain, says Dr. Saxby.

Blink a lot. Each blink soothes and moistens the eyes and eases tight eye muscles, says Silvia Orengo-Nania, M.D., assistant clinical professor of ophthalmology at Baylor College of Medicine in Houston.

Wet 'em. Eyes tend to get dry when they're strained and, vice versa, dryness can cause eyestrain, says Dr. Orengo-Nania. Next to blinking, artificial tears—available over the counter at any drugstore—are the easiest way to remoisten your eyes and ease the strain. Avoid certain eye products like Murine and Visine—they're decongestants and can dry your eyes out further.

Take a break. To give your eyes a chance to refocus, once or twice an hour, take a five-minute break from whatever you're doing—reading, doing needlework or staring at the computer screen, says ophthalmologist Kathleen Lamping, M.D., associate clinical professor of ophthalmology at Case Western Reserve University in Cleveland. "Look across the room or out the window, get a cup of coffee or take a short walk."

Turn up the contrast on your computer. The words and numbers on your screen are formed by fuzzy beams of light that are much harder to read than print on a page. To minimize the strain on your eyes, set the

WHEN TO SEE A DOCTOR

Resting your eyes usually relieves eyestrain—unless you're peering through an outdated eyewear prescription (or don't realize that you need glasses to begin with).

Ophthalmologist Kathleen Lamping, M.D., associate clinical professor of ophthalmology at Case Western Reserve University in Cleveland, suggests that you see an eye specialist if you experience the following problems:

- Your eyes are strained all the time or don't respond to home remedies.
- Your eyes are extremely sensitive to light (if you have to shut them when you go out into the sun, for example).
- You don't see as well as you used to.

monitor contrast knob on high, says Dickie McMullan, M.D., an ophthalmologist in private practice in Atlanta.

Get out of the glare. "If you can, position your computer screen so that window light doesn't bounce off and create glare," says Dr. McMullan. Some experts recommend placing an antiglare shield on the screen.

Tone down your attire. "Bright, white clothes will reflect off the screen and create glare that can tire your eyes," says Dr. McMullan. A white blouse may be the worst, but wearing it with a tan jacket or muted scarf reduces the glare.

You may need reading glasses. "If you're age 40 or so and suddenly have trouble reading or seeing up close, it may be time for bifocals or reading glasses," says Dr. Saxby. If you have 20/20 distance vision, check out the reading glasses in your corner drugstore. Start with the lowest power and find a pair that fits. If you're nearsighted—that is, if you can't see well at a distance—see your optometrist.

Don sunglasses year-round. Whether you're swimming, skiing or just running errands, the sun's ultraviolet rays can make you squint, straining the facial muscles around your eyes. Buy yourself a good pair of sunglasses—ones specifically labeled as blocking out as much ultraviolet light as possible, says Dr. Saxby.

And wear a wide-brimmed hat. The cool thing about baseball-style caps is that, along with sunglasses, their wide brims help shade your eyes, reducing glare and squinting, says Dr. McMullan. So if you have one, wear it—bill forward.

Fatigue

Boost Your Energy—Today

*I*f you feel like falling asleep on your feet right now, you're not alone. In fact, eight out of ten people who are referred to sleep specialists don't have trouble getting to sleep—they have trouble staying awake. Doctors guess that about one out of every ten people (many of them women) may be troubled by daytime fatigue.

The cause? Sometimes fatigue stems from elusive factors such as sleep problems, any of a number of medical conditions, the side effects of medication or something as simple (yet little-known) as not drinking enough water. More often the likely cause is more predictable: lack of exercise, an unbalanced diet, stress, smoking, drinking alcohol and (of course) not getting enough rest.

HELP FOR THE WEARY WOMAN

For women, having too much to do ranks high on the list of possible causes. "Many women are simply juggling too many responsibilities, and that's what makes most of us feel so tired," says Susan Schenkel, Ph.D., a clinical psychologist in Cambridge, Massachusetts, and author of *Giving Away Success: Why Women Get Stuck and What to Do about It.*

If you suspect that you have plain old too-much-to-do-and-not-enough-time-to-do-it fatigue, women doctors offer these strategies.

Count the hours in your day. If you're like a lot of women, you may have an unrealistic idea of how long it takes to perform your daily chores, and you might be trying to accomplish more than is humanly possible, leaving you exhausted.

"To take stock, write down everything that you do each day," says Dr. Schenkel. "Next to each task, estimate how much time that each task truly takes. Don't leave anything out from the moment you rise until bedtime. Then add up the hours. If you're trying to do 23 hours' worth of work in 16 waking hours, adjust your efforts downward."

Do one thing at a time. Dr. Schenkel adds, "Many women handle several jobs at once—they sort the laundry while they cook dinner. They think that they're saving time, yet often in reality they're just doing too much and will feel fatigue as a result."

WHEN TO SEE A DOCTOR

If you've made every effort to work less and sleep more and you still feel tired, make an appointment with your doctor. "Unexplained fatigue can be a symptom of many different illnesses," says Anstella Robinson, M.D., a fellow at the Stanford Sleep Disorders Clinic and Research Center in Palo Alto, California. "But it can also be a symptom of some easily corrected sleep disorders."

Wake at the same time every day. "Don't give in to the urge to sleep in on weekends," cautions Anstella Robinson, M.D., a fellow at the Stanford Sleep Disorders Clinic and Research Center in Palo Alto, California. "It will disrupt your body's clock."

Aim for eight. "Give yourself a period of two weeks during which you successfully get eight hours of sleep every night," suggests Dr. Robinson. "Lights should go out at 10:00 or 11:00 every night and on again at 6:00 or 7:00 every morning."

Watch the caffeine. "Coffee or other caffeinated beverages mask how tired you really are," says Dr. Robinson. "Gradually wean yourself off caffeine to determine your actual level of fatigue."

Another reason to forgo the coffee is its tendency to cause stomach upsets in some women, which can disturb sleep quality.

Substitute exercise for work. If your exercise program has fallen by the wayside under the crunch of work and household demands, you're missing out on one proven way to energize. "Working toward a higher level of fitness is the best way to battle fatigue problems, says Peggy Norwood-Keating, director of fitness at Duke University Diet and Fitness Center in Durham, North Carolina. So head for the gym, trail, cycling path or pool—and make it a priority, at least three times a week.

Get the blood circulating. Tired right this minute? "If you've been sitting for hours, get up and walk around your chair. Better yet, energetically stomp around your chair a few times," says Norwood-Keating. "Just sitting and sitting for hours takes a toll on your energy."

Feeling Left Out
Take the Initiative

*T*he opportunities for being left out are essentially endless. No tree house, school yard, university, sorority house, bowling league or home is big enough to accommodate everyone.

"One of life's difficult lessons is that you can't be included in everything," says Susan Seidman, Ph.D., a psychologist and associate professor at Fordham University in New York City. "At one time or another everyone feels left out."

Simply recognizing this often assuages the hurt, momentary self-doubt and disappointment of being left out.

Some of us, though, are more sensitive to rejection than others and take it harder, notes Dr. Seidman. If family members didn't reassure us when we were left out during childhood, or if our self-esteem now needs shoring up, we're more vulnerable.

"Self-esteem is generally a good indicator of how you handle rejection," says Dr. Seidman. "If you're very secure, being left out won't make such a dent."

Overall, women may be more sensitive to rejection than men—we're more likely to internalize it, says Dr. Seidman. If a woman doesn't pass an entrance exam, for example, she's more apt to tell herself, "I'm not smart enough," while a man is more inclined to say, "I didn't study long enough." Thinking that you lack the necessary smarts hurts more than thinking that your social schedule was too packed to allow for the necessary cramming.

Rejection, if acute and frequent enough, can be depressing, even hazardous, to your health. A sense of belonging, studies show, contributes to quality of life and helps you manage stress.

WELCOME ADVICE

Luckily, anyone can either minimize rejection or, given the inevitable, handle it better. Here's how.

Reach out. You won't be included if no one knows that you're around, notes Myrna Shure, Ph.D., professor of psychology at Allegheny University of the Health Sciences in Philadelphia. So circulate. Instead of eating lunch at your desk, join your office mates in the cafeteria. At home, don't hole up inside by yourself. If your neighbors are out playing catch with their kids, go out for a chat.

"The more you reach out to other people, the less likely you are to be left out," says Susan Heitler, Ph.D., a clinical psychologist in Denver and author of the audiotape, *Anxiety: Friend or Foe?*.

Advertise your interests. Let people know that you're interested in doing things with them. If the gang at the water cooler is talking about in-line skating, say, "If you ever plan to go as a group, I'd love to come with you," says Dr. Heitler.

Assess your style. If you're letting people know that you're interested but you're still getting left out a lot, the problem may be your style, says Dr. Shure.

"In general, people like to be with other people who are happy, pleasant, well-groomed, interested in others and who don't criticize or complain or talk about others in a negative way," says Dr. Heitler.

If you're not sure that you fit that description, check with someone you trust.

"You might say, 'I was surprised, or a little confused, when I wasn't included in such and such,'" suggests Dr. Heitler. The response that you get will help you identify the underlying problem. Maybe you're too retiring or too domineering. And it will remind the other person that you'd like to participate.

Be a better listener. If, on the other hand, you tend to dominate every conversation, other people will start to resent it and begin to exclude you, cautions Dr. Shure. So before jumping into a conversation, listen first.

Interview others. Changing the topic to one that focuses more on you and your interests may turn people off, says Dr. Heitler. Instead, develop the art of asking questions. The more you invite others to talk about their activities and concerns, the more eager they will be to include you. Let yourself be curious about their worlds. (But don't offer unsolicited advice.)

Give others equal time. Monitor conversations, says Dr. Heitler. "Make sure that everyone has spoken at least once before you speak again." If you are utilizing more than an equal share of the airtime, switch from talking to asking questions, she suggests.

Be brief. Especially if several people are trying to speak, limit yourself to three sentences at a time, says Dr. Heitler.

Choose differently. Still having problems? Perhaps, you're trying to fit into the wrong group. Accept the fact that some groups are closed to new members or have a style that's different from yours.

Issue the invitations. Plan events and get-togethers yourself—you're guaranteed an invitation, says Dr. Shure. Like to read? Start a book discussion group. You're a movie buff? Invite a neighbor to the movie house. Play tennis? Ask a colleague to join you for a game of singles.

"You might still be rejected," says Dr. Shure. "Keep trying different tactics until something clicks."

Fever

From Barbecue-Hot to Cucumber-Cool

*L*ately, it seems that your co-workers have been sick more often than not. And now it's your turn—you feel sweaty, tired and achy. So you pop a thermometer in your mouth and sure enough, you have a fever.

Normal body temperature is 98.6°F. "But women don't necessarily have a fever until it reaches 100.4°F," says Pamela Tucker, M.D., assistant professor of medicine in the Division of Infectious Diseases at Johns Hopkins University School of Medicine in Baltimore. "The most common causes of fever, other than heatstroke, are a flu virus or bacterial infection."

Besides the above-average temperature, typical symptoms of fever include chills, sweating, headache, dry mouth, muscle aches, fatigue and sleepiness.

A fever is not a disease; it is your body's natural defense mechanism against invading organisms. So whether or not you should treat a fever is a matter of ongoing debate. "In small studies of people who had fever from an upper respiratory tract illness, such as the flu, those who treated their fevers didn't get well any quicker than those who didn't treat them," notes Dr. Tucker.

Her advice? "Treat a fever only if it makes you feel uncomfortable," says Dr. Tucker.

What Women Doctors Do

The Old-Standby, Ginger Ale

Pamela Tucker, M.D.

Sooner or later, everyone gets a fever, and experts in infectious disease are no exception.

"I usually get a fever with the flu," says Pamela Tucker, M.D., assistant professor of medicine in the Division of Infectious Diseases at Johns Hopkins University School of Medicine in Baltimore. "If I really don't feel well, I take acetaminophen. Besides fighting the fever, acetaminophen makes me feel better overall—it reduces body aches and eases sore throat pain.

"I also go to bed for a few days and drink lots of fluids—either water or ginger ale. For me ginger ale is a comfort food—it was a special treat when I was growing up. The only time that my mother gave it to us was when we would get sick."

The higher your temperature, the more you should consider treating a fever, says Dr. Tucker.

THE OPTIMAL STRATEGY

Here's what women doctors say that you can do to cool your sweated brow.

Step into a tepid bath. "If you feel hot and sweaty, taking a lukewarm bath will help your body cool off at the right pace," says Dr. Tucker. "A cold bath or shower will chill you too quickly and make you shiver."

Combine baths with a fever reducer. "Aspirin, acetaminophen or ibuprofen will all help reduce a fever," says Dr. Tucker. "They're antipyretics; that is, they work by blocking production of prostaglandins—hormones that among other functions play a key part in causing fever."

"I recommend that you take a fever reducer every four hours and a tepid bath every four hours," says Susan Black, M.D., a board member of the American Academy of Family Physicians. "For example, you can take the fever reducer at noon, then a tepid bath at 2:00 P.M. Then, at 4:00 P.M., take the fever reducer and at 6:00 P.M., take another tepid bath. That way, you'll be doing something every two hours to treat that fever."

Chugalug. "Drinking fluids is important when treating a fever—especially if you're sweating and perspiring—in order to prevent dehydration," says Dr. Tucker. "Aim for six to eight glasses of liquids a day. Drink water, but drink orange juice and other fruit juices high in vitamin

WHEN TO SEE A DOCTOR

Women doctors say that you should consult you physician if:
- You have a fever of 101°F or higher.
- You are over age 60 and have a fever of 100.4°F or higher.
- Your fever doesn't break in two days.
- Your fever is accompanied by a stiff neck, severe headache, rash, confusion, back pain, excessive vomiting, excessive diarrhea or painful urination.
- You have been prescribed medicine (such as prednisone) that affects your ability to fight infection.
- You have an underlying illness, such as diabetes or heart or lung disease.

"A fever can aggravate these conditions," says Pamela Tucker, M.D., assistant professor of medicine in the Division of Infectious Diseases at Johns Hopkins University School of Medicine in Baltimore. "When you have a fever, for example, your heart beats faster. This could mean trouble for someone with a heart condition."

C, too." Research suggests that vitamin C may help boost your immune system by preventing the formation of free radicals in your body—substances that weaken immune function.

Reach for a sports drink, not a diet soda. "You can also drink sports drinks and regular (not diet) soft drinks," says Dr. Black. "When you have a fever, your body's metabolism is speeded up, and you burn extra calories," notes Dr. Black. "Skip the diet sodas until your fever breaks; your body needs calories."

Take your temperature in the afternoon. "Your body temperature varies throughout the day; it's lowest in the morning and highest in the afternoon," explains Dr. Black. "So if you stay in bed the first day of your fever and take your temperature the next morning, your reading will be down, and you may think that it's okay to go to work. But your temperature will be up again later in the day."

Take your temp under your arm. "If you have a cold or flu and breathe through your mouth because of a stuffy nose, a temperature taken by mouth may be inaccurate," says Dr. Tucker. "To get your accurate body-core temperature, place the thermometer under your armpit for three minutes, then add one degree to the reading shown."

Call in sick. "Because a fever uses up energy, it can be very taxing on the body," says Dr. Tucker. "I recommend bed rest for a day or two. Besides, staying in bed can also keep you from infecting other people."

Dr. Black echoes that advice. "If you exert yourself, you're going to prolong the illness. Stay in bed until your fever has been broken for 24 hours."

Ask for help. "When women run a fever, they should ease off on the household responsibilities," says Dr. Tucker. "It's okay to ask your spouse or family to pitch in with dinner, or a friend to take care of the kids so you can take care of yourself."

Fibromyalgia
Help for a Painful Malady

Feel like you've gone ten rounds with the heavyweight champ—and lost—every day for the past few months? You know—you hurt all over and feel too tired to perform the most basic daily activities. In fact, specific spots are exquisitely tender to the touch, and you are unable to sleep at night. That's the hallmark of fibromyalgia.

Medically, fibromyalgia is described as a pain syndrome. Textbooks call it a painful, non-joint-related condition that predominantly involves the muscles and connective tissue called fascia. Fibromyalgia puzzled doctors for years. But Susan Ward, M.D., clinical assistant professor of medicine and associate director of the Jefferson Osteoporosis Center at Thomas Jefferson University Hospital in Philadelphia, believes that fibromyalgia is related to not sleeping well.

"Normally, when people sleep, they enter the stage-four sleep, which produces deep relaxation, and their muscles naturally 'turn off,'" says Dr. Ward. "But people with fibromyalgia don't enter stage-four sleep. As a result, their muscles don't rest properly and they ache."

Doctors can treat fibromyalgia with antidepressant medications

221

WHEN TO SEE A DOCTOR

"The women who do best with fibromyalgia are those who have had the symptoms for less than six months and who have received immediate care," says Elizabeth Tindall, M.D., clinical associate professor of medicine in the Division of Rheumatology at Oregon Health Sciences University in Portland. So she urges anyone who has symptoms to see a doctor promptly.

According to Dr. Tindall, the classic symptoms of fibromyalgia are:

- Chronic pain
- Profound fatigue
- General debilitation

that normalize sleep patterns, says Dr. Ward. So if you think that you might have fibromyalgia, see your doctor.

EASING THE ACHE

If in fact you do have fibromyalgia and not a similar condition such as chronic fatigue syndrome, these at-home strategies can enhance comfort.

Get moving, even if you hurt. "It's hard to tell a patient who's hurting all over that the most effective treatment is exercise, but it's true," says Elizabeth Tindall, M.D., clinical associate professor of medicine in the Division of Rheumatology at Oregon Health Sciences University in Portland. "The good news about the pain of fibromyalgia is that the pain has no purpose. That means that even though you hurt, exercise won't do any damage. Exercise can significantly control the pain of fibromyalgia."

Start slowly and set realistic goals, says Dr. Tindall. Try for a brisk five-minute walk, then gradually increase the time and intensity until you're walking briskly for 20 minutes three times a week.

Try warm-water exercise. "Many women avoid aquatic exercise because the thought of getting into a cold pool is too much. Check with your local Y or with the health clubs in your area about special therapeutic 'aqua-cize' programs held in heated pools," says Dr. Tindall. Water at body temperature—that is, between 90° and 100°F—is best.

Hop into a hot tub. "Heat can soothe the pain of fibromyalgia," says Sharon Clark, R.N., Ph.D., a family nurse practitioner and associate professor of nursing at the School of Nursing and assistant professor of medicine at the School of Medicine Division of Arthritis and Rheumatic Diseases at Oregon Health Sciences University School of Medicine in Portland. "Try a long soak in a hot bath, or use a hot tub with a gentle whirlpool if one is accessible. This would also be a good time to do some gentle stretching."

Flatulence

Shut Down Your Gas Engine

Why does it always happen in a crowded elevator? No one knows.

What doctors do know is that everybody thinks they pass too much gas. Chances are, though, that you're all well within the normal range. On any given day, your average Jane releases gas 14 times.

If you pass more, it doesn't mean that something is wrong. Most likely, the culprit is in what you eat. Or in your lifestyle. Or it's just plain bad luck. (Some people are just more prone to giving off gas than others.)

DIMINISHING WINDS

If you're tired of sounding like the little engine that could, here are some ways to lower your octane level.

Quick! Buy some activated charcoal. If you can feel gas building up, and there's a crowded elevator in your immediate future, stop off at a drugstore and try Charcoal Plus, an over-the-counter remedy that can help absorb gas trapped in your colon, says Jacqueline Wolf, M.D., a gastroenterologist, assistant professor of medicine at Harvard Medical School and co-director of the Inflammatory Bowel Disease Center at Brigham and Women's Hospital in Boston.

Chew your food. "The more slowly you eat, the less air you swallow, and the better your food is broken down, so the less likely you are to suffer from gas," says Barbara Frank, M.D., gastroenterologist and clinical professor of medicine at Allegheny Universtiy of the Health Sciences MCP–Hahnemann School of Medicine in Philadelphia. Taking more time at meals can prevent future gas attacks.

Watch for gas producers. "Among the top culprits are cabbage, corn and beans," says Linda Lee, M.D., assistant professor of medicine in the Division of Gastroenterology at Johns Hopkins University School of Medicine in Baltimore. In fact, many fruits and vegetables are big gas producers. (But they're also high in fiber and low in fat, and they've been shown to reduce rates of colon cancer, the second biggest cancer killer in the United States.)

In other words, high-fiber foods are good for you. So before eliminating them from your diet, see how you react when you eat them. If they bother you, try eating smaller amounts or substitute other high-fiber foods (like whole-wheat cereal or bran flakes) that may be easier for you to digest, says Dr. Lee. Complete elimination is not desirable, so try different high-fiber foods to find the ones that you tolerate best.

Degassing the beans. Indigestible sugars in beans are notorious gas producers. If you elect to keep high-fiber beans in your diet, help is at hand, says Dr. Wolf. Before cooking, soak dry beans overnight in a potful of water with a couple of tablespoons of vinegar to reduce gassiness.

Sprinkle on the enzyme mix. Beano, an over-the-counter liquid enzyme that breaks down the indigestible sugars in beans, works well on dense beans like limas or lentils, says Dr. Lee. Just sprinkle several drops right on the beans just before eating. Or buy Beano in tablet form and take two tablets before you eat.

"Unfortunately, Beano doesn't work as well on high-fiber, high gas–producing vegetables like cauliflower and broccoli," Dr. Lee says.

Stay away from sugarless. Few women realize that sorbitol, a natural sugar used in sugarless gums and candies and many diet sodas, is hard to digest and causes gas, says Dr. Lee. So park the gum and see if circumstances improve.

Uncarbonate your life. The bubbles and fizz in carbonated beverages such as soda, beer, champagne and sparkling water produce lots of gas, says Dr. Lee. She advises women who complain of gas to drink water or low-calorie, low-sugar fruit juices instead, especially with large meals.

"Eating a lot and then adding beer or soda bubbles is an invitation for gas," says Dr. Frank.

Cut out the caffeine. "Caffeine irritates the colon," and an irritated colon is often a noisy, gassy one, says Dr. Lee. And remember, cutting out coffee alone is not enough: Tea, chocolate and most sodas also contain caffeine.

Exercise. "Moving around keeps your bowels on the move and prevents gas from getting—and staying—trapped," says Robyn Karlstadt, M.D., a gastroenterologist at Graduate Hospital in Philadelphia. Getting just 30 minutes a day three times a week of any kind of aerobic exercise—the kind that gets your heart pumping, like walking, swimming or cycling—will help defuse the gas.

(For practical ways to manage lactose intolerance, which can also cause flatulence, see page 336.)

Food Cravings
The Absolute Best Approach

*Y*ou just gotta have it—chocolate chocolate-chip ice cream with hot fudge sauce and nuts on top. But you can't. You know you can't. It has fat. It has sugar. Calories galore. But you're on a diet. You know what's good for you. Chocolate chocolate-chip ice cream with hot fudge sauce and nuts is definitely not it. Okay, the nuts have protein, but . . . no, no, no, no, no.

So you go for the carrot sticks, the celery, the low-fat dressing. You skip the butter on your bread. And then you go home and eat two gallons of ice cream.

Sometimes cravings occur when your body lacks nutrients—including vitamins and minerals—during pregnancy, says Helene Leonetti, M.D., an obstetrician/gynecologist in private practice in the northern suburbs of Philadelphia. But the funny thing is, we rarely crave a nice big bowl of steaming butternut squash. More like pumpkin pie. And that's where we can get into trouble.

"Food cravings are the body's natural cravings gone awry," says Dori Winchell, Ph.D., a psychologist in private practice in Encinitas, California.

"That happens because women often won't allow themselves the

225

Pickles Helped Nausea

Helene Leonetti, M.D.

Among the pregnant women she counsels, few experience the sort of food cravings often associated with pregnancy, says Helene Leonetti, M.D., an obstetrician/gynecologist in private practice in the northern suburbs of Philadelphia. When cravings do hit, she says, they could be caused by a physiological need or, less commonly, simply triggered by suggestion.

"If we hear that women crave pickles during pregnancy, then we'll crave pickles," says Dr. Leonetti.

And crave them she did when she was pregnant.

"When I got pregnant in adulthood, I was nauseated, and the tart-sour taste of pickles made me feel better," she recalls. When her nausea went away, so did her pickle craving.

Along with her craving for pickles, Dr. Leonetti developed an aversion to coffee. "While I was pregnant, I couldn't even be in the same room with coffee," she says.

food they need. Instead, they skip breakfast, eat a tiny salad for lunch and then go home and head for the chips, fries and chocolate bars," says Jan McBarron, M.D., a weight-control specialist and director of Georgia Bariatrics in Columbus, Georgia.

TINY TACTICS FOR BIG CRAVINGS

If you're in perfect health and satisfied with your weight, cravings may be harmless. But if you suspect that giving in to cravings for food high in fat, sugar or excess calories may be to blame for a recent weight gain or a jump in your cholesterol levels, or that food cravings are jeopardizing other aspects of your health, here's what women doctors suggest.

Suck a sour pickle. "If you are about to pig out, suck a sour pickle to eliminate the craving for sweets," says Maria Simonson, Sc.D., Ph.D., director of the Health, Weight and Stress Clinic at the Johns Hopkins Medical Institution in Baltimore.

Juice it. A really strong craving for sweets can often be stifled by eating a peppermint washed down by a few ounces of fruit juice or a few nibbles of fruit, such as an apple or pear, says Dr. Simonson.

Fool your sweet tooth with spice. "Cinnamon, vanilla and nutmeg can satisfy a sweet tooth, since these spices add a sweet flavor without the calories," says Elizabeth Somer, R.D., author of *Food and Mood* and *Nutrition for Women*. Add cinnamon, vanilla or nutmeg to yogurt or steamed milk, Somer says.

Grab something absorbing. Instead of reaching for a bag of chips, reach for the op-ed page of the newspaper—or whatever else you might find engaging. "Once you're absorbed in an interesting or playful activity, your craving is likely to fade away," says Susan Olson, Ph.D., a clinical psychologist in Seattle and co-author of *Keeping It Off: Winning at Weight Loss*.

Take your minerals. Food cravings are often generated by a lack of the mineral chromium, complicated by bad eating habits—namely, starving yourself during the day and overeating at night. One way to quickly get your nutrient intake back in balance and send cravings packing, says Dr. McBarron, is to go to a health food store, ask for a complete multivitamin-mineral supplement that includes chromium and take one a day.

Give in—occasionally. "If you absolutely require potato chips or some other food that you feel guilty about eating, build it into your diet deliberately to decrease the anxiety," says Dr. Olson. If you must have ice cream, plan ahead. Decide just how much and how often you will eat it. Then, when you're ready to fulfill your longing, go out and buy just what you want. Don't set yourself up for cravings by keeping a half-gallon ready at hand in your freezer.

Foot and Heel Pain

Feel-Good Strategies for Aching Feet

*W*ith every step that she takes, the average woman, going about her daily business, puts 500 pounds of pressure on her feet. Multiply that times 10,000 steps a day—more or less—and it's no wonder that feet hurt sometimes. As a matter of fact, it's a wonder that your feet don't hurt all the time.

Running Shoes Save Her Feet

Kathleen Stone, D.P.M.

Hairdressers, waitresses, nurses and yes, even women podiatrists have benefited from relaxed dress codes that make cushy running shoes acceptable attire in many workplaces, says Kathleen Stone, D.P.M., a podiatrist in private practice in Glendale, Arizona.

"I always wear running shoes, not dress shoes, on days when I am going to be on my feet a lot," she says.

The doctors's take-home lesson: Think comfort and save the pumps for all-day sit-down meetings.

When shopping for running shoes, your best bet is an athletic shoe store. A skilled salesperson can size up your feet and help you select the right shoe.

Look for a fixed heel counter at the back of the shoe and flexibility at the ball of the foot.

Women podiatrists report that women tend to have more foot pain than men, or at least they tend to consult doctors for the problem more than men do, says Kathleen Stone, D.P.M., a podiatrist in private practice in Glendale, Arizona. "That's because traditionally, women's shoes have been designed for fashion, not comfort," she says. "Once women switch to better-designed footwear—which many have done—they have fewer foot problems."

AT-HOME FOOT THERAPY

Here's what women podiatrists and other "foot therapists" tell women bothered by sore heels, aching arches, cramped toes and other everyday foot and heel complaints.

By performing these simple exercise, you may minimize or prevent continued progression of stiffness, says Phyllis Ragley, D.P.M., vice president of the American Academy of Podiatric Sports Medicine who practices in Lawrence, Kansas.

Play footsie with an orange juice can. If the arch of your foot hurts, you may have a touch of plantar fasciitis, or inflammation in the plantar fascia—the tough, gristly sheet of connective tissue that stretches from your heel to your toes. To soothe it, take a seat and—barefooted—

roll your arch over a can of frozen juice concentrate for five to ten minutes, suggests Marika Molnar, P.T., director of West Side Dance Physical Therapy in New York City. "The cold helps reduce inflammation, while the massage helps loosen the tense tissues." Mark the juice can, keep it separate from juice that you plan to drink and reuse it as needed.

Stretch like a dancer. For a super-duper stretch, give this dancer's technique a try, suggests Helen Drusine, a massage therapist who works with professional ballet and Broadway dancers in New York City. Kneel on the floor or on a rug, with the balls of your feet on the floor, tucking your spread-out toes under to stretch the arches of your feet. Sit back on your heels so that most of your body weight presses your toes against the floor. Do this for a few seconds, slowly increasing your time as it becomes more comfortable.

"Tucking the toes this way helps people who use their feet a lot, because it keeps the plantar fascia and the tendons stretched," says Drusine.

Do not do this stretch, however, if you have sore tendons, says Dr. Ragley. Try a light massage of your feet and toes instead.

Do the follow-up stretch. Next, says Drusine, perform the same exercise with the tops of your feet flat on the floor. Again, do not do this exercise if you have sore tendons.

Loosen up your calf muscles. Tight calf muscles can hobble your feet, interfering with their ability to properly strike the ground and roll forward, says Dr. Ragley. That, in turn, can cause heel or arch pain as tissues in your feet are unduly stretched to make up for tight calves.

To stretch your calf muscles, stand barefoot facing a wall, with your arms straight out in front of you and your palms flat against the wall. (*Hint:* To maximize the stretch, says Dr. Ragley, point your feet inward slightly.) Keep your heels on the ground, tuck your buttocks so that your body remains straight (do not bend forward at your waist), bend your elbows and lean into the wall until your cheek touches the wall.

"You should feel the stretch in your calves," she says. "If you don't, you are either standing too far from the wall and bending at the waist to lean into it, or too close." How far you need to be from the wall depends on your height and how flexible your calf muscles already are. "I'm about five feet six inches. For a good stretch, I stand about 1½ feet from the wall when I do this."

Hold the stretch for as long as you feel comfortable. Then repeat (five times to start), this time with your knees slightly bent. "This helps stretch the soleus—the small muscle that leads directly into the Achilles tendon," Dr. Ragley explains.

WHEN TO SEE A DOCTOR

If you change footwear and try home remedies for a week or two and your feet still hurt, see a podiatrist for diagnosis. If there is some swelling, drainage, discoloration or history of injury, you should go sooner. Certain problems, such as broken bones, inflamed tendons, pinched nerves or gait problems, can only be corrected with medical attention.

Tip: Take broken-in shoes with you when you go the podiatrist, says Phyllis Ragley, D.P.M., vice-president of the American Acadamy of Podiatric Sports Medicine who practices in Lawrence, Kansas. She may be able to determine what's causing your foot or heel pain by looking at wear patterns on your shoes.

It's best to stretch after you've warmed up a bit from easy walking or after a warm shower or bath.

EXERCISE YOUR "FOOT FINGERS"

"Normal walking does not do much to strengthen or stretch the small muscles in the feet," says Carol Frey, M.D., of the Orthopedic Hospital in Los Angeles.

To keep your toes loose and flexible and to isolate and strengthen the small muscles in your feet, Dr. Frey suggests the following exercises.

Play pickup. Use your toes to pick up marbles from the floor and drop them into a bowl. Or place small corks or pencils between your toes and squeeze them for five seconds.

Stretch and release. Wrap a thick, taut rubber band around all the toes on one foot, then spread your toes and hold the stretch for five seconds. Repeat ten times.

Try a golf-ball massage. Roll a golf ball under the ball and arch of your foot for two minutes.

MORE HELP FOR THE HURTING

It should be no big surprise that changing the kind of shoes you wear—or how you wear them—is a big part of foot comfort. Here's some additional advice from experts who counsel women with foot pain.

Buy running shoes, even if you don't run. If your feet hurt, they need all the support they can get, says Dr. Ragley. So forget flimsy canvas shoes, flip-flops, moccasins and slippers. Instead, wear running shoes whenever you can, everywhere but in the bed and bath. "These provide the cushioning, arch support and proper heel that reduce stretch on the plantar fascia."

Cup your heel. If your plantar fascia is tight, you can develop heel spurs—bony deposits where the tissue connects to the heel bones. "That area can become inflamed, causing acute pain in the middle and inside rear of the heel first thing in the morning and after prolonged sitting," says Pamela Colman, D.P.M., a podiatrist in private practice in Bethesda, Maryland.

A heel cup, available at most drugstores, will stabilize your heel and slightly control the rolling-in of the foot (pronation) that can contribute to the pain.

Forgetfulness
Quick Fixes for Memory Lapses

*W*ho among us hasn't forgotten a name in the middle of an introduction or spent the better part of an afternoon searching a shopping mall parking lot for a misplaced car?

Don't worry. Minor bouts of forgetfulness like these don't mean that you're losing your memory. The truth is, your ability to recall should stay sharp well into your sixties, says Elizabeth Loftus, Ph.D., professor of psychology at the University of Washington in Seattle and author of *Memory*.

Although natural changes occur with the memory process as we age, there is usually no cause for alarm. As we get older it is the increased anxiety about memory lapses that distorts and exaggerates our perception of memory loss, says Danielle Lapp, a memory training specialist and researcher at Stanford University and author of *Don't Forget!* and *(Nearly) Total Recall*. Some women do complain of temporary spells of forgetfulness during menopause—possibly because night sweats keep them from getting enough sleep.

IT'S NOT ALZHEIMER'S

"No matter what your age, you can improve your memory," says Lapp. But first, some emergency advice on what to do when you draw a blank.

Wait 30 seconds. If you can't remember someone's name, don't let on right away, says Lapp. Rather, just continue talking. More often than not, it will occur to you soon enough, especially if you're not stressed.

Backtrack. Circling the shopping mall parking lot looking for your car? Stop circling and mentally switch into reverse, says Irene Colsky, Ed.D., adjunct professor of psychology and education at Miami-Dade Community College and president of the Colsky Associates, a firm offering learning and memory seminars.

If you replay the trip to the mall in your head, you're likely to hit upon some key information that triggers a memory of where you left your wheels. For example, visualize what you saw when you left the driveway, headed west on Elm and pulled into the South View Plaza, and you're likely to recall seeing the Good Friend Pharmacy right in front of you. Great. Now look for your car around the drugstore.

Backtracking also helps when you walk into a room—your bedroom, for example—and can't remember why, says Dr. Colsky. Ask yourself, "Where was I before I walked in here and what was I doing?"

TRAIN YOUR MIND TO REMEMBER

So much for instant recall. Here's how to prevent future memory lapses.

Pay attention. If you don't attend to what you're doing, reading, watching or hearing, you won't remember it later. Lapp's advice is to pause before you do something, become aware of your surroundings and mobilize your senses: Look, listen and feel. If you're parking at the mall, notice landmarks, listen for telltale sounds, check the temperature. Then make a mental note of what your senses tell you. Say mentally to yourself, "I'm parking the car so that it's facing the drugstore. The parking space is near the playground—I can hear the kids shouting nearby. It's hot, because there are no shade trees around." Processing information visually and verbally leaves the best memory trace and yields the best results, says Lapp.

Avoid distractions. "Make a mental note of what you're going to do before you do it," says Dr. Colsky. "It will minimize distraction, which makes you forget why, for example, you walked into the living room. You head for a room to find something in particular, but as you enter, something else gets your attention."

So tell yourself, "I'm going into the living room to get the photo album," for example, and you will be less likely to get distracted by the magazines and papers on the coffee table.

Make meaningful connections. To remember things like street addresses or a shopping list, says Lapp, make up a story or a sentence that links that information in a meaningful way. To remember someone's address, for example—say, 65 South Street—tell yourself, "Sixty-five is retirement age, and many people move South after they retire."

Or, to remember to buy milk, eggs and four cans of bug spray on the way home, turn the list into an acronym: MESSSS (M for milk, E for eggs and the four S's for the four cans of bug spray.)

Paint a mental image. Concrete visual images can help connect new names and faces, says Dr. Loftus. Assume that you meet a prospective boss, Ms. Saucer, at a job interview, and her most striking feature is her green eyes. Envision saucers painted to look like huge green eyes. So later in the conversation, or the next time that you meet her, her eyes will remind you that her last name is "Saucer."

Increase your intake of the "memory minerals." Studies suggest that deficiencies of iron, zinc and boron can interfere with concentration and recall. To assure adequate intake, say researchers, you need to eat at least three servings of red meat (a good source of both iron and zinc) each week and at least five servings per day of fruits and vegetables (for sufficient boron).

Sharpen your memory with exercise. In one study researchers found that volunteers who got an hour of aerobic exercise three times a week performed better on memory tests than those who didn't work out. Exercise, they speculate, may increase oxygen flow to the brain and speed glucose metabolism, improving recall. Exercise can also reduce stress, which can interfere with memory.

Frown and Laugh Lines

Wipe Out the Imprints

*R*emember when you got the first inkling that all was not right with *The Stepford Wives*?

Ten to one it was the moment that you sat in your theater seat and realized that the faces on the screen were registering absolutely no emotion. They didn't laugh, they didn't smile, they didn't frown. They simply looked out over the audience like Barbie dolls that had come to life.

In real life, women register all the emotions of which the human species is capable. And after 35 years or so, we register them visibly on our faces, says D'Anne Kleinsmith, M.D., a staff dermatologist at William Beaumont Hospital in Royal Oak, Michigan.

Laugh and smile a lot, and a series of tiny lines may appear along the corners of your mouth—along with single, slightly deeper lines that will eventually extend from the corners of your mouth to your nose. Frown a lot, and you may also get a few lines between or above your brows or even extending down from the corners of your mouth to your chin.

Although these expression lines are initiated by our emotional responses to life, how deep and how noticeable they become as our skin ages depends on two additional factors, says Dr. Kleinsmith. One is the bone structure that we've inherited from our families, and the other is how much sun has been allowed to damage the elastic fibers in our facial skin.

A TWO-PRONGED STRATEGY

Superficial expression lines can be minimized or prevented with the following strategies recommended by women doctors.

Try a glycolic acid moisturizer. "A moisturizing cream or lotion that contains glycolic acid (one of the alpha hydroxy acids, a synthetic version of acids that occur in fruit and other plants) will help eradicate lines that are not deep," says Margaret A. Weiss, M.D., assistant professor of dermatology at the Johns Hopkins Medical Institutions in Baltimore.

Your best bet is to try a moisturizer that contains 8 or 10 percent glycolic acid, adds Allison Vidimos, M.D., a staff dermatologist at the Cleveland Clinic Foundation. The glycolic acid will loosen old cells on the skin's surface and swap them for fresher cells underneath—a process that will lessen or eradicate fine lines.

Smooth on a sunscreen. "Minimizing sun exposure is the most important thing that a person can do to prevent facial lines," says Dr. Weiss.

So after your glycolic acid moisturizer has had a moment or two to dry, smooth on a sunscreen that has a sun protection factor, or SPF, of at least 15, says Dr. Kleinsmith. If your skin is prone to acne, use a gel; if you have dry skin, use a lotion or cream.

A sunscreen will prevent any further damage to the elastic fibers that keep your skin taut and smooth, effectively halting new wrinkles from forming and old ones from deepening.

If your skin is sensitive, says Dr. Kleinsmith, avoid potentially irritating sunscreens that contain PABA or oxybenzone and use one that contains particles of titanium dioxide instead. It is less likely to irritate.

Reapply according to package directions, adds Dr. Kleinsmith. Most sunscreens will work all day under your makeup. But if you're going swimming, make sure that you use a waterproof sunscreen and reapply it hourly.

Gallstones
Head Off Repeat Attacks

*I*f your gallbladder is acting up, you'll know it.

"Women who have had gallstone attacks say that they are as bad as labor," says gastroenterologist Grace Elta, M.D., associate professor in the gastroenterology division of the University of Michigan in Ann Arbor. Attacks are painful and can last for hours.

WHEN TO SEE A DOCTOR

Women who are experiencing a gallstone attack rarely need to be coaxed to go to the doctor or hospital. While the degree of discomfort varies from person to person, the pain can sometimes be excruciating.

If you feel steady, severe pain in your upper abdomen and have a fever or persistent vomiting, call your doctor or go to the hospital immediately.

When it's not giving you grief, the gallbladder quietly goes about its business, which is to store and concentrate bile, a yellow-brown fluid containing cholesterol, fats, salts that break up fats and a pigment that gives bile and stools their color. The main function of bile is to help digest fats. Gallstones form when there is too much cholesterol or pigment in the bile.

Gallstones can be as small as a grain of sand or as large as a golf ball. The gallbladder may develop a single large stone or as many as several thousand smaller, pebble-size stones.

In fact, most people have "silent" gallstones, which may never require treatment.

When gallstones do cause trouble, you may be more apt to think that you're having a heart attack rather than suffering from an overdose of bile, because the usual sign of an attack is pain in the right upper abdomen traveling to the shoulder or back, often accompanied by nausea and vomiting, says Colleen Schmitt, M.D., a gastroenterologist with the Galen Medical Group in Chattanooga, Tennessee.

LESSEN THE RISK

Once your gallbladder is causing symptoms, surgery is the best option, says Dr. Elta.

And, because no one knows what causes gallstones, very little is known about how to prevent them. But women doctors offer some key advice that should lessen your risk.

Stay trim. Though slender women get gallstones, too, obesity is a common link to gallstones, says Dr. Schmitt. "To prevent gallstones, try to stay as close to your ideal weight as possible," she says.

Doctors no longer adhere to a set weight that women should be at any given height. Instead, medical professionals believe that women with a high ratio of muscle and bone to fat are likely to avoid health problems. So concentrate on burning off fat by taking a brisk 30-minute walk daily rather than starving yourself down to the bone.

Slenderize gradually. Rapid weight loss actually increases your risk of developing gallstones, says Melissa Palmer, M.D., a gastroenterologist in private practice in New York City.

Aim to lose only one or two pounds a week, says Wanda Filer, M.D., a family practice physician in York, Pennsylvania.

"If you need to take off weight, try to do it slowly. If for some reason you need to fast or lose weight quickly, do so only under a doctor's supervision," says Dr. Palmer.

Eat only lean. Though there is no proof that fatty foods lead to gallstones, some doctors believe that they can contribute to gallstone formation. So to be on the safe side, and because it's better for your general health, avoid fatty foods such as butter, burgers and fries, says Dr. Palmer. Instead, choose lean cuts of meat, vegetables, fruits and salad with fat-free dressing.

Focus on grains and beans. "Some studies have shown that vegetarians have a lower risk of developing gallstones, possibly because of the higher fiber content of a meatless, plant-based diet," says Dr. Palmer.

Gastritis

More Than Just a Sour Stomach

Next time you take an aspirin for a headache or ibuprofen for menstrual cramps, pay attention: Do you develop a slight burning sensation below your breastbone? Or a wee bit of indigestion—like you just ate something that disagreed with you?

Perhaps you experience the discomfort for no apparent reason. Either way, you may have gastritis—inflammation of the stomach lining.

WHEN TO SEE A DOCTOR

Symptoms of gastritis include indigestion or burning pain below the breastbone, which may waken you at night. Symptoms may resemble an ulcer, and the only way to tell for sure if you have gastritis is by biopsy (examining the stomach tissue under a microscope).

Uncontrolled, gastritis can damage your stomach lining. So see a doctor whenever you have sharp, dull, gnawing or burning abdominal pain or black stools.

Once diagnosed, gastritis takes as long as four to six weeks to heal. If you're not better in six weeks, call your doctor again.

Gastritis can be silent—or feel like an ulcer. The symptoms of both are alike: indigestion or abdominal pain, sometimes so sharp that it wakes you up at night. The difference: "If you have an ulcer, your stomach will develop raw, craterlike spots," says Susan Dimick, M.D., an internist in private practice at Presbyterian Hospital in Oklahoma City. "It gets red and oozy and inflamed with little red capillary spots, and it can bleed profusely." So ulcers are much more serious.

Not to sound alarming, but since many women with gastritis eventually get ulcers, it's prudent to control gastritis when it first occurs, says Dr. Dimick.

SPICY FOODS NOT THE PROBLEM

Like ulcers, gastritis can sometimes result from irritation by aspirin or other nonsteroidal medications, not from eating a lot of spicy foods or overeating, says Marie L. Borum, M.D., assistant professor of medicine in the Division of Gastroenterology and Nutrition at George Washington University Medical Center in Washington, D.C.

Aspirin and other anti-inflammatory medications such as ibuprofen can cause gastritis, because they interfere with the stomach's ability to fight against excessive stomach acid, says Barbara Frank, M.D., gastroenterologist and clinical professor of medicine at Allegheny University of the Health Sciences MCP–Hahnemann School of Medicine in Philadelphia. Women often take aspirin and nonsteroidal medications for menstrual cramps.

More often, though, a bacteria called *Helicobacter pylori*, or *H. pylori*, is associated with gastritis. This spiral-shaped bacteria burrows through the protective mucous lining of the stomach and may allow the stomach lining to become inflamed, which can lead to gastritis and often ulcers, says Dr. Borum.

HELP IS AT HAND

If your doctor has confirmed that your problem is gastritis, and not something else, there are a few comfort measures that you can take to minimize symptoms and prevent recurrent episodes.

Go aspirin-free. "If you need to take painkillers, switch to acetaminophen to minimize symptoms," says Dr. Frank. It doesn't irritate the stomach the way aspirin does.

Suppress the acid. Acid-suppressing drugs known as H$_2$ (histamine 2) blockers (some include Tagamet HB and Pepcid AC) reduce production of stomach acid at its source. Once available by prescription only, acid-squelching drugs are now available at your drugstore at about half the prescription dose. Talk to your doctor about the advisability of trying nonprescription medications and about the amount that's right for you. Some women physicians who treat gastritis feel that it's okay to buy H$_2$ blockers over the counter, but you may have to take higher than the recommended doses for them to work as well as the prescription medications.

If you're not better in six weeks, go back to your doctor.

Get your calcium through supplements, not milk. Once thought to soothe the sharp pains of gastritis, doctors now know that milk triggers the release of acid and can make your symptoms worse, says Melissa Palmer, M.D., a gastroenterologist in private practice in New York City.

Kick the habit—please. Nicotine and other toxic substances consumed when you smoke cigarettes and other tobacco products erode your stomach's protective lining and increase your chances of getting gastritis, Dr. Palmer says.

Choose nonalcoholic brew. Alcohol makes your stomach burn more, says Dr. Dimick.

If it bothers you, don't eat it. Though doctors no longer believe that any particular foods or spices cause or worsen gastritis, if you feel that you have a flare-up every time you eat, say, pickles or chili or anything else, stop eating the offending food, says Dr. Palmer.

Genital Warts

Get Rid of Warts for Good

They're not a pretty sight, these little red bumps, some of them growing in cauliflower-like clusters. Not that you can easily see them, since they're in the area of your vagina or anus. But you sure can feel them—you're probably literally itching to be rid of them. They might even be extremely painful.

Genital warts, also called venereal warts or condyloma, are caused by the human papillomavirus (HPV), of which there are more than 50 known types. These troublemakers are contagious, a form of sexually transmitted disease (STD) passed from one person to another primarily during sexual or otherwise intimate physical contact. Once contracted, the virus is pretty much your constant companion. Even after warts are removed by your doctor, the virus often remains beneath the surface, ready to reemerge. Worse yet, genital warts are not mere irritants or an interpersonal embarrassment. Some varieties of HPV appear to be linked to cancers of the cervix.

DO'S AND DON'TS

Resist the urge to use any over-the-counter wart removal products, all of which are formulated for nongenital warts. "Some of these products can severely burn and irritate you," warns Kimberly A. Workowski, M.D., assistant professor of medicine in the Division of Infectious Diseases at Emory University in Atlanta. Other less caustic products aren't strong enough to do the job. Instead, see your doctor: She'll either elect to remove your warts with medication, freeze them with liquid nitrogen or remove them surgically.

Assuming that you've been diagnosed with genital warts, here's what women doctors say that you can and should do to relieve symptoms and hasten healing.

Wash off wart removers. Prescription wart removers containing powerful substances like podophyllin, applied only by your doctor, and podofilox, are applied by your doctor or by yourself at home under your doctor's supervision, often several times over the course of two to four

WHEN TO SEE A DOCTOR

If you or your sexual partner show signs of genital warts, see a doctor. It may take from 8 to 18 months after infection for warts to become apparent, so if your partner has them and you don't notice any, you may still have the virus.

Genital warts should be promptly removed, says Kimberly A. Workowski, M.D., assistant professor of medicine in the Division of Infectious Diseases at Emory University in Atlanta. If your sexual partner has genital warts, he too should see a physician and have them removed. If you prefer to consult a specialist in the diagnosis and treatment of sexually transmitted diseases (or infections), try your gynecologist, the county or city health department Sexually Transmitted Disease clinic or Planned Parenthood Clinic. Call 1-800-230-PLAN for the Planned Parenthood clinic nearest you.

weeks. They cause warts to gradually shrivel up and fall off. So powerful are these medications, however, that they can also burn and cause severe irritation to neighboring tissues, says Dr. Workowski. To protect your sensitive skin, she advises washing off these medications within four to six hours after each application. Dabbing the area repeatedly with a warm, wet washcloth should do it. Better yet, take a warm, relaxing bath.

Keep the area clean and dry. In the event that your doctor opts to use liquid nitrogen or laser surgery, you should expect that there will be some local skin or mucous membrane irritation, says Judith O'Donnell, M.D., assistant professor of medicine in the Division of Infectious Diseases at Allegheny University of the Health Sciences in Philadelphia and a medical specialist for the Sexually Transmitted Disease Control Program at the Philadelphia Department of Public Health. "Immediately after the procedure, keep the area clean and dry so the skin heals," she says. Take a daily bath or shower and wash with a gentle soap. Then gently and thoroughly pat yourself dry with a soft towel.

Soak in an oat bath. "Taking an oatmeal bath can be extremely soothing for genital itchiness that may occur from warts," says Dr. Workowski. She recommends Aveeno bath treatment, available at drugstores. The product contains a finely powdered oatmeal called colloidal oatmeal, which is a good antidote to itching and won't clog your bathtub drain.

241

Gingivitis
Act Now for Healthier Gums

*T*he next time you brush your teeth, look at your toothbrush. Are the bristles red? Look in the mirror and smile. Are your gums puffy and swollen or losing their pink glow? If so, you probably have gingivitis.

Scary as it may sound, gingivitis is a fancy word for gum disease. It occurs when a sticky film of dental plaque (a gluelike film of bacteria, food and saliva) invades the warm and inviting crevasses at and below your gum line. There it hardens into tartar (sometimes called calculus), triggering inflammation and infection.

In other words, if plaque and tartar collect on your teeth, you get cavities. If they sneak into your gums, you get gingivitis.

THE HORMONE LINK

Woman are at increased risk for developing gingivitis during pregnancy, says Rita D. Zachariasen, Ph.D., professor of physiology at the University of Texas Health Science Center at Houston. According to Dr. Zachariasen, estrogen and progesterone (female hormones produced by your ovaries) seem to enhance conditions for growth of certain types of plaque-forming bacteria, while reducing the ability of your gums to heal once gingivitis occurs. Therefore, you should pay special attention to cleaning your teeth during pregnancy and whenever you are taking oral contraceptives, since ovarian hormones are elevated at these times.

Pregnancy's flood of hormones can be especially hard on the gums, with scientists estimating that 60 to 75 percent of pregnant women will have gingivitis, says Dr. Zachariasen. Prevention is the key. Studies show that women who are plaque-free when they enter pregnancy or start taking oral contraceptives can avoid swollen, bleeding gums, or at least minimize the problem.

DON'T GET SCARED, GET BUSY!

Some women tend to pull back from their dental hygiene routine when they see bleeding or experience sore gums, says Caren Barnes,

R.D.H., professor of clinical dentistry at the University of Alabama School of Dentistry in Birmingham. But that's when simple steps can do the most good.

"We can stop gum disease, but we can't reverse it," she warns. So make cleaning your teeth and gums a priority now, and you can put the brakes on before you have full-blown periodontitis, where bacteria from the dental plaque actually undermines the bone and structures that hold your teeth in their sockets. Women doctors say that it's never too late to treat gingivitis.

Don't wait until your gums hurt, say women doctors. Here are some home tips to help you on the road back to healthier gums.

Brush and floss. You probably already own the two simplest tools for fighting gingivitis: a toothbrush and dental floss (thread specifically designed to clean between the teeth). "Used properly and regularly, they can thoroughly remove the plaque and bacteria from your teeth and gums at least once a day," says Barnes.

Brushing should be done a minimum of twice a day, says Mahvash Navazesh, D.M.D., associate professor and vice-chair in the Department of Dental Medicine and Public Health at the University of Southern California School of Dentistry in Los Angeles. Flossing should be done at least once a day.

If you're pregnant, brush and floss thoroughly and carefully after each meal, says Dr. Navazesh.

Lighten up. "Some people think that the harder you scrub, the more plaque you remove," says Diane Schoen, dental hygienist, clinical assistant professor and coordinator of the Preventive Dentistry Program at the University of Medicine and Dentistry of New Jersey in Newark. But brushing your teeth isn't like scrubbing a floor. Plaque is sticky like jelly, not sticky like glue, she says. "It adheres to teeth softly, so you don't need to scrub hard—it just needs to be mechanically broken up." Schoen recommends a soft-bristled toothbrush, held at a 45 degree angle to the gum line.

Start with an ultrasoft brush. If your gingivitis has left your gums sore and inflamed, keep brushing. But go with an ultrasoft brush until your dentist-directed healing program takes hold, says Schoen.

Pick up a tiny tool. A special brush called an interproximal brush has tiny bristles that go below the gum line, where floss can't reach. They can remove bacteria in the pockets formed by periodontal disease and can be helpful to use in conjunction with normal brushing and flossing, says Barnes. "One such tool is the Proxabrush, found in the toothbrush aisle."

Use no-frills floss. Dental floss or tape works whether you use waxed or unwaxed, regular gauge or extra-fine, thread or ribbon, looped or un-

WHEN TO SEE A DOCTOR

If you feel pain or notice bleeding when you brush, don't wait until your next scheduled appointment to see your dentist: Unchecked, serious gum disease can undermine the tissues that support your teeth and lead to tooth loss.

If you're pregnant, be sure to schedule several prenatal visits with your dentist, says Mahvash Navazesh, D.M.D., associate professor and vice-chair in the Department of Dental Medicine and Public Health at the Universty of Southern California School of Dentistry in Los Angeles. Hormonal changes during pregnancy leave pregnant women especially vulnerable to gum disease.

looped, plain or mint-flavored, says Barnes, as long as you use it. You don't need anything elaborate. Barnes and her associates compared gingivitis in men and women who used traditional dental floss to those who tried out an electromechanical flossing device that can fit between tightly spaced teeth. After a month both groups had benefited from flossing, but the new device offered no better results than ordinary floss from the drugstore.

Swish as you style. At least once a day, swish mouth rinse around your mouth for about a minute (maybe while drying or styling your hair) after brushing and flossing, advises Heidi K. Hausauer, D.D.S., instructor of operative dentistry at the University of the Pacific Dental School in San Francisco and a spokesperson for the Academy of General Dentistry. Look for rinses that say "antiplaque" on the label. They kill bacteria that causes gingivitis and can be quite effective when combined with brushing, flossing and regular checkups, says Dr. Hausauer.

Buy a crate of oranges. You don't hear much about scurvy these days. But the fact remains, the hallmark of a textbook case of vitamin C deficiency—or scurvy—is rampant gum disease, leading to tooth loss. Vitamin C benefit is essential to healthy connective tissue, including gums, says Carole Palmer, R.D., Ed.D., professor and co-head of the Division of Nutrition and Preventive Dentistry in the Department of General Dentistry at Tufts University School of Dental Medicine in Boston.

"If you don't get enough vitamin C, your gums will be less able to resist bacterial infection," says Dr. Palmer. She recommends eating fresh fruits and raw or lightly steamed vegetables. "And it won't hurt to take a multivitamin, too."

Swallow two aspirin, and call your dentist in the morning. If your gums are really sore, rinsing with saltwater or taking over-the-counter analgesics such as aspirin or ibuprofen may help. But don't make the mistake of putting your aspirin where your pain is—directly on your gum. "I see this all the time, but aspirin is acidic," notes Dr. Hausauer. "It can really burn your gums."

Gout

Little Ways to Relieve Big Pain

*G*out is a one-of-a-kind sort of ailment, best known for triggering a big pain in your big toe and striking in the middle of the night.

Plus, gout has one of two distinct causes. A genetic error (present at birth) prompts the body to make too many purines—a naturally occurring by-product of protein metabolism that the body converts into uric acid. Or the kidneys aren't able to excrete as much uric acid as the body requires, says Elizabeth Tindall, M.D., clinical associate professor of medicine in the Division of Rheumatology at Oregon Health Sciences University in Portland. Either way, uric acid slowly begins to accumulate in the blood. Eventually, the acid precipitates out of the blood and into fluid in a joint—commonly the big toe—in the form of uric acid crystals.

NATURAL PROTECTION

It usually takes about 20 years of gradually accumulating uric acid before the first gout attack occurs, says Dr. Tindall. But once the crystals form, your body defends itself by attacking the crystals with white blood cells. The result is an inflammation that causes the toe to swell, turn purple and hurt like the dickens.

Women may also be protected by the female hormone estrogen, says Audrey Nelson, M.D., a consulting rheumatologist at the Mayo

Clinic in Rochester, Minnesota. While men build uric acid levels from puberty, women apparently do not accumulate uric acid until after menopause.

If uric acid levels only begin to build in women when estrogen levels drop—around age 50—women may not live long enough to develop gout.

COUNTERATTACK

If everyone in your family has gout, you may be one among the minority of women who experience gout. Women who are overweight, have high triglyceride levels or are being treated with medications to fight cancer or reduce blood pressure may be at a slightly higher risk, says Dr. Tindall.

Most attacks last about seven to ten days, says Dr. Tindall. Here's what women doctors say you can do.

Pack your toe in ice. You can reduce pain temporarily by packing your toe in ice, says Nancy Becker, M.D., a rheumatologist in private practice in Kansas City, Kansas. Loosely fill a plastic bag with crushed ice, wrap a towel around the bag, then wrap both around the toe, making sure the towel lies between your toe and the bag of ice. Leave the ice pack in place for 20 minutes (you can refill the bag with fresh ice if it melts too quickly). You may ice your toe up to three times daily.

Stay off your feet. Any movement is bound to aggravate the pain, says Dr. Tindall. She advises sitting with your foot propped on a footstool or staying in bed.

GOUT-FIGHTING DIET STRATEGIES

Once an attack has passed, women doctors offer this advice for keeping future attacks at bay.

Limit alcohol. To prevent repeat attacks of gout, limit your alcohol intake to no more than one drink a day of beer, wine or liquor, says Dr. Tindall. Alcohol triggers gout attacks in people predisposed to gout. And if you don't drink at all, so much the better.

"Even just a couple of drinks can push you over the edge into pain," says Dr. Tindall.

Avoid purine-rich foods. Forget organ meats such as liver, heart, kidney and sweetbreads, says Dr. Tindall. They're all loaded with purines and can precipitate an attack.

Experiment with a vegetarian diet. The higher the amount of protein in your diet, the more purines you're likely to get, says Agatha

WHEN TO SEE A DOCTOR

A first-time gout attack will generally resolve itself within seven to ten days whether or not you do anything about it, says Nancy Becker, M.D., a rheumatologist in private practice in Kansas City, Kansas.

But if you have had recurring attacks, it's best to see your doctor to get treated early; otherwise, the attack could last weeks or even months, says Dr. Becker. Your doctor can prescribe medications (such as colchicine) that can reduce the pain and shorten the length of the attack. There are also medications such as allopurinal (Zyloprim) that can minimize your body's production of uric acid as well as medications such as probenecid (Benemid) that will maximize your kidney's ability to excrete it.

Thrash, M.D., a preventive medicine specialist and pathologist with Uchee Pines Institute in Seale, Alabama. So she suggests that women with gout adopt a diet based on vegetables, fruits and grains. In her experience, says Dr. Thrash, once meat, poultry, eggs and fish are out of the diet, women with gout can frequently live without another attack.

Try the 1,200-calorie-a-day plan. Since those who get gout tend to be overweight, women who have experienced gout pain and are carrying even a few extra pounds should cut their calorie intake to around 1,200 calories a day until they reach a healthy weight, says Dr. Thrash.

"I usually recommend a breakfast of fruits and whole grains with a lunch of vegetables and whole grains," says Dr. Thrash. "You can add a handful of nuts to either meal, then have a light supper of fruit." When you've lost all the weight you want, keep eating the same mix of grains, fruits, vegetables and nuts, but add enough calories so that you maintain a healthy weight.

Although this eating plan is somewhat limited, women who have experienced gout pain are more than willing to follow it, says Dr. Thrash—especially after she tells them that no woman who has followed the diet has ever had gout return.

Whatever you do, don't fast or crash diet, says Dr. Tindall. Going without food for 24 hours or more or eating less than 1,000 calories a day causes the body to break down protein so fast that uric acid levels will soar.

Gray Hair
Sort through Your Color Options

*I*f you're like a lot of women, when you notice more than a few gray hairs, you head for the nearest drugstore to check out the seemingly endless aisle of hair-coloring products. You pick up one box after another, look at the color chart—and leave the store more confused than when you arrived.

Everyone's hair turns gray eventually. When you turn gray is determined by genes passed on to you by your parents, explains Patricia Farris Walters, M.D., clinical assistant professor of dermatology at Tulane University School of Medicine in New Orleans and a spokesperson for the American Academy of Dermatology. The timing is different for everyone.

"I began graying in my early twenties," says Dr. Walters. "Although both of my parents were significantly gray in their sixties, no one in our family grayed as prematurely as I did."

Hard numbers are difficult to come by, but somewhere around two-thirds of women stay au naturel when their hair turns gray and one-third reach for a coloring product, says Ellie Steuer, vice-president of Revlon in New York City.

Many women who turn gray don't do anything radical, adds Steuer. They seem to prefer products a shade or two different than their natural color, designed to color only the gray. The result is a natural two-tone effect in which the gray appears to simply be a lighter shade of the natural hair color. Others decide that this is a good opportunity to find out what they'd look like with a completely different hair color and go from brown to blond, red or black.

TEMPORARY OR PERMANENT?

Experts say that your choice depends on how much of your hair has turned gray and how often you're willing to recolor your hair, among other factors.

Try a two-week product. If you're just beginning to gray, and you're not sure whether you want to keep your gray or get rid of it, try a semipermanent rinse, suggests Clancey Callaway, the Atlanta-based head of hair technology at Vidal Sassoon North America. A semipermanent product designed for home use is Clairol's Loving Care.

Callaway calls semipermanent rinses no-commitment colors. Unlike more permanent coloring products, semipermanent rinses deposit color on the hair's outer cuticle only. It never penetrates to the cortex of the hair shaft itself, says Callaway. The color is gradually washed away in 6 to 12 shampoos. If, like most women, you wash your hair every day or two, semipermanent color will last anywhere from one to three weeks.

Semipermanent rinses can't lighten your hair—they can either match your natural color or darken it. Nevertheless, semipermanent rinses give you just enough color to help you decide whether or not you like yourself with—or without—gray hair.

Study the instructions. Home coloring products are tested so well that they're just about foolproof—provided that you follow the directions, says Steuer. Also, always do a patch test to make sure that the dye won't irritate your skin. Follow the instructions included with the colorant. Patch-testing usually requires that a small amount of color be applied to an area of tender inner-arm skin for 48 hours to check for irritation prior to coloring.

Brave it with a harmonizer. If your hair is up to 50 percent gray, and you're pretty sure that you want to ditch the gray, you may want to try what the industry calls a longer-lasting semipermanent product, suggests Steuer. Also called tone-on-tone products or harmonizers, Revlon's Shadings, Clairol's Natural Instincts and L'Oreal's Casting are all longer-lasting semipermanent hair-color products marketed for home use. They don't begin to fade until after four to six weeks, and they leave no hard, telltale demarcation at the root line.

For the most natural-looking results, Steuer suggests that you choose a harmonizer one shade lighter than your own natural hair color.

Tint your hair. If you're more than 50 percent gray, and your mind is made up to ditch the gray for good, Steuer suggests that you color your hair with a permanent hair color. One advantage to permanent color is that if you wish, you can go lighter or darker or change your color completely, while covering 100 percent of your gray. Keep in mind, however, that this type of color won't wash out—your hair will remain the new color until it grows out, and the roots will be more obvious.

Play it safe—or go wild. When you find a hair color that you like, look at the swatches on the back of the boxes or read the instructions to see what results you can expect for your original hair color. "Remember that all hair color results are determined by a user's own natural color," says Steuer.

Gynecological Exam Jitters

Ways to Ease the Dread

*Y*our heart is pounding and you can barely breathe. Your mouth is dry, muscles tense, palms sweaty. You're embarrassed, consumed with fear, counting the minutes until your doctor finishes taking a Pap smear, looking at and touching your genitals, feeling your breasts for abnormalities, checking your rectum . . . until finally, mercifully, she utters those wonderful words, "All done. You can get dressed now."

At least one out of ten women find a gynecological exam to be a traumatic experience, says Charanjeet Ray, M.D., an obstetrician/gynecologist and associate professor in the Department of Obstetrics and Gynecology at Rush Medical College of Rush University and attending physician at Illinois Masonic Hospital, both in Chicago. "I see it in the same women year after year. They turn pale. Some have even passed out."

Your doctor needs to see you at least once a year to detect problems in your reproductive organs and elsewhere in the pelvic area, along with breast lumps and signs of sexually transmitted disease as well as for a general health checkup. Yet some women avoid the pelvic exam entirely because of a bad experience, says Lila A. Wallis, M.D., clinical professor of medicine and director of "Update Your Medicine," a series of continuing medical educational programs for physicians, at Cornell University Medical College in New York City. Consequently, she says, health problems that need attention go undetected.

A NECESSARY RITUAL

If you dread going to the gynecologist and tense up before she even touches you, here's what women doctors say you can do to keep calm.

Time it right. Some women experience breast tenderness right before or during their menstrual periods, says Mary Lang Carney, M.D., medical director of the Center for Women's Health at St. Francis Hospital in Evanston, Illinois. Schedule your exam right after your period so you won't jump when the doctor does your breast exam.

Empty your bladder. Urinating before your exam makes you more comfortable, says Dr. Wallis. It also makes it easier for your doctor to feel your uterus, ovaries (which produce eggs) and fallopian tubes (which carry eggs to the uterus) and enhances the reliability of her findings.

Keep your socks on. If your feet are cold and uncomfortable in the heel rests, wear socks or slip a folded paper towel between your heel and the metal of the heel rest. In addition, wearing shoes with heels allows you to effectively grip the heel rests. Finally, says Dr. Wallis, ask your doctor to adjust the heel rest brackets to allow the most comfortable bend in your knees. Also, many doctors' offices have knee rests on their examining tables, which may make it more comfortable for some women, she adds.

Admit that you're uneasy. If your doctor knows you have the jitters, she can do her best to be even more reassurng and gentle than usual, says Dr. Ray.

Breathe in. Breathe out. Repeat. For many women, the worst part of the exam is the insertion of a speculum, a metal or disposable plastic device that opens the vagina to allow the doctor to examine it and obtain a tissue sample. This can be a rather strange sensation, says Dr. Ray. Tense pelvic muscles make insertion of a speculum difficult, if not impossible, says Dr. Carney. This, in turn, drags out the exam. But relaxing isn't always easy. "Lying back and taking a few deep breaths may help," Dr. Carney says.

Relax your muscles. Put your hand on your tummy muscles, which are often really tight at exam time. When you get a sense of how hard those muscles are, you can begin to relax them, says Dr. Carney.

Dr. Wallis suggests this taut muscle antidote: Tighten the muscles you use to control urination and then relax them. Repeat several times before your doctor inserts the speculum.

Escape the stirrups—mentally. Focusing on the exam only makes matters worse, says Dr. Ray. Instead, imagine that you're sunning on a beach in Hawaii or doing something else you enjoy.

If it hurts, say so. Your doctor is not a mind reader. Let her know if something she is doing hurts, says Dr. Ray. Inserting a speculum may tug on your pubic hair, for instance. Tell your doctor, and she may suggest that you help guide the insertion. Recognize, too, that telling your doctor something hurts may provide her with valuable information about the state of your health.

Count on it being quick. "It helps to realize that the whole process doesn't take long," says Dr. Carney. "A Pap smear takes just a few seconds." It'll be over before you know it.

Hair Loss
Not Only a Male Problem

Somewhere around her 38th birthday, Sara began to notice that there were more hairs caught in her brush than usual after she brushed her hair. She also noticed that there was more hair trapped in the bathtub drain after she showered. And even more alarming, she was also beginning to find hair here, there and everywhere. It was turning up on sweaters, pillows, coats, hats—even on her car seat.

What was going on?

"The most common cause of hair loss in women is a shift in the growth cycle," says Rebecca Caserio, M.D., clinical associate professor of dermatology at the University of Pittsburgh. In other words, at any given time, some of your hair is growing and some of it is done growing. Most hairs have a life expectancy of three to six years, even if you get a haircut—or several—in the meantime. These hairs go into a resting stage for three months and fall out, and then new hairs are produced from the same roots.

NO BALD CATS

In other words, a certain amount of hair loss is normal. Think about it: Your cat probably sheds hundreds of hairs a day without going bald.

"We normally shed somewhere between 50 and 100 hairs every day," says Dr. Caserio. "But there are a whole host of life events—namely, hormone shifts from birth control pills, pregnancy and menopause—that affect growing conditions, so that we can sometimes lose hundreds of hairs a day." Rapid weight loss, severe dandruff, iron deficiency and a low protein intake can also speed up the normal rate of hair loss by forcing hairs into a rooting stage. A serious illness or a physical stress, such as childbirth, can trigger dramatic (but temporary) hair loss of up to 50 percent, but this only occurs in extreme circumstances, says Dr. Caserio.

"Hair loss—particularly when it occurs at the crown—can also be caused by genetics," adds Dr. Caserio. Hereditary baldness is not just a male problem, she points out. Women can inherit a predisposition toward baldness from either parent.

252

WHEN TO SEE A DOCTOR

Although a certain amount of hair loss is normal, it can sometimes suggest that something is wrong somewhere in your body—especially if hair loss is accompanied by an increase in facial hair, abnormal periods or a deepening of the voice.

If hair loss seems to be on the increase, or is accompanied by these symptoms, talk to your doctor.

If your problem isn't overall sparseness, but noticeable thinning at the crown (female pattern baldness), you may benefit from use of either a prescription or over-the-counter version of minoxidil (Rogaine), says Rebecca Caserio, M.D., clinical associate professor of dermatology at the University of Pittsburgh. Check with your doctor to see if you're a candidate for medication.

"Hair loss takes an enormous emotional toll on people, especially women," says Diana Bihova, M.D., a dermatologist in New York City and author of *Beauty from the Inside Out.* "We invest so much in our appearance. Although hair loss is not something that we're going to die of, it affects our self-esteem."

SLOWING—OR REVERSING—HAIR LOSS

If your doctor has ruled out medical causes for accelerated hair loss, women doctors say that there's plenty you can do to hang on to what hair you have and encourage healthy regrowth. Their advice will be of special help to women who experience hair loss after childbirth.

Be gentle. Treat your hair like a baby's, says Dr. Bihova. Use baby shampoo and shampoo no more than once a day. Lather up only once when you do and rub your scalp gently. Then spritz your hair with a detangling conditioner.

Air-dry your hair. Avoid drying vigorously with a towel, says Dr. Bihova. Also, if you must use a blow-dryer, keep it on a low setting.

Style when dry. Grooming wet hair can cause it to stretch and break, says Dr. Bihova. So don't comb or brush your hair until it's dry.

Switch shampoos with the season. Change your brand of shampoo at the beginning of every new season—summer, winter, spring and fall, suggests Dr. Bihova. In her experience, it seems to prevent some shedding.

253

Don't tease. Even women who aren't losing their hair should avoid teasing or back-combing, says Yohini Appa, Ph.D., director of product efficacy at the Neutrogena Corporation in Los Angeles. "It is one of the worst things that you can do to your hair." Teasing breaks the hair and contributes to the appearance of hair loss.

Perm and color carefully. When perming and coloring your hair, follow product instructions carefully, says Elizabeth Whitmore, M.D., assistant professor of dermatology at Johns Hopkins University School of Medicine in Baltimore. Neither perms nor color causes hair to fall out, she adds. But both, when done incorrectly, do cause hair to break. And when the break is very close to the scalp, it can make you look as though hair has fallen out.

NUTRITIONAL HELP

So much for treating hair loss externally. To address possible internal causes, try these strategies.

Get adequate protein. Eat a couple of three- to four-ounce servings of fish, chicken or other lean sources of protein every day, even if you're dieting, says Dr. Whitmore. Protein is needed by every cell in your body, including the cells that make the hair. Without adequate protein, the cells in your body don't work efficiently and can't make new hair to replace old hair that's been shed.

Maintain iron levels. Since iron-deficiency anemia can also cause hair loss, make sure that you eat a well-balanced diet that includes a daily serving or two of iron-rich foods, says Dr. Whitmore. Good sources of iron include lean red meat, steamed clams, cream of wheat, dried fruit, soybeans, tofu and broccoli.

Take vitamin B_6. "I have no idea why it works, but 100 milligrams a day of vitamin B_6 seems to decrease hair-shedding in some people," says Dr. Caserio. Just don't take any more than that without consulting a doctor, she cautions. Larger amounts can be toxic, especially over a prolonged time.

Hair Texture Problems

Solutions for Coarse or Fine Hair

We all have about 100,000 hairs on our heads, but if you're a woman with fine, silky hair, you may feel like you have half that much. And if you have a full head of coarse, frizzy hair, chances are that you have more than you care to deal with.

The texture of your hair—be it coarse or fine—is inherited, says Elizabeth Whitmore, M.D., assistant professor of dermatology at Johns Hopkins University School of Medicine in Baltimore. Hair with a thicker shaft tends to feel coarse and rough, while hair with a thinner shaft tends to feel fine and silky. And what makes the difference between coarse and fine hair are those cellular blueprints that your parents passed along.

Fortunately, the entire hair-care industry has devoted itself to figuring out how to help women with hair texture problems make the most of they have.

COARSE HAIR: WORK WITH IT

Here's what experts advise for coarse hair.

Moisturize. If you have coarse hair, make sure that you follow every shampoo with a moisturizing conditioner, says Elizabeth Hartley, the West Coast creative director for Vidal Sassoon in San Francisco. It will help subdue your hair's tendency to curl by adding a little weight.

Since coarse hair reflects little light, use a conditioner to resurface your hair, says Hartley. Any conditioner will slick down your hair's cells into a flat, highly reflective surface, whether it contains silicone, oil or lanolin. Try them all and pick the one that works best for you.

Let it air-dry. If you have coarse hair, comb a conditioner through your locks, then let it air-dry, says Hartley. The more you handle coarse hair in the drying stage, the more it tends to frizz.

Keep it short. Coarse hair can be shaped to lie a little flatter and straighter when it's short than it would if left long. So if your hair is coarse, a short cut is better, says Hartley.

255

FABULOUS FIXES FOR FINE HAIR

Experts have equally practical advice for women with fine hair.

Crop it. Fine hair looks thicker and chunkier when cut short, says Hartley.

Let it swing free. Fine hair reflects lots of light, so styles that let your hair hang free alongside your face show off the shine, says Hartley.

Use a clarifying shampoo. Fine hair tends to go limp when the residues of various hair products are added to its own tendency toward oiliness, says Hartley. To free your hair to swing, she advises shampooing fine hair with a clarifying shampoo containing a strong detergent base, such as sodium lauryl sulfate, to remove heavy buildup from gels, sprays or detanglers.

Mousse it. If you have fine hair, add volume by moussing your roots, says Hartley. Lean forward from your waist, squirt a quarter-size poof of mousse into your palm, rub your hands together, then smudge the mousse through your roots. When it's well-distributed, throw your hair back and shake it.

Avoid using gels on fine hair, Hartley adds. They're so heavy that the weight will make your hair collapse.

Let wet hair rest. If you have fine hair, after it has been washed and moussed, comb it into place and then leave it alone for at least ten minutes, says Hartley. Get dressed, put on your makeup or putter around your home. Your hair needs an opportunity to rest, or it will go limp and flat.

Coax your hair dry. Fine hair does not like rough handling, says Hartley, so don't style it with a blow-dryer set on high. Use a lower speed, and don't manhandle it: Instead of pulling on the ends with a brush, use your fingers to push or twirl ends into shape. The result will be more bounce and curl.

Coat with color. Coloring your hair may thicken it, says Diana Bihova, M.D., a dermatologist in New York City and author of *Beauty from the Inside Out*. The color penetrates the hair's cortex during coloring and causes it to swell. The result is thicker hair.

Hangnails

Be Your Own Manicurist

*B*ecause hangnails are dead skin and are therefore painless, you may not even realize that you have one until you snag your panty hose.

"A hangnail occurs when the cuticle around your nail grows out onto the nail plate," says Phoebe Rich, M.D., clinical assistant professor of dermatoloty at Oregon Health Sciences Center in Portland.

Don't try to chew off a hangnail with your teeth or pick at it, says Loretta Davis, M.D., associate professor of dermatology at the Medical College of Georgia School of Medicine in Augusta. When removed improperly, hangnails can cause an unsightly bloody mess on your finger. Or they can get infected.

WISE ADVICE

"With proper cuticle care, hangnails don't have to ever become troublesome," says Dr. Rich. Follow this expert advice.

Keep it under wraps. It takes willpower to resist the urge to tear or bite off a hangnail, says Dr. Davis. "So it's a good idea to have a bandage or two in your cosmetic bag for this very purpose. If you discover a hangnail, put the bandage over it to keep yourself from picking at it until you can treat it properly."

Cream your cuticles. "The first line of defense is a good manicure," says skin-care specialist Lia Schorr, owner of Lia Schorr Skin Care Salon in New York City. "It's also very helpful to smooth around the nail with cream and to buff the whole nail area."

Soak, then clip. "Don't cut cuticles when they're dry," says Trisha Webster, a hand model with the well-known Wilhelmina Modeling Agency in New York City. "I recommend softening them first by soaking them in warm water and olive oil. Since the idea is to remove only the dead skin that makes up the hangnail and not to injure the living tissue around it, clip closely without going too far down. You don't want to leave anything to play with."

Dab on some antibacterial ointment. If a mishandled hangnail gets infected, apply an over-the-counter antibiotic cream and keep it bandaged, says Dr. Davis.

257

Hangover
Revive Yourself

*L*ast night you and a male co-worker went out for drinks after work. You were feeling great when you got home. Now you're shaky and headachy. Your stomach is heaving (or feels as though it's about to), your heart is racing and your mouth is dry—the rebound effects that your body feels after an evening of excessive drinking. What happened?

"Too much alcohol depresses the nerve cells in your brain," explains Anne Geller, M.D., neurologist and chief of the Smithers Alcoholism Treatment and Training Center at St. Luke's-Roosevelt Hospital Center in New York City and past president of the American Society of Addiction Medicine. "When the alcohol leaves your system, the nerve cells are no longer sedated, so you become anxious and irritable." Plus, alcohol irritates your stomach lining (explaining the queasies) and dilates the blood vessels in your head (explaining the headaches).

Meanwhile, your drinking buddy is fine. What gives?

Women react more intensely to alcohol than men do. Within seconds of drinking the same amount of beer, wine or liquor as your male companion, your blood alcohol content is higher than his. And the toxic effects of what you drank more quickly attack sensitive organs like your liver and brain.

One reason that women suffer worse hangovers than men may be because of differences in body fat and water in the body. Since women have a higher percentage of body fat and a lower percentage of water in their systems, alcohol is less diluted with water when it reaches your brain, liver, kidneys and other organs.

GETTING BACK TO NORMAL

If you have a hangover, you won't need a doctor to diagnose what's wrong with you. As for what to do about it, Dr. Geller advises that you treat a hangover in its earliest stages instead of waiting until later in the day. "Without question, the earlier you get active and start treating your hangover, the better you're going to feel." Here's her advice.

WHAT WOMEN DOCTORS DO

The Medical School Cure

Anne Geller, M.D.

Currently a neurologist and chief of the Smithers Alcoholism Treatment and Training Center at St. Luke's-Roosevelt Hospital Center in New York City and past president of the American Society of Addiction Medicine, Anne Geller, M.D., doesn't get hangovers anymore. But like a lot of people, she profits from previous experience.

"I used to get hangovers when I was in medical school," says Dr. Geller. "Women today are lucky—back then, we didn't know very much about how to treat a hangover. But I did know enough to drink two large glasses of water the next day. I also knew that I couldn't stay in bed; that would be counterproductive. Since I had an irritated stomach with my hangover, I never felt inclined to eat very much, so I just kept it light."

Today, that's the same basic advice that Dr. Geller gives other women who find themselves suffering from the aftereffects of overimbibing.

Fill up on fluids. "Alcohol stimulates the kidneys to produce more urine," says Dr. Geller. "Consequently, you're dehydrated, and you need to replace the lost fluids. So as soon as you get up in the morning, drink two eight-ounce glasses of water." It doesn't hurt to drink some water before you go to bed the night before, either.

Get up and get out. "Exercise is the best thing to do when you have a hangover," says Dr. Geller. "Excessive alcohol depletes your body's supply of endorphins, or mood-elevating hormones."

You can boost your body's supply of endorphins with light to moderate exercise for 20 minutes. Dr. Geller recommends taking a brisk walk, working out at the gym or going for a light jog.

Soothe an upset stomach. "Too much alcohol can inflame the stomach lining," says Dr. Geller. "If you have stomach upset, reach for an antacid. Follow label directions."

Eat light. "Most women aren't interested in eating a heavy meal when they have hangovers," notes Dr. Geller. "If you feel like eating, stick to light foods that are bland and easy to digest—such as melba toast, white rice and pretzels—and sip beverages like ginger ale and bouillon."

Peel a banana. "Excessive alcohol can diminish carbohydrate levels," says Dr. Geller. "Bananas are a nutritious source of complex carbohydrates and provide energy, which is sorely lacking the morning after."

Tame that throbbing head. "If you have a headache, take enteric-coated aspirin, which is formulated to digest in the intestines, rather than in your already upset stomach," says Dr. Geller.

AND NEXT TIME...

If you have a wicked hangover, you've probably resolved to drink less next time (or not at all). Here are some tips to make sure that your current hangover is your last hangover.

Know your limits. "Your body gets rid of alcohol at the rate of three-quarters of a drink per hour," says Dr. Geller. "One drink is one five-ounce glass of wine, one can of beer or one shot of gin, bourbon, whiskey or other hard liquor. For women, more than three drinks per hour will put them over the legal limit."

Pace yourself. "Alternate alcoholic with nonalcoholic drinks over the course of an evening," suggests Dr. Geller. Or skip the alcohol and stick to ginger ale.

Hay Fever
Take a Recess
from Congestion and Sneezing

*U*nfortunately, the same sunny, breezy days that make spring, summer and fall so great also cause ragweed, trees and grasses to release their pollen into the air to make you miserable. It doesn't seem fair. While other folks are enjoying the last few weenie roasts before Labor Day, you're battling hay fever, which causes stuffy noses and sneezing fits.

Actually, the word "hay fever" is a misnomer: The condition is caused by ragweed that pollinates during what used to be known as hay pitching season, but not by hay itself. Hay fever now refers to both fall allergies (caused by ragweed) and spring and summer allergies (caused by grasses and trees). And there's no fever involved. The medical term for hay fever is *allergic rhinitis*: In plain English, it means your nose is stuffed up and running, and you're sneezing because of something you're breathing other than air.

Approximately 1 in 20 people suffers from this outdoor-related allergy, which can also cause sore throats, red eyes, earache and headache.

A FEW HANDY STRATEGIES

Women doctors offer these tips for minimizing the bothersome symptoms of hay fever.

Crank up the AC. If you suffer from hay fever, the ideal strategy is to stay indoors, keep your windows closed and use an air conditioner, which filters out the pollen, says Helen Hollingsworth, M.D., associate professor of medicine at Boston University School of Medicine and director of allergy and asthma services at Boston University Medical Center Hospital. (In the event you anticipate buying a new car in the near future, Dr. Hollingsworth suggests you consider a make and model—such as Ford or Saab—that has filters in its air conditioning. "Check with the dealers," she says.)

Cut the A.M. workout. Pollen counts are at their highest early in the morning, between 5:00 and 8:00 A.M., when plants release pollen, so try to exercise later in the day, notes Carol Wiggins, M.D., clinical instructor of allergy and immunology at Emory University in Atlanta. "Working out during your lunch hour is fine. Or wait until later in the day. If you must exercise in the morning, you may want to use a treadmill and do more indoor things," she says.

Wear a special mask. Wearing a face mask while mowing the lawn or exercising outdoors is a good way to keep those nasty allergens from reaching you, says Dr. Hollingsworth. Using a surgical mask isn't the best method, though, because it doesn't completely fit against your face and block everything out. Instead, go for the fiber-fill cuplike masks with a foam face seal—some of which have an exhale valve that opens with the force of your breath and shuts as you inhale. You can find these at hardware stores.

Rinse your eyes. To soothe stinging red eyes, wash them out, notes Rebecca Gruchalla, M.D., Ph.D., assistant professor of internal medicine and chief of the Division of Allergy and Immunology at the University of

When to See a Doctor

If your hay fever lingers long after ragweed season or if at-home strategies and over-the-counter medications don't control your symptoms, it's time to go to the doctor, says Rebecca Gruchalla, M.D., Ph.D., assistant professor of internal medicine and chief of the Division of Allergy and Immunology at the University of Texas Southwestern Medical Center at Dallas.

Don't worry that if you see an allergist, she'll automatically say you need allergy shots, says Dr. Gruchalla. Prescription medications or intra-nasal medication may suffice.

Texas Southwestern Medical Center at Dallas. "Get an over-the-counter eyewash solution and just wash the eye out over a sink," she says. "That will get some of the allergen out of the eye." Do it at least a couple of times a day—especially when you're coming in from outside.

Take an antihistamine at night. Although many people shy away from antihistamines because of their grogginess-inducing side effects, taking them at night is usually fine, notes Dr. Wiggins. "At least if you take one at night, you'll be able to get a good night's sleep and be able to fight the allergy that much better," she notes.

Beware of melons. People allergic to ragweed could get an itchy mouth when eating cantaloupe, honeydew and other melons, notes Kathy L. Lampl, M.D., an instructor in the Department of Medicine in the Clinical Immunology Division at Johns Hopkins University School of Medicine in Baltimore. Interestingly, allergies to birchwood can cause the same mouth-itching reaction to chamomile tea, apples and pears. This is known as oral allergy syndrome. "It's not life-threatening, it's just uncomfortable; but you'll want to be aware," she says.

Be extra diligent. Indoor allergens could increase your sensitivity to outdoor allergens, says Dr. Lampl. "If you're already congested, it may take only 10 pollen grains to stir up a reaction, where it might have taken 50 or 100 grains of pollen before," she says. Keep pets out of the bedroom and make sure the house isn't humid, so it won't be home to dust mites and mold.

(For other practical tips on managing allergies, see page 9.)

Hearing Problems
Listening Skills for the Volume-Impaired

*A*re you asking people to speak up or repeat themselves more often these days? Are you wondering who keeps turning down the volume on your TV? Or why your husband or friends whisper? Perhaps everyone has suddenly decided to tone it down. More than likely, though, your hearing isn't what it used to be.

"What?" you say. "Hearing loss at my age? I'm too young!"

Don't bet your Grateful Dead posters on it.

"We're seeing hearing loss typical of 60-year-olds in 20-year-olds," says Kathy Peck, executive director of H.E.A.R. (Hearing, Education and Awareness for Rockers) in San Francisco. "Noise-induced hearing loss is showing up in younger people more frequently than ever before"—and much of it, she believes, is caused by powerful sound technology in full use at rock concerts.

Other possible causes of hearing loss include day-to-day exposure to loud noise levels, earwax buildup, side effects of medication or blows to the ear. If the cause is temporary (earwax or medication), hearing loss is correctable. When caused by noise, hearing loss is permanent, caused by nerve damage to the inner ear.

PROTECTION IS THE NAME OF THE GAME

To prevent noise-induced hearing loss—or prevent it from getting worse—take the following expert advice.

Invest in a pair of ear protectors. According to Harriet Kaplan, Ph.D., professor of audiology and director of clinical services at Gallaudet University (a one-of-a-kind liberal arts university for the deaf located in Washington, D.C.), you're asking for trouble when you are hearing 85 decibels of sound continually for eight hours.

How loud is that? In the same range as a vacuum cleaner, power lawn mower or a blender.

"When you're mowing the lawn, working or playing around loud machinery or other noises, wear ear protectors (padded cuplike protectors are available at home improvement centers, and earplugs can be

263

WHEN TO SEE A DOCTOR

If you experience sudden and dramatic hearing loss in one ear or both, have your ears checked by a professional.

Whatever you do, don't panic," says Barbara Hopson, R.N., certified nurse practitioner at the Veteran's Administration Medical Center Occupational Health Unit in Dallas. The problem could be simply too much earwax, rather than a serious ear problem.

But don't procrastinate, either. "Would you put up with fading eyesight without having an eye exam? Probably not," says Carol Flexer, Ph.D., an audiologist and professor of audiology in the School of Communicative Disorders at the University of Akron in Ohio. "There's no reason to put up with fading hearing, either."

Start with an audiologist, who is trained to evaluate hearing losses, says Dr. Flexer. He or she can prescribe a hearing device, fit you with custom-made ear plugs, or refer you to a medical specialist if necessary.

"Today's high-tech hearing devices offer hope for many kinds of hearing loss," says Dr. Flexer.

found at drugstores) to muffle the sound," says Carol Flexer, Ph.D., an audiologist and professor of audiology in the School of Communicative Disorders at the University of Akron in Ohio.

Plug 'em up. Rock concerts (and some home stereo systems) are much louder these days. Smart rockers know that good earplugs are a must when it comes to concerts—either playing or attending, says Peck, a former musician who has significant hearing loss. "If music is so loud that you can feel it, wear earplugs."

Earplugs can be custom-made by an audiologist or purchased over the counter, says Peck. The custom-made plugs are best and cost up to $100. They weaken sound but allow you to hear high, middle and low frequencies at the same rate and allow for truer sound transmission. But you can substitute inexpensive ear plugs made from putty or spongy material available at drugstores.

Stick to your workout routine. Research shows that physically fit people have half the hearing loss of people who aren't fit—and you don't have to run marathons to qualify for the benefits. A study co-authored by Helaine M. Alessio, Ph.D., associate professor of physical education and sport studies at Miami University in Oxford, Ohio, showed that people who exercised briskly three or four times a week boosted their hearing power and actually reversed a certain amount of hearing loss.

Exercise training may allow more oxygen-rich blood to be pumped to distant small areas such as the inner ear, says Dr. Alessio. There was also an increase in circulating proteins that defend the inner organs of the ear against stressors, so they hold up longer.

Skip the headset. Or at least make sure that you can hear someone talking when you play it, especially if you're power-walking, jogging or biking while wearing a personal headset, says Kathleen Hutchinson, Ph.D., an audiologist at Miami University in Oxford, Ohio, and study co-author.

Any exposure to noise for a prolonged period of time can ultimately damage your ears, says Dr. Hutchinson.

Heartburn

Douse the Inner Fire

Digestive juices usually follow the law of gravity. But if stomach acid takes an unbidden upward swing back into your throat when it's supposed to be heading to your stomach, that's heartburn.

You feel like you're on fire. Your insides are burning, and you feel pressure under your ribs and an acid taste in your mouth from partially digested food.

It's a most unpleasant, but all too common, sensation. About one out of four pregnant women suffer from heartburn. For them, heartburn is a double whammy: Higher hormone levels relax the esophageal muscle that's supposed to keep stomach acid where it belongs, and at the same time, the growing baby presses up against the stomach.

Other culprits? Certain foods (like chili), smoking cigarettes, drinking alcohol, severe overweight or just lying down or bending over right after a meal.

WHEN TO SEE A DOCTOR

Heartburn and chest pain can feel pretty similar. But if pain from your chest radiates to your shoulders, neck or back, or if it doesn't stop or it is exercise-induced, see a doctor immediately. You could be having a heart attack or angina. Don't be shy. So what if it turns out that you've rushed to the emergency room for heartburn? It's better to be safe than sorry.

NOW WHAT?

For most of us, certain simple dietary and lifestyle changes will cool down the burning under our rib cages and send our meals straight to our tummies. And women doctors say that with the exception of over-the-counter acid-blocking medications, their remedies can work well even if you're pregnant.

Stand up. "When gravity is on your side, what goes down will stay down," says Barbara Frank, M.D., gastroenterologist and clinical professor of medicine at Allegheny University of the Health Sciences MCP–Hahnemann in Philadelphia. Whatever you do, don't bend over or lie down, or the churning contents of your stomach are more likely to fly upward.

Beg, borrow or buy an antacid. Over-the-counter antacids such as Mylanta or Maalox ease the pain by neutralizing stomach acids, says gastroenterologist Grace Elta, M.D., associate professor in the gastroenterology division of the University of Michigan in Ann Arbor.

For some women, liquid antacids break down acid faster, but for others, chewable tablets stay in the esophagus longer. Experiment to find out which works better for you, says Dr. Frank.

Try an acid suppressor or two. If antacids are not helpful, you can try an acid-suppressing medication known as H_2 (histamine 2) blockers. Once available only by prescription, Tagamet HB and Pepcid AC can decrease the release of acid in the stomach, says Marie L. Borum, M.D., assistant professor of medicine in the Division of Gastroenterology and Nutrition at George Washington University Medical Center in Washington, D.C.

They're available over the counter in your drugstore or supermarket. The dose is half of what you'd get if your doctor prescribed the medication. So if the suggested dose isn't enough to soothe your inner flames, take twice as much but no more, says Dr. Elta.

Dr. Borum cautions against using an H_2 blocker during pregnancy. Although they are considered safe, regular antacids may be even safer.

KEEP YOUR HEARTBURN ON ICE

Women doctors say that a few simple changes in the way that you eat and sleep can douse heartburn.

Eat no chocolate, drink no brews. The road to heartburn is almost always paved with alcohol, chocolate, fatty foods, mint and coffee (even decaffeinated coffees contain irritants that can affect your stomach and esophagus), says Dr. Elta. All are capable of weakening the lower esophageal sphincter.

Eat like Jack Sprat, not his wife. Fat takes longer to digest than anything else, which gives acid even more time to head back up before digestion is complete, says Dr. Frank.

Plan meals around veggies and lean cuts of meat and fish, not foods like cheeseburgers and fries, she says.

Cut out the citrus. Another common flame-bearer for many people who get heartburn is citrus fruits (such as oranges or grapefruit) and tomatoes, says Dr. Frank.

Pregnant? Skip spicy seasonings. Spicy seasonings are hard to digest, says Jennifer Niebyl, M.D., professor and head of obstetrics and gynecology at the Hospitals and Clinics at the University of Iowa in Iowa City. And when you're pregnant, the increase in the hormone progesterone slows down your digestion so much that it takes longer to digest a meal. The harder food is to digest, the more likely you are to get heartburn. "So eat bland foods such as rice and bananas and avoid cayenne and other types of chili peppers," she says.

Eat a small dinner. Large meals sit in your stomach longer, which gives stomach acid more chance to head back up to your mouth, says Melissa Palmer, M.D., a gastroenterologist in private practice in New York City.

"Don't make your evening meal your heaviest meal," says Helen Greco, M.D., obstetrician/gynecologist at Long Island Jewish Medical Center in Hyde Park, New York.

Fast before sleeping. "Try not to eat or drink anything for two or three hours before you go to bed," says Robyn Karlstadt, M.D., a gastroenterologist at Graduate Hospital in Philadelphia. That way, all your food should be emptied from your stomach before you go to bed.

Don't exercise right after a meal. Your mother was right—you shouldn't exercise for at least an hour after a meal. "The movement of exercise defies gravity and brings up acid reflux," Dr. Frank says.

Keep off the pounds. Try to get to and stay at your optimal weight, says Dr. Frank. Obesity and heartburn have long been linked, because excess weight loosens the esophageal sphincter.

Kick the habit. Stop smoking, Dr. Elta says. Cigarettes increase the rate of stomach acid production and weaken the esophageal sphincter that keeps food down.

Heart Palpitations
Calming Strategies for Skipped Beats

It's long past midnight and you're lying in bed, wide awake and frightened. You can't fall back to sleep because something seems to be wrong with your heart. It skipped a beat when you first woke up, and now you're lying in the darkness, waiting to see if it'll fall into that distinctive rhythm—*fwop, fwop, f—WOP!*—again.

It does.

So now you worry that (a) you're having a heart attack, (b) you're going to die or (c) you'll die of embarrassment if you go to the emergency room and find out that nothing is wrong after all.

Chances are, none of the above will occur.

"Skipped heartbeats—generally referred to as palpitations—are incredibly common," says Vera Bittner, M.D., associate professor of medicine at the University of Alabama School of Medicine in Birmingham. And they're not cause for panic.

NOTICEABLE, BUT NOT DANGEROUS

Any odd heartbeat that occurs once or twice and attracts your attention qualifies as a palpitation, says Dr. Bittner. The heart isn't actually skipping a beat; what you feel is a less forceful beat followed by one with more force than you're used to. Whether your heart seems to be skipping,

WHEN TO SEE A DOCTOR

If your heart seems to skip a beat "more than just momentarily" or "more than once in a while," you should see a doctor, says Vera Bittner, M.D., associate professor of medicine at the University of Alabama School of Medicine in Birmingham. Medical attention is also in order if your heart skips a beat and:

- You feel as though you are about to pass out.
- You also have swollen ankles or shortness of breath.
- You have any form of heart disease.
- You have chest pain or pressure.

flipping or leaping into your throat, you probably aren't in danger.

"People frequently notice what feels like a skipped beat when they wake up after a bad dream, especially if they've been lying on their left side," says Deborah L. Keefe, M.D., professor of medicine at Cornell Medical Center and a cardiologist at Memorial Sloan-Kettering Cancer Center, both in New York City. "Your heart is close to the chest wall on the left, and if you're lying on that side, you're more likely to notice a skipped beat."

QUIETING A FLIGHTY HEART BEAT

What can you do to prevent these frightening but harmless palpitations from recurring? Here's what women doctors say.

Take a deep breath. Some palpitations are caused by anxiety, says Dr. Bittner. Sometimes just taking a deep breath and slowly exhaling will relieve tension and discourage future skips.

Recondition your heart with exercise. Spending too little time at exercise (like walking) or other active pursuits (like gardening) can cause palpitations simply because your heart—which is, after all, a muscle—is out of shape, says Dr. Bittner.

To put your heart in peak condition, the American Heart Association suggests that you exercise three or four times a week for 30 minutes. You should work your body at 50 to 75 percent of its aerobic capacity. Translation? If you're walking, walk fast enough so that you can talk but not sing.

Keep alcohol to a minimum. Drinking too much alcohol can cause palpitations, says Dr. Bittner. Overindulgence leads to what doctors have dubbed "holiday heart"—irregular heartbeat experienced by those who overindulge at holiday parties and then end up in the emergency room. But it can happen any time of the year.

There's no way to tell exactly how much alcohol it takes to interfere with your heartbeat, says Dr. Bittner. Nor can doctors tell in advance who will develop alcohol-induced palpitations and who won't. So to help keep your heart on an even keel, experts advise against drinking more than one or two drinks a day, tops. A drink is generally considered to be one shot of hard liquor or its equivalent in a mixed drink; one 12-ounce can, bottle or mug of beer or 5 ounces of table wine.

Cool the caffeine. Caffeine is what gives coffee, tea, chocolate and even some over-the-counter drugs—headache remedies, for example—their stimulating effects, says Dr. Bittner. So if you're bothered by palpitations, it makes sense to avoid anything containing caffeine.

Don't even think of lighting up. Nicotine and other chemicals in cigarette smoke can constrict arteries and encourage heart palpitations, says Dr. Bittner. So if you smoke, quit.

If all else fails, ignore skipped beats. If you exercise regularly, don't overindulge and your doctor has determined that you don't have heart disease, yet your heart seems to occasionally skip a beat, chances are that your palpitations are nothing to worry about, say Drs. Bittner and Keefe. If you don't dwell on them, you're less apt to notice repeat episodes.

Heat Exhaustion
Self-Rescue Pays Off

It's late Saturday morning, and you burst out of the house for your usual jog. The weather is unusually hot and humid for this time of year, but that doesn't stop you. You're trying to get in shape and can't afford to skip your workout. Before you know it, you're hot, sweaty and incredibly thirsty. But you press on until you begin to feel sick, have goose bumps and feel nauseated.

Chances are, you have heat exhaustion. Fluid lost through perspiration can lead to dehydration.

"Humidity plays a major role in heat exhaustion," explains Amy Morgan, Ph.D., an exercise physiologist at the Noll Physiological Research Center at Pennsylvania State University in University Park. "If the weather is really humid, the sweat on your body will not evaporate, and you will not cool as quickly."

A PERIL OF WORK OR PLAY

Typical symptoms of heat exhaustion include chills, fatigue, light-headedness, thirst, nausea, confusion, feeling faint, weakness and headache. Women are at risk for heat exhaustion if they exert themselves in the summer heat—playing tennis or tackling yard work, says Dr. Morgan. You're also at risk if you work in a warm building with poor air circulation, like a factory, for hours on end.

If this process continues, heat exhaustion can develop into a potentially life-threatening type of heat illness: heatstroke, which requires emergency medical attention. So women doctors and exercise physiologists say that you should take immediate action to counter heat exhaustion (or better yet, prevent it in the first place).

Here's what you can do to chill out.

Get out of the heat. "Stop what you're doing and get into the shade or an air-conditioned room as soon as possible," says Dr. Morgan. "A cool environment will lower your body temperature quickly." If you're too far from home to get back fast, duck into the nearest shopping mall, supermarket, convenience store, movie theater or other public building until you feel better.

Grab a drink A.S.A.P. "Aside from getting out of the heat, one of the very first things that you should do when you have heat exhaustion is drink plenty of liquids, to hydrate your body and increase blood flow to your skin, which will help increase cooling," says Susi U. Vassallo, M.D., assistant professor of surgery in the Division of Emergency Medicine at New York University School of Medicine in New York City and a fellow of the American College of Emergency Physicians.

"How much to drink depends on how hot and humid the weather is, and how much you were exerting yourself," says Dr. Vassallo. She recommends drinking to quench your thirst as soon as you start to feel uncomfortable and following up with additional fluid as frequently as possible throughout the day. (Dr. Vassallo, for example, drinks 32 ounces of liquid.)

271

WHEN TO SEE A DOCTOR

You should see a doctor if you experience any of the following:
- Fainting
- Vomiting
- Nausea

The following symptoms are signs of heatstroke, which is more serious than heat exhaustion and is, in fact, a medical emergency. See a doctor at once if:
- You are confused.
- Your speech is slurred.
- Your behavior is odd (like incoherence).
- Your pupils are dilated.
- You're having muscle spasms.
- You stop sweating. (By this time you are critically ill.)

If you take measures to relieve heat exhaustion and your symptoms get worse or don't improve, get medical help without delay. If you have heatstroke, 24 hours is too long to wait.

If you have heat exhaustion, waiting 24 hours isn't ideal, but it's not as crucial.

Drink a low-carb sports drink. Some experts recommend rehydrating with sports drinks, while others believe that water is just as good.

"Some research suggests that sports drinks help you hydrate more quickly than water alone," explains Dr. Morgan. "By intent, sports drinks tend to be high in carbohydrates—namely, the sugars fructose, glucose and sucrose. They also contain sodium and other electrolytes that you may lose through sweat.

"The sodium and carbohydrates are put in the sports drinks to help your body absorb the fluid from your stomach into your bloodstream perhaps more quickly than it absorbs water alone. This gets the fluid into your bloodstream sooner to help relieve dehydration," she says. "The downside is that too many carbohydrates may slow the release of fluids from your stomach to your bloodstream."

Since studies have yet to prove whether or not sports drinks are helpful, Dr. Morgan advises checking labels and choosing sports drinks lowest in carbohydrates (measured in grams). Water will also relieve dehydration and will suffice if you don't like the taste of sports drinks or if they are not available.

Spritz and catch the breeze. If you can, spritz yourself with a water sprayer. Focus the spray on your head and neck and sit in front of a fan, suggests Dr. Morgan.

Chill that scalp. "Your head contains many blood vessels," explains Dr. Vassallo. "When you make your head cold, the chilled blood circulates and cools the rest of your body." She recommends placing a bag of ice or a wet washcloth or something very cold on your head or the back of your neck until you feel better.

Fashion a cool head wrap. You can also cool your head fast by plunging a bandanna, a terry cloth sweatband or a towel in icy water and leaving it on your head, says Dr. Morgan. You could exercise with this on to keep your body from overheating.

Relax and put your feet up. "Elevating your feet will bring more blood flow back to your brain, which could help stop you from feeling dizzy," says Dr. Morgan. "Lie down with your feet one to two feet higher than your head." For example, lie down on the floor with your feet propped up on a sofa or a chair.

WHAT WOMEN DOCTORS DO

An Icy Head Wrap Helped

Susi U. Vassallo, M.D.

Playing tennis after a long layoff and pushing to get back into shape led to heat exhaustion for Susi U. Vassallo, M.D., assistant professor of surgery in the Division of Emergency Medicine at New York University School of Medicine in New York City and a fellow of the American College of Emergency Physicians. She used her ingenuity and did exactly what doctors advise for heat exhaustion.

"I left the court and sat in the shade under a tree," she says. "I drank a lot of ice water. But I also dunked a towel in the ice water and wrapped it around my head.

"And oh, yes—I quit playing tennis for the rest of the day," she adds.

Other remedies for heat exhaustion include drinking a low-carbohydrate sports drink, spritzing yourself with a water sprayer and sitting down with your feet elevated.

Heat Rash
Not Limited to Athletes

*A*thletes aren't crybabies, but they're prone to something that makes little babies cry—heat rash.

The trouble happens when those sleek bicyclists and runners speed along roads wearing tight spandex gear. While they look like the personification of good health, their tights may be posing a hazard.

The problem is the sweat trapped under the fabric. Normally, sweat regulates your body temperature, cooling your skin as it evaporates. Trapped underneath clingy fabric, however, perspiration can't escape, and your skin heats up and breaks out into itchy pink or red bumps—heat rash.

Heat, sweat and constricting clothes are almost guaranteed to produce heat rash, say women doctors. "The skin swells and blocks the sweat pores. The sweat backs up and causes that itchy rash," explains Karen S. Harkaway, M.D., clinical instructor of dermatology at the University of Pennsylvania School of Medicine and a dermatologist at Pennsylvania Hospital, both in Philadelphia.

When heat rash is severe, it's called prickly heat. And heat rash isn't limited to athletes, either. If you have large breasts or if you are a large woman, you have probably noticed that your skin itches when it's hot, says Toby Shaw, M.D., associate professor of dermatology at Allegheny University of the Health Sciences MCP–Hahnemann School of Medicine in Philadelphia. That happens when skin rubs repeatedly against skin, whether it's breasts against abdomen or skin folds against each other. Too much sun can provoke heat rash, too, she adds.

BREAKING FREE OF THE BREAKOUT

No matter what you call it, heat rash is fairly easy to alleviate. Here are some tips.

Apply a cold washcloth. "With simple cases of heat rash, you need to cool the skin down," says Diane L. Kallgren, M.D., a dermatologist in private practice in Boulder, Colorado. A simple cool compress relieves and refreshes heated skin. Dip a washcloth in cool water, wring it out and let it sit on your skin for five to ten minutes.

WHEN TO SEE A DOCTOR

"Heat rash is dangerous only if it's associated with heatstroke, which can destroy many sweat glands," says Diane L. Kallgren, M.D., a dermatologist in private practice in Boulder, Colorado.

If heat rash is accompanied by nausea, dryness, thirst, headache and pallor, move into an air-conditioned setting, drink fluids and seek medical help as soon as possible.

Simple heat rash should clear up in a week or less. If not, you may have some other kind of problem, such as eczema.

Call your doctor if:

- Red bumps turn into white pustules.
- Your rash continues for more than a week or two.

Ice is nice. When skin is angry, there's nothing like ice to reduce swelling, says Dr. Harkaway. Throw some ice cubes in a sealed plastic bag, wrap in a kitchen towel and apply for five minutes at a time.

Smooth on mentholated cream. Dr. Shaw's favorite heat rash remedy is Sarna, a mentholated cream that calms down hot-and-bothered skin. Follow the directions on the package.

Dust with talcum powder after bathing. Talc is cooling, says Dr. Harkaway, and it absorbs the moisture that is part of the problem—a good practice to add to your regular summertime routine.

Take a liking to cotton. If you are an active woman prone to heat rash, retire your jazzy bike shorts and running tights until fall. "They look nice, but the best clothes for working out in the heat are loose cotton T-shirts and gym shorts," says Dr. Harkaway.

"Tight fitness gear causes pressure on the skin and promotes heat rashes," says Mary P. Sheehan, M.D., chief of pediatric dermatology at Mercy Hospital in Pittsburgh. Synthetic fabrics allow sweat to lay on your skin, too, but cotton absorbs it.

Heavy Thighs
Thinner, Trimmer, Slimmer

Randomly poll any group of women about their least favorite body part, and chances are that a majority will point to their thighs.

It's the weight of heredity: If your thighs are heavy, chances are that your mother's are, too. The bad news? "You can't lose weight in a single body part," says Mary Ellen Sweeney, M.D., obesity researcher at Emory University School of Medicine and an endocrinologist and director of the Lipid Metabolism Clinics at the Veterans Affairs Medical Center, both in Atlanta.

BEST BETS FOR SHAPELIER THIGHS

The good news: If you work at losing weight and exercising, you can slim down and tone up your thighs, Dr. Sweeney says.

And there are a few specific exercises that may help bring out the best in them, says Kathleen Little, Ph.D., exercise physiologist and professor at the University of North Carolina at Chapel Hill.

Trim fat and trim your thighs. "Fat is fat," says Dr. Sweeney. If you want to get rid of the fat on your thighs, you'll need to reduce your overall body weight and body fat.

Start by getting most of your calories from low-fat or high-carbohydrate foods such as vegetables, chicken breasts and whole-grain, unbuttered bread.

Limit your fat intake to 20 to 30 percent of your daily calories. (If you eat 2,000 calories a day, that's between 400 and 600 calories from fat.) It's not complicated. Just cut back on fried foods, rich desserts, fatty meats and high-calorie salad dressings, Dr. Sweeney says.

The aerobic guarantee. "If you lose weight all over your body, you will lose it in your thighs," says Dr. Sweeney. She says that the best way to burn off the most fat is to get 20 to 60 minutes of aerobic exercise—in other words, activity that increases your breathing and heart rate, such as brisk walking, bicycling, step aerobics or running—at least three times a week.

Add weights, subtract inches. "The best way to work off weight and flab is to combine aerobic exercise with resistance training," says Dr.

Sweeney. Aerobic exercise burns off fat, while resistance training improves muscle tone and strength and firms up your thighs, and the flab goes away. Develop a regimen that includes both types of exercise, says Dr. Sweeney, and you'll be on your way to slimmer, sleeker thighs.

Dr. Little concurs: Specific resistance-training exercises can firm your thighs; they'll look smoother and jiggle less.

If you have access to a gym, work your thighs on a leg press or leg-extension machine, says Dr. Little. If you don't, Dr. Sweeney suggests leg lifts or semi-squats.

To do a leg lifts, lie on your side with your legs straight. Rest your head flat against your outstretched arm or cradle it in your hand with your arm bent. Slowly raise your top leg about 12 to 14 inches from the floor 10 to 12 times, explains Margot Putukian, M.D., team physician at Pennsylvania State University in University Park and assistant professor of orthopedic surgery and internal medicine at the Milton S. Hershey Medical Center in Hershey. Remember to breath out as your leg is raised and breath in as you lower it. Repeat three times for each leg at least three times a week.

To do semi-squats, stand sideways at your kitchen counter or next to a chair with your feet spread about shoulder width apart. While grasping the counter or chair with your hand, slowly squat down until your knees are bent to 90 degree angles, says Dr. Putukian. Keep your back straight and your shoulders and knees in line above your toes. Then come back up. Use the counter or chair for balance only and make your legs do the work. Do 10 to 12 repetitions three times a week.

OTHER SLIMMING TRICKS

Here are a couple of additional tricks for creating the illusion of thinner thighs.

Disguise it with dress. If your thighs are heavy, body-hugging knits—miniskirts, tube skirts and leggings—are not your best fashion options. Instead, opt for soft, flowing skirts in flattering fabrics such as wool crepe or silk, which direct attention away from your thighs, says Susan Bornstein, a wardrobe and fashion consultant at Nordstrom near Seattle.

Wear neutral colors. To cast a slim, thin-thigh silhouette, wear solid navy blue or black skirts or small patterns that don't scream out for attention, Bornstein says. Avoid plaids, large patterns or horizontal stripes.

Hemorrhoids
Nix the Itch and Burn

Bowel movements aren't supposed to be as hard to pass as the state bar exam. So if you spend a lot of your bathroom time straining, you could end up with painful, swollen hemorrhoids.

Hemorrhoids are swollen blood vessels in and around the anus and lower rectum—sort of like varicose veins in your legs. In addition to straining, they are frequently caused by forceful bowel movements brought on by bouts of constipation or diarrhea.

Pregnant women often develop hemorrhoids—both the pressure of the fetus on the abdomen and hormonal changes cause blood vessels around the anus to enlarge.

IMMEDIATE RELIEF FOR STRAINED VEINS

About half of all women develop hemorrhoids by age 50, but they will usually come and go away on their own, lasting only a few days. Here's what you can do to reduce the misery.

Draw a bath. Sitz baths are a tried-and-true method of easing hemorrhoidal aches and pains, says Robyn Karlstadt, M.D., a gastroenterologist at Graduate Hospital in Philadelphia. Fill your bath with three to four inches of warm—not scalding hot—water. "Don't add anything to the water—no Epsom salts, no bubble bath, no bath oils—all of which can irritate your bottom," she says. Lie back in the tub for 30 minutes if you can, or 10 minutes at a minimum, several times a day as long as you ache.

Soothe the itch. After your sitz bath a hemorrhoidal cream or suppository (available in supermarkets and drugstores) can stem the itch as you go about your daily activities, says Barbara Frank, M.D., gastroenterologist and clinical professor of medicine at Allegheny University of the Health Sciences MCP–Hahnemann in Philadelphia.

Or ice it. Applying an ice pack to the irritated area can reduce swelling, says Dr. Frank.

When you gotta go, go. One major source of the constipation that causes hemorrhoids is "holding it in when you need to go," says Joanne A. P. Wilson, M.D., a gastroenterologist and professor of medicine at

WHEN TO SEE A DOCTOR

For most women, hemorrhoids will respond to home remedies—or go away on their own—within a few days. If they don't or if they get worse, consult your doctor—they may need to be surgically repaired or removed, says Robyn Karlstadt, M.D., a gastroenterologist at Graduate Hospital in Philadelphia.

And see your doctor immediately if your rectum bleeds, she says. You may be suffering from something besides hemorrhoids.

Duke University Medical Center in Durham, North Carolina. If you need to get rid of body wastes, take the time to go to the bathroom to prevent straining later.

But go easy. Moving your bowels can take some time. You should schedule up to 15 minutes a day to sit on the pot, because trying to force out hard, dry stools is likely to cause the straining that leads to hemorrhoids, Dr. Wilson says.

(For practical ways to manage constipation—a common cause of hemorrhoids—see page 138. For additional ways to relieve rectal itching, see page 464.)

Herpes
Make the Pain Go Away

One in five people has genital herpes, and most of them don't even know it," says Kimberly A. Workowski, M.D., assistant professor of medicine in the Division of Infectious Diseases at Emory University in Atlanta. Only about one-fourth of the estimated 50 million Americans infected experience any symptoms. Worse yet, whether or not you have a single symptom, herpes is sexually transmittable.

WHEN TO SEE A DOCTOR

Symptoms of herpes, should you experience them, include a burning or tingling feeling in the genital area followed by the eruption of painful small red blisters that rupture and form shallow ulcers. Particularly with the initial infection, other symptoms may include:

- Fever
- Headache
- Swollen lymph glands
- Abnormal vaginal discharge

If you exhibit these symptoms, see your family doctor, gynecologist or a specialist working in a sexually transmitted disease (STD) clinic. Planned Parenthood also offers specialized services for some STDs.

Herpes is caused by herpes simplex virus type II (HSV-2). (Another strain, HSV-1, is the type responsible for cold sores, but it also sometimes causes genital infections.) Once you've contracted the virus, it's with you for a lifetime, living in nerve cells at the bottom of your spine. If you do have symptoms, they usually consist of a tingly or burning sensation in your genital area, followed by the appearance of small red blisters. These grow into larger pimplelike blisters and are often itchy and painful, with a watery yellow center that eventually ruptures and grows a crusty skin.

EXIT PAIN AND SUFFERING

Medical treatment is aimed at relieving symptoms. Your doctor will probably treat your initial outbreak and perhaps recurrent outbreaks as well with the antiviral drug acyclovir. Gradually, outbreaks often weaken and may disappear altogether. Meanwhile, here are some ways to make yourself more comfortable.

Keep blisters clean and dry. "You don't want blisters to become superinfected from bacteria on surrounding skin," says Judith O'Donnell, M.D., assistant professor of medicine in the Division of Infectious Diseases at Allegheny University of the Health Sciences in Philadelphia and a medical specialist for the Sexually Transmitted Disease Control Program at the Philadelphia Department of Public Health. "Bathe or shower daily with a gentle soap and water, or just water alone."

Take an oatmeal bath. A warm bath helps relieve genital irritation, says Dr. Workowski. And if you have sores, it can also help relieve itching. Best of all is a soak in an oatmeal bath, she says. She recommends Aveeno bath treatment, available on your drugstore shelf. The product contains a finely powdered oatmeal called colloidal oatmeal that's very soothing to itching skin.

Wear loose-fitting clothes. Squeezing into panty hose, tight underwear or other form-fitting clothes will further irritate sensitive herpes sores, says Dr. Workowski. "You'll get chafing, which can be extremely painful." Opt for loose-fitting clothing until your sores heal.

Take a nonprescription painkiller. Acetaminophen, ibuprofen or aspirin might help relieve blister pain, says Dr. Workowski. Follow the directions on the label.

Make love later. Having sex during a herpes outbreak is a bad idea for a variety of reasons, says Dr. O'Donnell. "The herpes outbreak is always associated with some level of pain and discomfort, and this will be made much worse during intercourse. As part of the herpes outbreak, patients may experience swelling of the lymph nodes in the groin. This swelling may cause some discomfort, or it may be painless," she says. Having sex during an active outbreak will put your partner at risk of developing a herpes infection and may place you at higher risk for contracting other sexually transmitted diseases, including HIV, she adds.

Use a condom. If you don't have herpes, but your sexual partner does, or if you have a new sexual partner and aren't sure, using a condom offers some protection against contracting the virus, says Dr. Workowski. Use a condom even if no blisters are apparent. "The virus is still there," she says. Experts recommend latex over animal-membrane condoms.

Best of all may be the female condom, according to Dr. Workowski. This device consists of two plastic rings connected by a polyurethane sheath. "The female condom covers the whole vulva," she says, protecting nearby areas that would otherwise expose the virus or be exposed to it.

Hiccups
Tricks to Stop the Spasm

*F*aced with an intractable case of hiccups, doctors employ the same home remedies that women have traded across the kitchen table for generations. "First, hold your breath," says Mary Jo Welker, M.D., a family physician and associate professor in the Department of Family Medicine at Ohio State University in Columbus. "Or take a spoonful of granulated sugar."

Hiccups are an involuntary contraction of the diaphragm, the sheet of muscle that separates the chest from the abdominal cavity and plays an important role in breathing. With hiccups, the normally smooth function of this muscle is shortcircuited by some type of irritation, and the muscle goes into spasm. As the diaphragm moves downward, the person hiccuping inhales quickly, and the vocal cords snap shut across the throat. That's what causes the "hic."

Anything that causes your stomach to expand upward to press against your diaphragm—gulping air, carbonated drinks, indigestion—can cause hiccups. "Some people find that eating on the run or eating while they're laughing and talking results in hiccups, while others never seem to determine any cause," Dr. Welker says.

FOLK CURES DO WORK

It seems like just about everyone has a pet remedy for hiccups. Certain tactics make a lot of sense and may be based on physiology as well as folklore. Here's what hiccup veterans recommend.

Take a deep breath and count to 30. Holding your breath increases carbon dioxide levels in the blood, which, apparently, decreases the sensitivity of the vagus nerve center in the brain, Dr. Welker says. "That might be enough to stop the transmission of the hiccups signal."

Try a spoonful of sugar under your tongue. "It's the first thing that I'd try, and it's what I have suggested to nannies and other child-care providers," says Becky Luttkus, a child-care educator in Denver. However, sugar can be a choking danger to a child who is under two years old, and you'll want to use only a quarter- or half-teaspoon for small children.

"Just put a bit under their tongues and let it dissolve slowly."

"No one knows exactly why sugar may help hiccups," says Marla Tobin, M.D., a family physician in private practice in Higginsville, Missouri. "Some doctors speculate that the granules stimulate the vagus nerve, a long nerve in the back of the throat that sends branches to many muscle groups, including those in the diaphragm."

Chew some papaya. Hiccups, along with belching, bloating and aftertaste, can be a sign of digestive problems, says Betty Shaver, an herb practitioner in Grahamsville, New York. "I have recommended that people chew papaya digestive tablets, and it always works to relieve their hiccups." Eating fresh papaya or pineapple will also help. Both fruits contain every digestive enzyme that the stomach needs.

It's true that digestive problems, including heartburn, can aggravate hiccups, Dr. Tobin says (although doctors are more likely to give an antacid such as Maalox or Mylanta or an acid reducer such as Pepcid AC or Tagamet HB, than digestive enzymes).

Plug your ears and drink up. When confronted with hiccups, Marsha Henderson, R.N., a school nurse in Yorktown Heights, New York, tells women to plug both ears with their fingers, then drink a glass of water through a straw.

"I've used this myself—I even keep straws on hand for it—and it has always worked when I've recommended it to others," Henderson says.

High Blood Pressure
Nondrug Strategies with Maximum Effect

Doctors aren't sure what causes blood pressure to increase above 140/90 mmHg (millimeters of mercury), considered a healthy upper limit. Diseases affecting the kidneys, adrenals or other glands can occasionally raise blood pressure—a condition that doctors call secondary high blood pressure, says Lois Anne Katz, M.D., professor of

283

clinical medicine at New York University School of Medicine and associate chief of nephrology and associate chief of staff for ambulatory care at New York Veterans Affairs Medical Center, both in New York City.

But 19 times out of 20, high blood pressure happens for no apparent reason, she adds.

The kidney plays a major role in blood pressure regulation, says Dr. Katz. "It's possible that sometime in the future we might find a gene that affects the kidney and causes high blood pressure."

All we really know for sure is that women who are overweight, have diabetes or are African-American carry the greatest risk of getting high blood pressure, she says. Women who take birth control pills also have a slightly increased risk, although no one is quite sure why.

"High blood pressure is very common among women," adds Dr. Katz. According to the American Heart Association, if you're between ages 35 and 55, chances are about one in four that you have it, while nearly one out of two women over the age of 55 have it.

Uncontrolled, high blood pressure increases your risk of heart disease, kidney failure and stroke. But, for most women, elevated blood pressure can be controlled before it has a chance to do any harm, says Dr. Katz.

THE NONDRUG ROUTE

In some cases, doctors prefer that women with high blood pressure try nondrug strategies first, says Dr. Katz. And here's what they suggest.

Drop extra pounds. "People who lose a considerable amount of weight—say 20 or 30 pounds—can sometimes bring their blood pressure down," says Dr. Katz. Losing excess weight may actually cause a chemical change in the body that alters metabolism, she says. It decreases the amount of insulin you produce, which can sometimes be a factor in triggering high blood pressure.

The best way to lose excess weight is to listen to your body's appetite signals, adds Dr. Katz. Eat only when you're hungry (not around the clock), stop eating when you're full and avoid foods that are high in fat or sugar (or both). Also, keep portions modest. Gradually, weight should come down.

Work fruit, beans and potatoes into the menu. Loading up on potassium-rich fruits and vegetables is an important part of any blood pressure–lowering program, says Linda Van Horn, R.D., Ph.D., professor of preventive medicine at Northwestern University Medical School in Chicago. Aim for potassium levels of 2,000 to 4,000 milligrams a day, she says.

WHEN TO SEE A DOCTOR

Even if you've never been told that you have high blood pressure, it's good to have it checked at least once a year, because early detection (and control) is the key to preventing untoward effects, like heart or kidney disease.

And you should definitely have your blood pressure checked if you become pregnant. "Sometimes blood pressure goes up during pregnancy," says Lois Anne Katz, M.D., professor of clinical medicine at New York University School of Medicine and associate chief of nephrology and associate chief of staff for ambulatory care at New York Veterans Affairs Medical Center, both in New York City. Because blood pressure normally declines in pregnancy, she explains, a rise is of great concern.

During pregnancy a small but significant increase in blood pressure could be a sign of pre-eclampsia (a serious complication requiring immediate medical attention) if accompanied by excessive weight gain and the presence of protein in the urine, says Dr. Katz.

No one knows exactly how potassium lowers blood pressure, but a study at the Johns Hopkins Medical Institutions in Baltimore found that those who took 3,120 milligrams a day lowered their systolic blood pressure (the top number of a blood pressure reading) an average of nearly seven points and reduced their diastolic pressure (the bottom number of the reading) an average of about two points.

Top sources of potassium are orange juice, potatoes, bananas, beans, cantaloupe, honeydew melon and dried fruits such as prunes and raisins.

Work that body. Aerobic exercise—activities that use your major muscles and raise your heart rate, like biking, running and swimming— also seems to bring down blood pressure, perhaps by keeping your blood vessels more flexible, says Linda L. Colle Gerrond, M.D., director of the Center for Women's Health at the Shawnee Mission Medical Center near Kansas City, Kansas. Regular exercise also burns fat and calories, making it easier to lose or maintain weight.

To help control your blood pressure, Dr. Gerrond recommends 30 minutes of aerobic exercise three times a week as long as your physician says that you're ready. For a successful long-term program, do the exercises you like best, she suggests.

Use salt judiciously. In most people, eating salt does not increase the risk of high blood pressure, says Dr. Katz. But for some reason, it may affect a few. So if you have high blood pressure, it doesn't hurt to use salt judiciously—don't add it to foods at the table, and limit super-salty foods like chips to a once-in-a-while indulgence.

"Keep daily salt to no more than one teaspoonful—or its equivalent (2,000 milligrams) in sodium from food," she says.

Take calcium supplements. Although not all doctors agree, some research suggests that calcium is an important nutrient in keeping blood pressure levels healthy in at least some women, says Dr. Gerrond. In a study at the University of Florida Health Science Center in Jacksonville, researchers found that 2,000 milligrams of calcium a day reduced the onset of high blood pressure in pregnant women by 54 percent. Doctors don't know the exact mechanism that seems to be at work. But experts say that women should be sure to get the optimum daily intake for calcium, which is:

- 1,000 milligrams a day if you're under age 50 or on hormone replacement therapy
- 1,200 to 1,500 milligrams daily if you're pregnant or nursing
- 1,500 milligrams a day if you're postmenopausal and not taking estrogen, or if you're over age 65

"Most women don't consume enough milk, yogurt or other food sources of calcium, presumably because they're worried about the calories," says Dr. Gerrond. Nonfat dairy products or calcium supplements (or a combination of both) can help assure you consume protective amounts.

Trash tobacco. For those just starting, the powerful chemicals in inhaled cigarette smoke prompt blood vessel walls to constrict temporarily, increasing pressure on blood coursing through the arteries, says Dr. Katz. In addition, smoking greatly increases your risk for stroke, often blamed on high blood pressure. So if you smoke, quit.

Save alcohol for special occasions (or don't drink at all). Drinking alcohol in excess tends to raise blood pressure, so doctors advise moderation or abstinence. If you enjoy drinking, Dr. Katz suggests limiting yourself to two glasses of wine or bottles of beer a day at the most. And if you don't drink, don't start.

High Cholesterol
Little Changes, Big Benefits

*Y*ou're not a big eater. A bagel with a smear of cream cheese for breakfast, an egg salad sandwich for lunch and a pork chop with a salad for dinner will make you a happy camper.

But your doctor is worried. Blood tests show that your cholesterol is a little high—especially the reading for low-density lipoprotein (LDL) cholesterol, a bad sort notorious for clogging arteries with a soft, waxy substance that can harden into plaque. And your doctor seems to think that a steady diet of your favorites from the meat and dairy world is paving the way for heart disease.

Given the fact that your arteries have had three or four decades to accumulate cholesterol, you may find yourself wondering, "Is there anything that I can really do?"

"Absolutely," says Valery Miller, M.D., medical director of the Lipid Research Clinic at George Washington University Medical Center in Washington, D.C. "If you lower your LDL cholesterol to less than 100 milligrams per deciliter (mg/dl), the soft stuff will come off your arteries."

Besides measuring LDL cholesterol, your blood test also measures high-density lipoprotein (HDL) cholesterol—the "good" stuff that escorts LDL cholesterol out of the body.

Both readings are important, says Dr. Miller. If you can drop your LDL cholesterol to below 130 mg/dl and increase your HDL cholesterol to around 55 mg/dl, your risk of heart disease is significantly reduced.

But what about total cholesterol?

"Worrying about total cholesterol is passé," says Linda L. Colle Gerrond, M.D., director of the Center for Women's Health at the Shawnee Mission Medical Center near Kansas City, Kansas. "The focus now should be on LDL, HDL and triglyceride levels."

Here's how women doctors say that you can reduce high levels of LDL cholesterol.

Declare your plate a low-fat, cholesterol-free zone. Cholesterol is only found in animal products. Avoid foods loaded with saturated fat and cholesterol, such as red meat, liver, butter, cheese and eggs, says Dr. Miller. Saturated fat raises blood levels of cholesterol. True, your body uses cholesterol to make hormones and cell membranes, but it can manufacture what it needs without dietary assistance. So every time you eat a food that contains saturated fat and cholesterol, chances are that it ends up contributing to blood levels of LDL cholesterol.

Trade fiber for fat. Gradually substitute high-fiber foods for high-fat foods, says Linda Van Horn, R.D., Ph.D., professor of preventive medicine at Northwestern University Medical School in Chicago. Foods high in soluble fiber, such as oat bran, oatmeal, barley and beans, have the wonderful ability to help decrease LDL cholesterol, especially as part of a low-fat diet. What's more, eating high-fiber foods can help decrease your cravings for fatty, high-cholesterol foods like cheese and bacon by filling you up.

"If you stick with a high-fiber, low-fat diet, you can see a change in LDL cholesterol in as little as three weeks," says Dr. Van Horn. Your taste for burgers, three-cheese omelets and cheesecake usually disappears in about the same amount of time, she says.

Start with breakfast. Read cereal box labels and pick one that's high in fiber (five grams per serving or higher) and low in fat (three grams per serving or, preferably, lower), says Dr. Van Horn.

Go for the grain. Whole-grain bread has more fiber than white bread. And be careful with other breads like rye and pumpernickel, since they are often just white bread with a small percentage of rye grain added, says Dr. Van Horn. When buying bread and rolls, make sure that the whole grain—like whole wheat, oats, rye or millet—is listed as the first ingredient on the label.

Don't fry—ever. Cooking food at high temperatures in oil, shortening, margarine or butter can increase the risk of raising LDL cholesterol, says Dr. Van Horn. Instead, steam, microwave and broil foods.

A spritz or drizzle will do. When you must use something slippery to keep food from sticking, use a vegetable oil spray—preferably canola oil or olive oil—that will leave just a whisper of fat, Dr. Van Horn says.

Load up on plant foods. Citrus fruits, yellow-orange vegetables and dark leafy greens are rich in fiber and antioxidants such as vitamin C. Antioxidants are naturally occuring vitamins, minerals and other substances that, among other benefits, seem to help prevent damage to artery walls. Soy foods have flavonoids, saponins and other natural substances known as phytochemicals that can also help lower cholesterol or reduce clogged arteries (or both), says Dr. Van Horn. For similar reasons she advises using garlic and onions liberally.

Scientists haven't yet figured out how much of any one food that we need to eat in order to get a therapeutic amount of a particular cholesterol-lowering substance, says Dr. Van Horn. So the best strategy is to make sure that your diet is rich in all these plant-based foods.

Sweat. Dietary changes alone tend to drop HDLs along with LDLs, says Dr. Gerrond. Luckily, exercise can preserve your HDLs. So after checking with your doctor about your regimen, be sure to get 30 minutes of aerobic exercise three times a week. Examples of aerobic exercise include walking, swimming, jogging and skipping rope. Choose an activity that you like.

Hives
Relief for the Maddening Itch

Hives are small red bumps on your skin that tend to occur for no apparent reason. Hives generally crop up singly or in clusters, itch intensely, give you the urge to scratch, then disappear within a few hours.

Occasionally, hives linger for an entire day or return for regular visits. And you may never figure out what triggered the outbreak, say doctors.

A BIG MYSTERY

"A million different things can cause hives," says Karen S. Harkaway, M.D., clinical instructor of dermatology at the University of Pennsylvania School of Medicine and a dermatologist at Pennsylvania Hospital, both in Philadelphia.

"The most common causes of hives are food and medication," says Helen Hollingsworth, M.D., associate professor of medicine at Boston University School of Medicine and director of allergy and asthma services at Boston University Medical Center Hospital. "For example, a frequent cause of hives is nonsteroidal anti-inflammatory agents such as over-the-counter pain relievers that women use all the time." No one is exactly sure why it happens. The most likely to trigger a reaction are aspirin, ibuprofen (such as Motrin and Advil) and naprosyn (Aleve)—the sort of drugs that women take for menstrual cramps, muscle strains and headaches.

Other causes of hives include fever blisters, allergies or infections,

289

WHEN TO SEE A DOCTOR

If you have hives that last for more than 24 hours or hives that leave a bruise when they go away, check with your doctor, says Helen Hollingsworth, M.D., associate professor of medicine at Boston University School of Medicine and director of allergy and asthma services at Boston University Medical Center Hospital. You may have an underlying problem such as thyroid disease that requires medication.

You should also go directly to an emergency room if you have hives around your eyes or in your mouth, or if you have difficulty breathing, says Karen S. Harkaway, M.D., clinical instructor of dermatology at the University of Pennsylvania School of Medicine and a dermatologist at Pennsylvania Hospital, both in Philadelphia. You may require a shot of epinephrine (a synthetic form of adrenaline) to prevent the hives from causing your throat to swell shut.

plus foods such as nuts, licorice, blue cheese and shellfish, says dermatologist Esta Kronberg, M.D., a dermatologist in private practice in Houston.

A hot shower, exercise or even a stressful event can also trigger hives, says Dr. Hollingsworth. Even pressure from a bra strap, tight shoes or a shoulder bag can cause hives in susceptible individuals.

Hives are formed when any of these triggers sends a flood of immune substances known as mast cells coursing through your blood vessels, squirting an inflammatory substance called histamine into your cells. The vessel will become swollen and leak, forming the red, itchy bump that you see and feel as a hive.

SOOTHE, DON'T SCRATCH

"Trying to figure out what caused hives can be bewildering," says Dr. Harkaway. "So doctors generally just initially prescribe antihistamine medication—to eliminate the itch and inflammation—and hope that the hives will go away." If the hives do not go away within six weeks, the doctor will do tests to try and determine the cause.

Home treatments for hives are also aimed at eliminating the itch. (Besides, scratching only makes hives worse.) Here's what women doctors suggest.

Put the hive on ice. To constrict the blood vessel involved, prevent further leakage and begin to shrink the hive, rub an ice cube over the hive—or hives—for several minutes, says Dr. Harkaway.

Soak in an oatmeal bath. To relieve the itchiness of hives, add Aveeno brand colloidal oatmeal (an over-the-counter bath powder available at your local drugstore) to a tub full of lukewarm water. It stays suspended in water, so it won't clog your drain. Soak yourself for 10 to 15 minutes, suggests Dr. Kronberg. But avoid using hot water—it can make hives worse.

Apply medicated lotion. After your bath, smooth Sarna lotion over your skin, says Dr. Kronberg. Follow package directions. Soothing ingredients such as menthol and phenols in Sarna reduce itchiness.

Moisturize your skin. Dry skin tends to cause itching, which can irritate hives and make them worse. So if your skin tends to be dry, apply a moisturizer to the area around the hives as well, says Dr. Hollingsworth.

Stay cool. Heat of any kind will make hives worse. So until your hives subside, you'll be more comfortable if you keep as cool as possible, says Dr. Hollingsworth.

Wear loose clothes. Pressure generated by tight shoes and clothes are known to cause hives, so be particularly careful to wear loose clothing when you have hives, says Dr. Hollingsworth. The last thing that you want to do is encourage them to proliferate.

Watch your diet. Be cautious about eating things like tomato sauce, citrus, strawberries and shellfish while you have hives, advises Dr. Hollingsworth. Although no one knows why, these foods frequently aggravate hives.

Take an antihistamine at bedtime. Taking an over-the-counter antihistamine such as Benadryl can prevent hives from getting worse, says Dr. Kronberg. The usual dose is 25 milligrams of Benadryl once a day. Benadryl tends to make you sleepy, so she recommends taking it at bedtime. That way, you get the medication's full therapeutic effects without having to put up with daytime drowsiness.

Hot Flashes
No More Flushes and Night Sweats

*D*id someone just turn up the heat to a toasty 500°F, or are you having a hot flash?

If your chest suddenly feels warm and the heat quickly spreads to your face and neck, and you're going through menopause, chances are that you're experiencing a hot flash. A hallmark of menopause, researchers theorize that the drop in production of the female hormone estrogen and other hormonal changes associated with menopause somehow disrupt the body's heat regulation system (at least for a few months). Blood vessels in your face and neck dilate, your heart races, your skin gets warm and you sweat like you just sprinted around the block on a 90° day.

RED-HOT CHICKS

Hot flashes are temporary—for most women, they persist for anywhere between 9 and 16 months, according to Liliana Gaynor, M.D., D.D.S., clinical assistant professor in the Department of Obstetrics and Gynecology at Northwestern University Medical School in Chicago. But they're bothersome and embarrassing. Women doctors say that these remedies can provide some relief.

Keep cool. "Heat itself can trigger hot flashes," says Mary Jane Minkin, M.D., associate clinical professor at Yale University School of Medicine and co-author of *What Every Woman Needs to Know about Menopause*. In hot weather, head for an air-conditioned environment. When it's chilly outside, keep rooms heated comfortably—not overly hot.

Avoid dramatic temperature swings. "Some women find that it isn't heat per se that aggravates hot flashes but dramatic temperature changes," notes Lois Jovanovic-Peterson, M.D., clinical professor of medicine at the University of Southern California in Los Angeles and author of *A Woman Doctor's Guide to Menopause*. "Going from blistering heat into an air-conditioned building or room (or vice versa) can provoke the onset of hot flashes." She suggests that you wait a few minutes in a semi-cool lobby before entering an air-conditioned or heated room.

Breathe Deeply

Suzanne Woodward, Ph.D.

Slow, deep breathing throughout the day is effective in lessening the intensity and frequency of hot flashes, says Suzanne Woodward, Ph.D., a psychologist and assistant professor of psychiatry at Wayne State University School of Medicine in Detroit. She and her colleague Dr. Robert Freedman concluded this from a study in which they trained menopausal women to breathe from their abdomens, inhaling and exhaling six to eight times per minute. They hypothesize that deep breathing slows the metabolism, or modulates body temperature, or the production of certain brain chemicals related to hot flashes.

"Practice as often as possible and do it particularly when a hot flash begins," Dr. Woodward advises. She successfully uses the technique herself when she is awakened by hot flashes at night. "It helps me relax and get back to sleep."

Dress for success. In sweater weather, wear a T-shirt underneath a long-sleeved shirt underneath a sweater, so you can peel down to the T-shirt if you have a hot flash and pile it all back on when you cool off, suggests Dr. Minkin. Cotton and other natural fibers and athletic-wear fibers like polypropylene are best, because they help release heat and moisture instead of keeping it against your skin.

Skip the spices. Hot tamales or curried chicken may taste great, but they tend to trigger hot flashes. "They probably set off the temperature regulation mechanism that's at the genesis of a hot flash," says Veronica Ravnikar, M.D., professor of obstetrics and gynecology and director of the Reproductive Endocrinology and Infertility Unit at the University of Massachusetts Medical Center in Boston. If they bother you, skip them.

Cut caffeine. Caffeine is a stimulant and can trigger hot flashes by raising your blood pressure and heart rate, says Dr. Ravnikar. You probably don't need to completely cut out caffeine, but try to go easy on coffee, tea and soft drinks containing caffeine.

Steer clear of sweets. Eating sugar boosts your metabolism and, in turn, generates heat, says Dr. Gaynor. So if you want to avoid hot flashes, put the sweets away.

Abstain from alcohol. Research has shown that right after consuming alcohol, a woman's estrogen levels go up dramatically, says Dr.

WHEN TO SEE A DOCTOR

The vast majority of women who get hot flashes don't find them debilitating, says Mary Jane Minkin, M.D., associate clinical professor at Yale University School of Medicine and co-author of *What Every Woman Needs to Know about Menopause*. But for others, hot flashes are quite bothersome, keeping them up nights and otherwise interfering with their day-to-day lives. If you are uncomfortable and want help, see your physician to discuss medical approaches, particularly the pros and cons of hormone replacement therapy.

Incidentally, you don't have to be menopausal to experience hot flashes. Some medications, including estrogen-controlling drugs prescribed for endometriosis (an abnormality of the uterine lining) and tamoxifen for breast cancer, can induce hot flashes.

Ravnikar. These temporary "spikes" may be followed by sudden drops in estrogen, which can lead to hot flashes.

Fill up with soy. Soybean products contain phytoestrogens—natural plant compounds that act like estrogen. "Researchers have found that women in Japan and other Asian countries—who eat something like 35 to 45 milligrams of plant estrogens a day in the form of tofu, soy milk and other soy products—seem to experience fewer hot flashes," says Margo Woods, M.D., associate professor of community health in the Department of Family Medicine and Community Health at Tufts University School of Medicine in Boston.

Researchers in Australia found that menopausal women who ate soy flour daily for 12 weeks showed a 40 percent decrease in hot flashes.

SLEEPING THROUGH NIGHT SWEATS

No, night sweats aren't workout clothes that you wear to bed. They're hot flashes that wake some women in the middle of the night, drenched in perspiration, while they're going through menopause.

"Night sweats are a real problem for women who can't take estrogen replacement therapy," says Suzanne Woodward, Ph.D., a psychologist and assistant professor of psychiatry at Wayne State University School of Medicine in Detroit. "There is no way to eliminate night sweats—but there are ways to make yourself more comfortable and minimize their disruption of sleep."

Here's what Dr. Woodward suggests that you do if a night sweat strikes.

Sip ice water. Keep a carafe of ice water on your night table and sip as needed.

Take nine or ten slow, deep breaths. Repeat for several minutes, until the night sweat passes.

Turn down the thermostat. Keep the bedroom cool—no warmer than 72°F. Sleep with a fan operating by your bed, even in winter. And use light blankets only.

Sleep in all-cotton night clothes and sheets. Synthetics or blends trap body heat and can trigger a night sweat.

Hyperventilation
Bag Bad Breathing

Take a nice long, slow breath. Now, take another one. There. Feel better? Most of us respond to deep, slow breathing pretty much the same way. We relax, and can feel the tension in our bodies drain away.

Breathing isn't something we normally have to think about—we inhale and exhale at a fairly steady pace, without much thought or worry over how we're doing. People who tend to hyperventilate, or overbreathe in rapid, shallow or deep, heaving breaths may get anxious, further preventing them from breathing normally, says Sally Wenzel, M.D., associate professor at the University of Colorado School of Medicine and a pulmonary specialist at the National Jewish Center for Immunology and Respiratory Medicine, both in Denver.

Hyperventilation sets off physical changes that can make people feel even more breathless, and they may feel as though they're suffocating, Dr. Wenzel explains.

People with lung problems such as asthma or emphysema also sometimes hyperventilate when they're feeling short on air. And women report hyperventilation more so than men, Dr. Wenzel says.

Here's how it works: Getting the right amount of oxygen into the bloodstream depends on a balance of carbon dioxide and oxygen in the blood. When you hyperventilate, you release extra carbon dioxide with each breath, which throws that balance off.

A drop in carbon dioxide levels in the blood also can cause other alarming symptoms: faintness; numbness; visual disturbances; tingling in the arms, legs and mouth; headaches and even chest pain.

"Women may think that they are having a heart attack, or going to pass out, which seldom happens," says Dr. Wenzel. Once they understand that the physical symptoms that can accompany hyperventilation aren't serious, they're less likely to panic when these symptoms occur.

EVEN-KEELED BREATHING

Here's what women doctors, respiratory therapists and even a yoga instructor advise for women who overbreathe.

Keep your mouth shut. "It's very hard to hyperventilate through your nose," Dr. Wenzel says. "You just can't move that much air."

Learn belly-breathing. People who hyperventilate typically are shallow breathers, filling only their upper chest when they inhale, says Dr. Wenzel. So they need to learn belly-breathing, or diaphragmatic-breathing. This technique makes them use their entire lungs to breathe, and it also slows their rate of breathing.

Here's how Jane Hunter, a Bound Brook, New Jersey yoga instructor teaches belly-breathing.

Sit on a hard, straight chair with your feet firmly on the floor. (If your feet don't fully reach the floor, prop them up on a book or footrest.) Keep your knees hip-width apart and sit forward on your buttock bones.

Keep your spine very straight, your belly relaxed and your mouth closed. Notice the flow of air in and out of your nostrils. Pay close attention to how your lungs feel. Just doing that slows your breath.

Each time you inhale, consciously relax your airways and breathe a little more deeply. Gradually lengthen your breaths. Feel the breath entering and leaving your lungs. Let your belly expand when you inhale and contract when you exhale. "And as your lungs begin to relax, you can actually control the rhythm of your breathing by expanding the belly muscles to make room for the lungs to move down," Hunter says.

And once you reach a point where you are breathing deeply from the bottom of your lungs, try to equalize your breath so that inhaling takes the same amount of time as exhaling does, she advises. "Smooth

WHEN TO SEE A DOCTOR

If you just can't seem to catch your breath, if you frequently feel tired and winded, or if you sigh a lot, see a doctor. You could have a heart or lung problem that requires medical attention, says Sally Wenzel, M.D., associate professor at the University of Colorado School of Medicine and a pulmonary specialist at the National Jewish Center for Immunology and Respiratory Medicine, both in Denver. Anemia, too, can produce feelings of breathlessness or shortness of breath, along with fatigue. Deficiencies of iron, vitamin B_{12} and folic acid can cause anemia.

If your doctor can find no physical reason for your breathing problems, you may want to see a psychologist. Look for one who offers help for anxiety disorders.

out your breath so that there are no huffs and puffs."

Practice belly-breathing for five to ten minutes at least once a day.

Breathe into a brown paper bag. This tried-and-true remedy works by making you rebreathe the carbon dioxide that you have exhaled, so blood levels of carbon dioxide rise, says Dr. Wenzel.

"Some of the people with breathing problems I see, especially those with anxiety problems, will feel better carrying around a bag with them for a while," says Betty Booker, a respiratory therapist and pulmonary rehabilitation coordinator at University Hospital in Denver. "It's better for these people to learn to breath properly from their diaphragms, however. Once they've learned that, they seldom need paper bags."

Loosen up. Your clothes, that is. Tight belts and waistbands, girdles, bras, skintight designer jeans, all can restrict diaphragmatic breathing and can make shallow, upper-chest breathing the only kind that you can manage, says Booker.

To take in a deep breath, your diaphragm must relax and drop downward. This creates a vacuum in your lungs that makes them automatically fill up with air, explains Dr. Wenzel.

Get a move on. "Aerobic exercise forces you to breathe properly," Dr. Wenzel says. "You can't run for long taking shallow breaths." Exercise can also counterbalance anxiety, she adds, which contributes to hyperventilation. If you haven't exercised for a while, start out gradually, walking or using a stationary bicycle. Increase to a pace that's comfortable but effective for you, Dr. Wenzel advises.

Incontinence
More Control, Less Worry

*Y*ou know the line: You laughed so hard ... You know the rest. But when a woman loses control of her bladder often enough to be a problem, it's not funny—it's urinary incontinence.

In women incontinence usually takes one of two forms: stress incontinence or urge incontinence. If you leak urine during exercise or when you cough, laugh or sneeze, most likely you have stress incontinence, says Margaret Baumann, M.D., associate chief of staff for Geriatrics and Extended Care at Veterans Administration West Side Medical Center in Chicago. Caused by weakness of the pelvic area muscles incurred during childbirth, abdominal surgery (such as hysterectomy or laparotomy) or by changes associated with menopause, stress incontinence is fairly common. Nearly half of all pregnant women experience some temporary bladder leakage.

If you have the urge to go to the bathroom but can't get there in time, you probably have what's called urge incontinence, Dr. Baumann says. Normally, your bladder sends signals to your brain that it's time to urinate, and then the brain tells the bladder to wait. Urge incontinence occurs when that pathway is damaged by urinary tract infections, changes in pelvic muscles associated with menopause, or neurological disorders, such as stroke or (rarely) multiple sclerosis.

BONA FIDE CURES

Doctors say that eight out of ten women with urinary incontinence can be helped. "If you know what to do, you can improve," says Dr. Baumann. Here's what to try.

Try the tampon fix. According to a study conducted by Ingrid Nygaard, M.D., assistant professor in the Department of Obstetrics and Gynecology at the University of Iowa College of Medicine in Iowa City, women with stress incontinence are helped by inserting a tampon in the vagina. "We had women insert a super-size tampon a little lower than if they were menstruating. For women with mild stress incontinence—who lose less than a teaspoon of urine per episode—the tampon worked really well."

298

Dr. Nygaard says that inserting a tampon works, because it pushes against the wall of the vagina and compresses the urethra (the duct that carries urine out of the bladder). She advises women to use the tampon fix for emergency situations only—a tennis match or a meeting, for example. "The vagina is drier without the menstrual flow, so place a few drops of water on the tampon before inserting it. And remember to remove the tampon by the end of the day to prevent toxic shock syndrome, a serious condition associated with leaving tampons in for too long."

Use Kegels to build pelvic muscles. Kegels, or pelvic-muscle exercises, build strength and endurance in the muscles of the bladder. According to women doctors, Kegel exercises are now the first-line approach in treating most types of incontinence.

To do Kegels, you quickly contract your pelvic-floor muscles (the ones that you use to control your urine stream) for one or two seconds, then relax the muscles between contractions to prevent muscle fatigue and spasticity, says Tamara G. Bavendam, M.D., director of the Female Urology Clinic at the University of Washington Medical Center in Seattle. Do ten repetitions three to five times per day. As you repeat the exercise, hold the contractions for 5 seconds and gradually increase to 15 seconds three to five times daily.

"Basically, it's like holding in gas," says Dr. Bavendam. "In fact, one woman told me that she purposely ate a whole can of beans so she could practice contracting these muscles—a creative approach."

"When done correctly, Kegels are just as effective as surgery and medication for mild to moderate stress and urge incontinence, minus the side effects," says Dr. Baumann.

Call up a Kegel coach. To do Kegels correctly, women doctors advise getting some coaching from health care practitioners.

"Of all the exercises that you can do, pelvic-floor exercises win the prize for the hardest to learn," says Kathe Wallace, P.T., a physical therapist in private practice in Seattle.

Practice Kegels in the shower. "It takes about eight weeks of intense Kegel training before you notice any improvement at all," says Dr. Nygaard. "Be patient. You're bulking up a muscle in your pelvis. And just like any other muscle-building exercise, it takes time. If you're trying to get strong arms, you don't do just one push-up now and then."

Once you've successfully treated your incontinence, you can do Kegels while you're in the shower, driving your car or watching TV or during other routine activities as part of your maintainence program, says Dr. Nygaard. One study found that women who practiced Kegels three times a week had the most success, even after five years.

299

WHEN TO SEE A DOCTOR

If you leak urine when you cough, laugh or sneeze, or if you leak urine before you can make it to the bathroom, see a doctor—preferably a urologist or gynecologist experienced at treating urinary incontinence in women, advises Margaret Baumann, M.D., associate chief of staff for Geriatrics and Extended Care at Veterans Administration West Side Medical Center in Chicago. Women doctors say that performing pelvic muscle exercises, called Kegels, is the single most important home remedy for urinary incontinence. But they also emphasize the importance of getting expert instruction to do Kegels correctly. "If home remedies have not helped eliminate the problem, seek help and don't give up," says Dr. Baumann.

Women doctors say that you should also consult a physician if you have any of these symptoms, to rule out a more serious contributing condition.
- Pain or burning upon urinating
- Voiding more than two quarts of urine a day
- Blood in your urine
- Change in bowel habits
- Pain during intercourse
- Numbness or weakness in your arms or legs
- Changes in vision

"Correct practice pays off," says Wallace. "So many women come in after a Kegels exercise training session and are surprised by the results. They wish they had sought help earlier."

Urinate every three to four hours. "Regular voiding prevents the bladder from getting too full," says Dr. Nygaard. "A lot of busy women find that they are going once in the morning, then not again until they get home at night."

Traveling? Hold the fluid. When traveling without easy access to rest rooms, drink no more than one quart of fluid a day, for convenience, and plan your last beverage for two hours before your trip, advises Dr. Baumann. At your destination, remember to choose liquids other than alcohol or caffeine beverages like coffee, which stimulate urine production and make you go.

Indecision
Make Up Your Mind

E at from the Tree of Knowledge of Good and Evil or serve the same old bananas for dinner? Stay in Camelot or run off with Lancelot? Stand by your man in the presidential campaign or run for the office yourself?

Women's lives have always been packed with tough decisions and, consequently, opportunities for indecision.

Tough choices—whether to break the rules, how to handle relationships, what to do for a living—call for serious deliberation. There are, after all, risks to consider. Make bad choices, and you risk ending up with the wrong guy, choosing a dead-end career or getting expelled, if not from Eden, from your co-op.

Sometimes the risks accompanying a decision are so intimidating that a woman can get bogged down in protracted indecision, taking an inordinate amount of time to decide something that should be resolved much more quickly.

"When you are overwhelmed by potential risks, you feel like you can't commit to a decision," says Linda Welsh, Ed.D., director of the Agoraphobia and Anxiety Treatment Center in Bala Cynwyd, Pennsylvania. Prolonged indecision can ultimately rob you of choice.

"In some situations, if you don't make up your mind, you lose the opportunity to decide," says Camille Lloyd, Ph.D., professor in the Department of Psychiatry and Behavioral Sciences at the University of Texas Medical School at Houston. While you're scratching your head, the price of that growth stock that you've been eyeing may climb out of sight. The deadline for applying to grad school may pass. The guy who proposed marriage may decide that he wants a more enthusiastic partner.

In general, the more that you worry about mistakes, the harder decisions can come, says Dr. Lloyd. With practice, however, decision-making gets easier. The next time that you have to make a tough call, decide to go with this advice from the experts.

Do your homework. To make a decision with confidence, first compile and consider the relevant data.

"If a guy asks you to marry him, and you've known him only six months, you might well decide to keep dating him another year so that you can clarify certain things," says Dr. Lloyd. "Or, if you've been offered a new job but don't know what to make of your prospective supervisor, you might try calling someone who used to work for the company and ask about her. If you're trying to decide whether or not to go on hormone replacement therapy, maybe you need to go to the library and look up the latest studies or get a second opinion." And so forth.

List the pros and cons. Once you have the raw data, analyze it. Get a piece of paper, divide it in half and write "pro" on one side and "con" on the other. Say that you're offered a job in Chicago, for instance. In column one list the good stuff about the job (more money, added responsibility and so forth). In column two list the bad stuff (higher cost of living, far from friends and family, for instance). It's a classic way to help clarify matters, says Dr. Lloyd.

Form a backup plan. For any option that you may be contemplating, ask yourself, "What is the risk involved? What is the worst possible outcome? How likely is that outcome?" Then see if you can come up with a contingency plan that you can fall back on if you make that decision and the worst actually does come to pass. You may be able to plan for what Dr. Welsh calls a "redecision," a possible follow-up choice that mitigates undesirable consequences. Knowing what you're afraid of, and if you can handle it, will help you decide which course to take.

Talk about it. If you're having trouble identifying risks, or pros and cons, talking about your options with a friend or family member can help, says Dr. Welsh.

Accept your choice. If you've made a decision and aren't happy with the way things turned out, don't berate yourself, says Dr. Lloyd. There is no such thing as a "perfect" choice. Sometimes you can't get all the information that you need in the time available, or you can't foresee all the potential outcomes.

"It may well have been impossible to foresee the particular outcome that you're unhappy with," she says. "Remember that you made a reasonable decision based on the information that you had at the time."

Infertility
An Action-Oriented Approach

Sometimes you wonder why you spent all those years worrying about getting pregnant, because now you *want* to have a baby, but nothing is happening. Infertility is of particular concern among women over age 35, the age at which the female reproductive system starts showing signs of decline, from having fewer healthy eggs to producing less of the female hormone estrogen. Infertility can be hard on your emotions, too. A group of women in one survey reported that they felt more depression and anxiety going through the experience of infertility than they had at any other time in their lives.

IF AT FIRST YOU DON'T SUCCEED . . .

Couples are considered infertile if they have been having unprotected intercourse for a year and no pregnancy results. The cause varies from couple to couple. Whether you're working with an infertility specialist or not, here are some things that women doctors say you can do to help yourself.

Buy a test kit. Knowing when your ovaries are about to release an egg will give you a clue as to the best time to try to conceive, says Susan Treiser, M.D., Ph.D., co-director of In Vitro Fertilization (IVF) New Jersey in Somerset and co-author of *A Woman Doctor's Guide to Infertility*. Your best bet is an ovulation test kit, available from a drugstore. Use it around the eleventh day of your menstrual cycle, and follow the directions on the package.

Mind your mucus. Another ovulation clue: Cervical mucus in your vagina is normally sticky and opaque. Around mid-cycle, it becomes stretchy and clear, similar to the consistency of egg whites. This is a signal that you'll ovulate within about 36 hours, says Marilyn R. Richardson, M.D., clinical assistant professor of reproductive endocrinology at the University of Texas Southwestern Medical School and in practice with Reproductive Medicine Associates, both in Dallas. Cervical mucus aids the process of conception by collecting sperm in a sticky reservoir within the cervix and then transporting it into the uterus and fallopian tubes on

303

something of a time-release basis, increasing the odds of fertilization.

You've probably seen cervical mucus when you wiped yourself after using the toilet, but just never paid attention to it. The best way to check on the status of your cervical mucus is to examine the toilet paper used after you urinate, says Charanjeet Ray, M.D., an obstetrician/gynecologist and associate professor in the Department of Obstetrics and Gynecology at Rush Medical College of Rush University and attending physician at Illinois Masonic Hospital, both in Chicago. Or take a piece of tissue and gently wipe yourself, whether you've urinated or not. If the mucus is clear and stretchy and there's a lot of it, you're probably about to ovulate, she says.

Try three days off and three days on. Inundating the cervix and fallopian tubes with sperm will increase the chances that one of these guys will fertilize an egg. So when you're about to ovulate, Dr. Treiser suggests having sex daily for three days. To increase the odds still further, abstain from sex for two or three days prior: That way, your partner's sperm levels will be higher than usual.

Use a new approach. A study at the National Institute of Environmental Health Sciences in Research Triangle Park, North Carolina, suggests that a woman's fertile time actually ends with ovulation. Researchers

WHAT WOMEN DOCTORS DO

Bond with Others

Bethany Hampton, Ph.D.

A few years ago, Bethany Hampton, Ph.D., associate professor of psychology at Texas Woman's University in Denton, experienced infertility herself. She joined RESOLVE, a national organization with local support-group meetings, where women share their experiences and feelings.

"For infertile women the world looks so fertile. It looks as though everyone is having babies, and it eats them up," she recalls. "It's important to see that other women who have gone through this are functioning well. I think that was critical to my getting through it."

Dr. Hampton has since become the biological mother of two. And she made some friends at RESOLVE with whom she is still very close.

For more information, Dr. Hampton recommends contacting RESOLVE at 1310 Broadway, Somerville, MA 02144-1731.

WHEN TO SEE A DOCTOR

Infertility tends to increase as you age. A woman is born with all the eggs that she will ever have, and their quantity and quality diminish with the passing years. Consult a physician if you are under the age of 35 and have tried unsuccessfully to conceive for a year, or if you are over 35 and have tried for six months.

Any woman with problems such as irregular menstrual periods, endometriosis, fibroid tumors or a history of a pelvic infection should seek assistance sooner rather than later, since these may reduce her chances of becoming pregnant.

Time is of the essence, says Susan Treiser, M.D., Ph.D., co-director of In Vitro Fertilization New Jersey in Somerset and co-author of *A Woman Doctor's Guide to Infertility.* "It's important that you seek the help of an infertility specialist."

found that the women who got pregnant during the course of the study conceived when they had intercourse during a six-day period ending on the day of ovulation.

Or, have sex every other day. If you're not tracking ovulation, have intercourse every other day—particularly on days 8, 10, 12, 14, 16, 18 and 20 after the first day of your last period—says Dr. Treiser. This will ensure that when you do release an egg, there is sperm (which can survive for up to three days) in your fallopian tubes.

Lie still after sex. Standing up or running to the bathroom right after intercourse allows some semen to run out, says Dr. Richardson. Instead, lie back and wait for at least 10 to 15 minutes.

Use over-the-counter drugs selectively, if at all. Nonsteroidal anti-inflammatory drugs such as ibuprofen may compromise ovulation as well as implantation of the embryo to your uterus, says Dr. Richardson. If you need a painkiller around that time of the month, take aspirin or acetaminophen instead. Steer clear of antihistamines and decongestants, too, as they may reduce secretion of cervical mucus.

Stay away from smoke. Smokers, on average, take longer to conceive and have a higher incidence of miscarriage, says Dr. Treiser. Also, their eggs are less likely to succeed in IVF, in which a woman's eggs are removed, fertilized in the laboratory and returned to her uterus.

(For more advice from women doctors about your biological clock, and on dealing with the emotional fallout of delayed conception, see page 55.)

Influenza
Help for Whole-Body Flu Misery

Yesterday you felt perfectly fine. Today you feel as though someone has handed you a large appliance and asked you to carry it for two blocks. You have the flu, and you feel miserable.

Flu viruses change from year to year, keeping the bugs one step ahead of our immune systems, says Carole Heilman, Ph.D., chief of the respiratory diseases branch at the National Institute of Allergy and Infectious Diseases, part of the National Instiues of Health in Bethesda, Maryland. Disease-fighting antibodies produced after exposure to a previous year's virus no longer recognize the next year's strain, so we have no defense from any previous exposure.

What Women Doctors Do

Go to Bed!
Carole Heilman, Ph.D.

The chief of the respiratory diseases branch at the National Institute of Allergy and Infectious Diseases, part of the National Institutes of Health in Bethesda, Maryland, once had the flu while attending a meeting in Hawaii.

Carole Heilman, Ph.D., figures that she must have picked up the bug on the plane from the recycled air. (Planes are notorious for spreading the flu.)

Dr. Heilman learned her lesson the hard way.

"Instead of taking care of myself, I pushed myself to go on to my next meeting, and I got a secondary infection—a miserable case of bacterial pneumonia," she says. "I was a mess. The doctor gave me very strong, very expensive antibiotics, and I was out of commision for weeks.

"I've learned my lesson," she says. "Now, if I get the flu, I stay in bed for two days, wait for the fever to break, drink plenty of fluids and then go back to work."

WHEN TO SEE A DOCTOR

If you're over age 65 or have a history of respiratory problems or other chronic diseases, including heart disease, diabetes and kidney disease, don't take the flu lightly. See your doctor as soon as possible. And get a flu shot every fall. But for healthy women, doctors say that you don't necessarily need to seek medical treatment unless you have any of the following symptoms.

- Shortness of breath
- Chest discomfort
- Prolonged high fever
- Painful breathing
- Phlegm tinged with blood
- Pain around your eyes or cheekbones
- Earache
- Irregular or rapid heartbeat
- Asthma attack or wheezing

As soon as these symptoms develop, contact your doctor, who can prescribe either amantadine or rimantadine, both antiviral medications. They're most effective if prescribed early on.

IF YOU HAVE THE FLU

If you've been bitten by the flu bug, there's plenty that you can do at home to feel better.

Pick one drug, not several. "We advise women against taking multiple over-the-counter drugs to treat multiple flu symptoms," says Dr. Heilman. "Say you have a splitting headache, a stuffy nose and a cough. You could end up taking a painkiller like acetaminophen for your headache, plus a decongestant that contains the same drug, and a cough syrup. Drugs interact. To avoid overmedicating, pick your most uncomfortable symptom—the painful headache, for example—and treat that. Skip the OTC decongestants or cough syrups."

Get vaporized. "Plugging in a vaporizer and resting in bed for two days is key to treating the flu," says Janet McElhaney, M.D., assistant professor of medicine at the University of Alberta in Edmonton. "A vaporizer can make you feel better by returning moisture to dry, cracked nasal passages and lips. It can also help relieve a painful sore throat and loosen dried mucus."

Take a hot, steamy shower. "The steam acts as a vaporizer, because it can provide a moist environment," says Dr. McElhaney.

Fill the cup and don't say when. Dr. McElhaney recommends drinking at least one quart of liquid a day. "When you have a fever with the flu, your body can get dehydrated, driving the fever up even higher." Reach for water, fruit juice, seltzer water, mineral water, decaffeinated soft drinks and decaffeinated coffee and tea. "Caffeine is a diuretic, which can speed dehydration," she explains.

Gargle with saltwater. To relieve a sore throat, Dr. Heilman recommends gargling with one teaspoon of salt mixed into an eight-ounce glass of warm water.

Go to bed early. If you must go to work, at least go to bed earlier than usual, says Dr. Heilman. This will lessen the stress on your body and help it fight the infection.

Listen to your body. "Your body will tell you what it needs," says Dr. Heilman. "If you feel tired, rest in bed for two days. Most women ignore the symptoms and put themselves last—they need to start putting themselves first. If you take care of yourself, you will get better faster."

Ingrown Hair
Straighten Out Wayward Fuzz

New, high-tech razors make shaving a dream. A little lather, and they give legs the closest shave ever. No stubble! But you do have a line of tiny blemishes on your left calf.

What did you do wrong?

"You probably shaved too close," guesses Esta Kronberg, M.D., a dermatologist in private practice in Houston. And the result is ingrown hair.

An ingrown hair occurs in one of two ways, doctors agree. When you shave too close, you can nick the top of the hair follicle and cause it to become partially obstructed. That forces the hair inside to grow at an angle. Eventually, instead of growing straight up through the hair follicle, the hair pierces the side of the follicle and buries itself in your skin—and

WHEN TO SEE A DOCTOR

Most ingrown hairs straighten out within a week or two. If an ingrown hair persists or becomes infected, check with your doctor. You may need medication to clear up the infection and prevent scarring.

your skin reacts by setting up an inflammation that may appear as a tiny red bump.

An ingrown hair can also occur when an individual hair grows straight up out of a follicle, then curls back down and reenters the follicle, says Dr. Kronberg.

Women with thick, curly hair are particularly prone to this later type of ingrown hair, says Dr. Kronberg. But anybody who shaves any part of her body, uses wax to remove unwanted hair or plucks—rather than trims—hairs that appear on her chin is also likely to get an ingrown hair.

"Ingrown hairs are also common around the upper, inner thigh (also known as the bikini line)," adds Mary Stone, M.D., associate professor of dermatology at the University of Iowa in Iowa City. "Sometimes, because of the rubbing that occurs in that area, the follicles close up a bit, which tends to encourage the hair to bend and grow through the side of the follicle rather than straight up through what's left of the opening."

TAMING ERRANT HAIRS

Fortunately, ingrown hairs can be cleared up within a week or two. Here's what doctors suggest.

Use an antibacterial bar. To help clear up the inflammation, wash the ingrown hair area twice a day with a Panoxyl bar, an antibacterial soap of 10 percent benzoyl peroxide found at your local drugstore, says Dr. Kronberg.

Dab on some cortisone cream. Apply an over-the-counter hydrocortisone preparation such as Cortaid around the ingrown hair according to package directions, says Allison Vidimos, M.D., a staff dermatologist at the Cleveland Clinic Foundation. It will soothe any inflammation and speed healing.

Change your blade. If ingrown hairs are inflamed and infected, change your razor blade each time you shave until the ingrown hair is gone, says Dr. Stone. Otherwise, you can reinfect yourself.

PREVENTING FUTURE PROBLEMS

As with many skin problems, preventing an ingrown hair is fairly simple. Here's what women doctors suggest.

Shave, don't wax. If you're prone to ingrown hairs, remove unwanted hair by shaving rather than waxing, says Dr. Stone.

"Waxing is traumatic," she explains. "It rips out your hair at an angle." When the hair grows back, it grows back at the same angle instead of growing straight up, piercing the side of the hair follicle instead of reaching the opening on the surface of your skin.

Moisten hair. Try to protect your hair follicles by keeping a barrier of moisture between you and the blade, suggests Dr. Kronberg. You can use the expensive foams and gels if you like, but a mild soap like Cetaphil will also do the job.

Ingrown Toenails
Tame Tortured Toes

Toenails are made to be as tough as, well, nails. So when a toenail happens to dig into the delicate flesh of your tender tootsies, the pain ranks right up there with, say, stubbing your toe or getting it run over by a cement truck.

An ingrown toenail occurs when a nail—usually the outside edge of the big toe—grows into the neighboring soft skin. People whose toenails are convex are more likely to develop ingrown toenails than people whose nails are rather flat. How you cut your nails and the style of shoes that you wear can also make a big difference. "Women who trim their toenails to the quick, then squeeze their feet into tight shoes, are most likely to complain of pain from ingrown toenails," says Theresa G. Conroy, D.P.M., a podiatrist in private practice in Philadelphia.

WHEN TO SEE A DOCTOR

If you have an ingrown toenail and it's hot, red or begins oozing, it's infected. See a podiatrist without delay. You should also see a podiatrist if the nail bed of your toe has been injured, making your nail grow crooked.

SOOTHING THE HURT

To ease the pain of an ingrown nail, women podiatrists share this advice.

Take the plunge, feetfirst. To help soften the nail, immerse your foot in warm water for five to ten minutes, suggests Cheryl Weiner, D.P.M., a podiatrist in Columbus, Ohio, and president of the American Association for Women Podiatrists.

Then pack it. Work a bit of loose cotton under the nail where it's biting into your flesh. This helps lift the edge of your nail so it can grow past the tissue it is digging into, explains Dr. Weiner. "You have to get a feel for how much cotton to use and how far to insert it; too much can be worse than too little." The packing should not hurt. Check and replace the cotton each day.

Don't cut too close. Dr. Weiner recommends cutting your toenails straight across, even with the end of your toe. If you have tough nails, soak them first to ease trimming.

Give your toes elbow room. Add ingrown toenails to the list of foot woes that women podiatrists blame on pointy toed shoes that put the squeeze on your toes, says Kathleen Stone, D.P.M., a podiatrist in private practice in Glendale, Arizona. Your best bet: round- or square-toed shoes with a high toe box. Your toenails will thank you.

Inhibited Sexual Desire

More Sex, More Often, More Fun

*R*obin was happy. She'd met a nice guy. They'd fallen in love. They got married.

Then came the wedding night.

"When they started having sex, she had a terrible time," says Kathleen Gill, Ph.D., a clinical psychologist and sex therapist in Wellesley, Massachusetts, and a lecturer at Harvard Medical School.

Robin (not her real name) confesses that she simply wasn't interested.

Her lack of sexual desire and the problems that it caused in her marriage eventually brought Robin to Dr. Gill for professional help. Through therapy, the root of the problem came to light. Because Robin's father had hit her when she was a girl, she grew up fearing men, and intimacy made her feel vulnerable. And as a result, Robin's sexual desire hovered around zero.

Robin experienced a textbook case of what psychiatrists refer to as inhibited sexual desire (or hypoactive sexual desire disorder). And some degree of inhibited sexual desire isn't uncommon among women, says Dr. Gill.

If deep-seated conflicts are to blame, seeing a sex therapist or psychologist is the first order of business, says Barbara Bartlik, M.D., a psychiatrist and sex therapist with the Human Sexuality Program at New York Hospital–Cornell Medical Center in New York City.

In less extreme cases women continue to have active sex lives but have lost interest in sex, says Dr. Gill. When desire has fizzled, the culprit is more likely something more temporary, like stress, fatigue, conflict with the woman's partner, or unhappiness with her partner's technique.

Hormonal changes triggered by birth control pills, premenstrual syndrome, pregnancy, nursing, menopause, hysterectomy or hormone replacement therapy can put the kibosh on desire as well, says Dr. Bartlik. So can periodic bouts with depression or anxiety.

Fortunately, there are plenty of ways to cultivate desire.

312

PUMP UP YOUR LOVE LIFE

Here's what women doctors say that you can do if your sex drive has hit an all-time low.

Ask yourself, what's changed? If interest has waned, ask yourself, "What has changed since I was interested?" Maybe you're angry with your partner because he is increasingly caught up in his work and seems to be taking you for granted. If so, tell him how you're feeling, advises Dr. Gill.

Compare likes and dislikes. Maybe your sexual needs and your partner's needs aren't identical.

"Say he wants intercourse more often than you," says Dr. Gill. "You might agree to set aside time to engage in some other intimate behavior—oral sex, kissing, back rubs or hugging. The important thing is that you work out a mutually satisfactory compromise. If you feel pressured to have sex, your desire can get even more inhibited."

Get in touch—with your body and his. "One reason why some women have low desire is that they never become aroused," says Barbara Keesling, Ph.D., a sex therapist in Orange, California, and author of *Sexual Pleasure* and *How to Make Love All Night.*

Since arousal gives rise to desire, therapists recommend practicing a form of sensual massage that leads to arousal.

You and your partner should make dates to practice this. Set aside a half-hour to an hour when you won't feel rushed or distracted. To start, the two of you should stroke your own bodies, all over, focusing on how it feels to touch and be touched. If stray thoughts crop up (like "I should pick up the dry cleaning tomorrow"), turn your attention back to what you're feeling. Do whatever feels good. The idea is to learn what feels best.

Once you're familiar with your own bodies, take turns stroking one another. When you touch your partner, pay attention to how your fingertips feel running across his skin. Don't worry about pleasing him, since this can make you anxious and interfere with arousal. Ask him to let you know if you do something that makes him feel uncomfortable. When he touches you, focus on the sensation of being stroked. If he does something that bothers you, tell him. Let him know how you would like to be touched.

"Use 'I' statements," says Dr. Gill. "For instance, tell him, 'This is what *I* really like.' " That way, you avoid saying something that your partner could misinterpret as criticism of his technique.

If touching leads to intercourse, enjoy it. "But remember, intercourse isn't your immediate goal," says Dr. Gill. "Your goal is to get to know one another and what you each enjoy."

Make time for intimacy. "Most people operate under the myth

WHEN TO SEE A DOCTOR

When it comes to sexual desire, there's no normal level, says Merle S. Kroop, M.D., a psychiatrist and sex therapist in New York City. Whether you're enjoying sex three times a week, three times a month or three times a year, as long as you and your partner are satisfied and in good health, there's no need to worry.

If you're not satisfied, and efforts at self-help fail, women doctors say that you should consult a doctor to rule out medical causes. Various illnesses, such as depression, kidney disease, epilepsy, Lyme disease, chronic fatigue syndrome and thyroid disease, can inhibit sexual desire, says Dr. Kroop.

If menopausal or postpregnancy hormonal changes are causing vaginal dryness that inhibits desire, your doctor may prescribe creams to restore vaginal lubrication. And if deep-seated conflicts about sex are to blame, seeing a sex therapist or psychotherapist can help.

that spontaneous sex is the best kind," says Dr. Keesling. "But if you're waiting for spontaneity and nothing is happening, planned sex is better than no sex."

So set dates for sex.

"If you make a date for 10:00 P.M. on Saturday, you don't have to have sex promptly at 10:00," explains Dr. Keesling. "At 10:00, though, set things up so that they're conducive to having sex. Make sure that you have enough privacy. Take the phone off the hook, and make sure that you've bathed and primped and are feeling relaxed."

Set the scene. If candles, incense, soft lighting, pretty sheets and romantic music help get you in the mood, by all means, use them, says Dr. Gill.

Make love to Puccini or Streisand. Whether classical or pop, music can be a powerful aphrodisiac. "Music's ability to arouse depends on two things: its similarity to your heart rhythms—more likely with classical—or the memories attached to a song," says Dr. Keesling.

Insect Bites

Soothe the Itch

Red, swollen bumps are the bothersome but harmless symptoms of most bites from many common insects, including flies and mosquitoes. Most bug bites are an uncomfortable nuisance, but not a health hazard.

Bugs bite you because they're hungry. Like mini-vampires, they want to suck your blood. Usually, you don't even know what bit you. They dine and dash before you even realize that they've visited. "Most people find out that they've been bitten belatedly, when they realize that something hurts," says Leslie Boyer, M.D., medical director of the Arizona Poison and Drug Information Center in Tucson.

Other persistent little buggers, like blackflies, horseflies and deerflies, aren't so subtle. They go for the all-out attack, making a deep puncture wound and lapping up blood until they've had enough, says insect specialist May R. Berenbaum, Ph.D., head of the Department of Entomology at the University of Illinois at Urbana-Champaign.

Either way, the swelling, itching and red welt that you experience are reactions to the foreign proteins that the insect injected into your skin, says Dr. Berenbaum.

CHOOSE YOUR WEAPON

Regardless of what bit you, the treatment is the same, says Dr. Boyer. Here's what women doctors advise.

Wash away the itch. Even if a bite is mild, take time to wash it with soap and water. "Cleansing removes germs and allergy-provoking substances from your skin's surface so a bite doesn't get worse," says Dr. Boyer. For mild bites, washing may be all that's needed—they'll heal on their own, she says.

Rinse with cool water. Still uncomfortable? "Rinsing a bite with cool water can help take the itch and swelling down," says Dr. Boyer.

Try some ice. "If the bite is uncomfortable because of swelling and itching, you can also apply ice to cool your skin, decrease inflammation and calm your urge to scratch," recommends Constance Nichols, M.D.,

315

WHEN TO SEE A DOCTOR

Most insect bites are minor annoyances and can be easily managed at home. The following situations, however, call for medical attention.

- You have redness or streaking around the bite, yellowish pus and fever. These are signs of infection.
- You suddenly have trouble breathing, develop body-wide hives or feel faint after being bitten. You may be having a body-wide allergic reaction to a bite, which causes your airways to swell shut. Call your local emergency medical number immediately or get to a hospital right away.
- You develop significant swelling—a local allergic reaction—and taking an antihistamine such as Benadryl doesn't help.
- You repeatedly have local allergic reactions to bug bites. Your doctor may prescribe shots or medications.

Still in doubt?

"In general," says Leslie Boyer, M.D., medical director of the Arizona Poison and Drug Information Center in Tucson, "you should call a physician or a poison control center any time you're bitten and develop an alarming reaction within 12 to 24 hours."

an emergency physician and associate residency director in the Department of Emergency Medicine at the University of Massachusetts Medical Center in Amherst.

Apply an ice cube on and off for a few minutes at a time (but not much longer, because you could get frost bite), says Dr. Boyer. You can continue this process throughout the day as needed. Or wrap ice in a towel to make a cool compress.

Don't scratch. The more you scratch, the more you'll itch, so try to resist, says Dr. Nichols. Plus, scratching a bite can cause a secondary infection, because bacteria and germs under your fingernails can get into the opening in your skin, she warns.

To lessen the tendency to scratch, trim your fingernails, says Dr. Boyer.

Dab on hydrocortisone cream. Gently rub bites with hydrocortisone cream to soothe swelling and redness. "Put a bit on your finger and rub it in until it disappears, so the medicine absorbs in," says Dr. Boyer.

"The gentle massaging also gives you the sense of satisfaction that you get from scratching—except that it's much safer."

For easy application, look for Cortaid FastStick, a convenient roll-on form of hydrocortisone. It's available in drugstores.

Swab with calamine. Dab insect bites with drugstore preparations such as that old pink standby, calamine lotion, or Burow's solution to calm the itching sensation, suggests Saralyn R. Williams, M.D., a toxicologist and emergency physician at the San Diego Regional Poison Center.

Soak in an oatmeal bath. To soothe itchy skin, Dr. Nichols recommends Aveeno bath treatment, a powdered oatmeal preparation that you pour into a lukewarm bath. You can find it at drugstores.

Insomnia
Toss and Turn No More

When everyone else in the house is asleep, do you find yourself taking a sheep census? Or watching *I Love Lucy* reruns? Or folding laundry to wear yourself out?

If you're like most people with insomnia, you'll do just about anything to get a few good Zzzs.

One-third of all adults can't sleep at one time or another. And as women get older, they're especially prone to insomnia. Once you turn 40, you are 40 percent more likely to experience some degree of insomnia, thanks to the midlife hormonal changes that precede menopause. During and after menopause, a common cause of insomnia is nights sweats, or hot flashes that occur during sleep. (For practical ways to manage night sweats, see page 292.)

CAN'T SLEEP? READ THIS

For most women occasional insomnia isn't much of a problem. But a wakeful night can leave you less than perky for the day at hand.

WHEN TO SEE A DOCTOR

"If you've tried everything and still can't sleep, then it's time to see your doctor," says Rochelle Goldberg, M.D., assistant professor of medicine and neurology and cardiopulmonary director of the Sleep Disorders Center at the Medical College of Pennsylvania Hospital in Philadelphia. "She may refer you to a sleep disorders clinic for further evaluation."

Here's what women physicians advise for those who crave some shut-eye.

Turn the clock to the wall. "Staring at the clock makes you more tense about getting back to sleep," says Rochelle Goldberg, M.D., assistant professor of medicine and neurology and cardiopulmonary director of the Sleep Disorders Center at the Medical College of Pennsylvania Hospital in Philadelphia. "Instead of checking the time, concentrate on restful thoughts."

Dial into your comfort zone. "Make sure that your bedroom isn't too hot or cold," says Naomi Kramer, M.D., associate director of the Sleep Disorders Center at Rhode Island Hospital and assistant professor in pulmonary medicine at Brown University, both in Providence. Many people sleep best in a cool room, so turn down the thermostat when you turn out the lights.

Get out of bed. "If you haven't gone to sleep after 20 minutes, you could try to head for another room and do something dull," says Margaret L. Moline, Ph.D., director of the New York Hospital–Cornell Medical Center Sleep-Wake Disorders Center in White Plains, New York. If you distract your brain with something boring and stop fretting over your wakefulness, you'll nod off.

AND TOMORROW...

To prevent future episodes of sleeplessness, follow this advice.

Take a morning walk outside. "Light exposure during the day helps keep your body clock regulated," says Mary A. Carskadon, Ph.D., professor of psychiatry and human behavior at Brown University School of Medicine and head of the sleep research lab at E. P. Bradley Hospital, both in Providence, Rhode Island. "An early morning walk in the daylight upon rising will help promote sleep at night."

Set a daytime worry hour. "Set a concrete time for worrying during the day," says Dr. Goldberg. "Be very focused about it: List each worry in writing with a plan for handling each one. When a worry wakes you, tell yourself that you have it covered and go back to sleep."

Resist the urge to nap. Napping during the day after a sleepless night will only throw your body clock off balance, says Dr. Goldberg. "You want to consolidate your sleep and get enough of it," says Dr. Goldberg.

Set a bedtime. "Adults need a regular bedtime, just like children," says Dr. Carskadon. "We have body clocks that synchronize our systems. Establish a set sleep and wake time, then stick to it every day. That tells your clock to make you sleepy at night and wakeful in the morning."

Wind down before you get into bed. "Giving yourself about 45 minutes of 'quiet time' before you get into bed signals your body clock that the day is done and sleep time is imminent," says Dr. Goldberg. "Listen to soft music, write a letter, read something boring—but do nothing that jazzes you up (and nothing work-related)."

De-stress your bedroom. "You probably don't sleep in your office. Conversely, you shouldn't work in your bedroom," says Dr. Goldberg. "Your bedroom is for two things only: sleeping and sex. So remove your computer, your office reading pile, your fax machine and even your phone, if you can. And put your TV back in the living room where it belongs."

Lose the booze. "If you need a good night's sleep, don't have a nightcap," says Dr. Kramer. "Though you may feel relaxed at first, the alcohol will disrupt your sleep later. Avoid drinking anything alcoholic within two hours of bedtime." And of course, avoiding caffeine is smart, too.

Forget the smokes. "There's solid evidence that smoking disrupts sleep," says Dr. Carskadon. Nicotine is a stimulant. It raises blood pressure, gets your heart going faster and makes your brain more active.

Intermittent Claudication

Relief for "Angina of the Legs"

*D*ressed in sweats and sneaks, you step outside and breathe in the fresh fall air. You head toward the neighborhood park for your daily walk. As you reach the first cross-street, you pick up speed, swinging your arms and striding confidently.

Ten minutes later, a cramp in your calf stops you cold. You massage your leg, wait a couple of minutes, then resume walking—but more slowly this time.

That scenario is familiar to women with intermittent claudication. The leg arteries carrying blood from the heart and lungs become so narrowed by cholesterol deposits that blood (with its energizing cargo of oxygen) has difficulty getting through. So you feel pain.

"It's like angina of the legs," says Pamela Ouyang, M.D., associate professor of medicine at Johns Hopkins University School of Medicine and a cardiologist at Johns Hopkins Bayview Medical Center, both in Baltimore. The oxygen supply to calf muscles is temporarily insufficient, causing a cramped feeling. Older men and women with heart disease are most susceptible.

Here's what you can do.

Rest. "Intermittent claudication is brought on by walking, and it's relieved by rest," says Deborah L. Keefe, M.D., professor of medicine at Cornell Medical Center and a cardiologist at Memorial Sloan-Kettering Cancer Center, both in New York City. Essentially, your legs have worked so hard to walk that they've run out of air. So all you have to do is stop walking for a minute or two, blood flow will be restored, oxygen will saturate your muscles, and the pain will disappear.

Then, keep walking. Contradictory though it may seem, exercise can actually build a small network of collateral blood vessels that bypass the clogged arteries in your leg and give muscles an alternate supply of oxygen, says Dr. Ouyang. So even though walking can trigger occasional bouts of intermittent claudication, you still need to walk to build a natural bypass.

The trick is to walk right up to the moment that you feel pain, stop

WHEN TO SEE A DOCTOR

Calf pain triggered by walking should be evaluated by a doctor but does not indicate an emergency. If you have calf pain with very little walking or if the pain occurs while you are at rest, you should see a doctor at once, says Pamela Ouyang, M.D., associate professor of medicine at Johns Hopkins University School of Medicine and a cardiologist at Johns Hopkins Bayview Medical Center, both in Baltimore.

You should consult your doctor if you know you have intermittent claudication and:

- Leg pain wakes you up at night.
- You suddenly develop cold, numb or painful feet or legs.

until the pain stops, then resume movement, says Dr. Ouyang. Building new blood vessels takes time, she adds, but walking every day, as often as you can, should eventually pay off. You'll find that in time you can walk further and do more before pain sets in.

Seek a smoke-free environment. Cigarette smoke reduces the amount of oxygen available to your muscles, triggering the onset of intermittent claudication, says Dr. Keefe.

Irritable Bowel Syndrome
Pacify Digestive Turmoil

Sometimes it's called the angry gut. That's because if you have irritable bowel syndrome (IBS), your insides often stir up a fuss. Your digestive tract roils, rumbles and rolls out gas. You may suffer from frequent diarrhea, diarrhea alternating with constipation or just constipation. Usually, you have abdominal pain. And it's also likely that you'll experience flatulence and bloating.

An irritable bowel episode can ruin your day, keeping you in the bathroom when you would rather be out and about or when you have an important meeting to attend. In fact, an irritable bowel can make you an expert on where to find all the public bathrooms in town.

IBS tends to be a chronic, long-lasting problem. No one knows what causes it, though diet and stress are known to aggravate symptoms.

SOOTHING THE RUMBLES

Thankfully, women doctors say that making some simple changes in your diet and daily habits may help you turn your angry gut into a laid-back bowel.

Use laxatives sparingly. If you wake up with painful constipation or diarrhea, and you're about to get on a plane or attend an important event, it's okay to take a chemically based laxative or anti-diarrheal medication, says Ernestine Hambrick, M.D., a colon and rectal surgeon at Michael Reese Hospital in Chicago. Just don't make it a habit.

"You end up with a yo-yo effect that doesn't touch the underlying syndrome," says Dr. Hambrick. You'll go from constipation to diarrhea and back and perhaps even develop a lazy colon that no longer works on its own.

For long-term relief, you're better off relying on natural solutions, say women doctors.

Eat a lot of fiber. Fiber is key to stabilizing IBS, because it bulks up and softens stool, helping your irritable bowel become regular, says Ann

More Fiber, Slowly but Surely

Dietary fiber, say women doctors, plays a big role in the relief of irritable bowel syndrome (IBS). Jacqueline Wolf, M.D., a gastroenterologist, assistant professor of medicine at Harvard Medical School and co-director of the Inflammatory Bowel Disease Center at Brigham and Women's Hospital in Boston, and the nutritionists at the center, offer these suggestions.

- Increase your intake of dietary fiber slowly to allow your body adequate time to adjust. Start with 8 grams a day (the amount in one-third cup of Bran Buds cereal or two pears) and increase your intake by 3 to 4 grams a day until you reach 30 grams daily.
- If you experience excessive gas, bloating or diarrhea, add fiber more slowly (two grams a day instead of four).
- Eat fiber-rich foods before trying supplements, which are more expensive than food.
- Choose fresh rather than canned fruits and vegetables whenever you can.
- Sprinkle bran over hot and cold cereals, applesauce and yogurt.
- Toss in bran when you're cooking meat loaf.
- Add bran when baking homemade bread or buy 100 percent whole-grain breads.
- Plan meals around legumes, such as pinto or lima beans, instead of meat.
- Snack on high-fiber cereals and nuts instead of sugary sweets.
- Drink at least eight eight-ounce glasses of water daily to help form softer, bulkier stools.

Ouyang, M.B., B.S. (the British equivalent of an M.D.), professor of medicine and chief of the Division of Gastroenterology at the Milton S. Hershey Medical Center of the Pennsylvania State University College of Medicine in Hershey. So if you're constipated, fiber will help you go more often, and if you have diarrhea, it helps make the bowel movements more solid.

A sample day's worth of fiber might include a bran-based cereal for breakfast, a sandwich on whole-wheat bread for lunch, and a baked potato, a half-cup of peas and a cup of strawberries for dinner, says

WHEN TO SEE A DOCTOR

Like clockwork, you have always gone once a day. Gradually, you pass stool only every three days. Or vice versa. Or you have alternating constipation and diarrhea. These changes, or any other changes in bowel movements, especially when accompanied by abdominal pain aggravated in stressful situations and relieved by passing stools, are the cardinal signs of irritable bowel syndrome, says Ann Ouyang, M.B., B.S. (the British equivalent of an M.D.), professor of medicine and chief of the Division of Gastroenterology at the Milton S. Hershey Medical Center of the Pennsylvania State University College of Medicine in Hershey.

Other symptoms may indicate a more serious condition. See your doctor if you have:
- Blood in your stool
- Unexplained weight loss
- Diarrhea that causes you to wake up at night
- Constipation, diarrhea, abdominal pain or any combination of the three so severe that you can't work for several days or engage in social activities

Jacqueline Wolf, M.D., a gastroenterologist, assistant professor of medicine at Harvard Medical School and co-director of the Inflammatory Bowel Disease Center at Brigham and Women's Hospital in Boston.

Sample a supplement. The downside of fiber-filled foods is that while you're incorporating them into your diet, they can make you feel really bloated and gassy. If you're not used to a lot of fiber, women doctors suggest that you try a natural fiber supplement, such as Fibercon, Metamucil or Citrucel. Of these, Citrucel usually leads to the least gas formation, says Dr. Hambrick.

Supplements soften hard, dry stools and bulk up watery, loose stools, so they are effective whether your chief complaint is constipation or diarrhea.

Supplements are available in supermarkets and drugstores in granular or wafer form, so you can choose the type most palatable to you. They all require drinking extra fluid throughout the day, however, for them to function properly. A good way to do this is to drink something every other hour, suggests Dr. Hambrick.

Pick up some pectin. Pectin, another source of high fiber, is found in fruits such as papayas, oranges and grapefruit or in apple pectin—a granular natural supplement found in most health food stores, says Dr. Wolf. You can sprinkle apple pectin on your food or dissolve it in liquid.

Order water—and make it a double. "Water helps food move through your system smoothly and bulks up your stool," says Dr. Wolf. Try to down six to eight eight-ounce glasses a day.

Decaffeinate your life. "Caffeine is a major bowel stimulant; it makes material move through the bowel too soon," says Dr. Hambrick. But just cutting out coffee isn't enough. Chocolate, tea and soda also contain caffeine, so eliminate them from your diet, too.

Keep a diet diary. If you can't figure out what specific foods bother you, keep a diary to track your symptoms. One caveat: "The food that you just ate might not be causing your symptoms," says Dr Wolf. Delayed reactions to certain foods may kick in hours after you eat, so even a diary isn't foolproof. But it can provide useful clues.

Steer clear of wheat and dairy products. Many people with IBS are sensitive to wheat as well as milk and milk products, says Dr. Wolf. If you have this sensitivity and eat prepared foods, you may not realize that wheat or dairy products are among the ingredients unless you read the label. So read before you ingest. (For practical ways to cope with lactose intolerance, which can contribute to IBS, see page 336.)

Eat at home. For some, dining out is often a culprit regardless of what they eat, says Sheila Crowe, M.D., gastroenterologist and assistant professor of medicine in the Department of Internal Medicine in the Division of Gastroenterology at the University of Texas Medical Branch at Galveston. Even in the nicest, cleanest restaurants, people with IBS sometimes find that a lovely meal leads to problems. The reaction may be caused by rich or spicy foods or food additives.

Shake your bootie. "Exercise contributes mightily to the normal function of the colon; it moves things along," says Dr. Hambrick. Do whatever you like—swim, run, walk—any kind of aerobic exercise, at least three times a week, and four or five times if you can.

De-stress. Stress aggravates the symptoms of IBS. To calm down your colon, try to find a relaxation method that works for you, whether it's listening to a relaxation tape, meditating, or just taking time for yourself, says Robyn Karlstadt, M.D., a gastroenterologist at Graduate Hospital in Philadelphia. "Unplug yourself for 20 minutes a day."

One hint: Be a realist, Dr. Karlstadt says. Maybe you can't take time out when the kids get home from school. But what about while they're upstairs doing their homework? Think through all your options.

Jealousy
Turn Resentment to Your Advantage

Your husband arrives home late one evening to announce that he has a new assistant—a former Miss Texas who shares his appreciation of beef jerky, his enthusiasm for football, his conviction that the Three Stooges were comic geniuses and virtually every other opinion that he voiced to her over lunch.

Admit it: You're jealous—caught by that nasty mix of resentment and helplessness that grabs you by the throat when you fear that you may lose something you value to someone else.

Jealousy is closely related to envy, a mix of inadequacy and anger that torments you when you covet something that someone else has, says Shirley Glass, Ph.D., a clinical psychologist and marital therapist in the Baltimore area.

You are more likely to suffer the slings and arrows of both envy and jealousy—and suffer them deeply—if your self-esteem is on shaky ground, says June Price Tangney, Ph.D., clinical psychologist and associate professor at George Mason University in Fairfax, Virginia, and co-author of *Self-Conscious Emotions*. But no one is immune.

"These are normal feelings—just like anger and boredom," says Harriet Lerner, Ph.D., a senior staff psychologist at the Menninger Clinic in Topeka, Kansas, and author of *The Dance of Intimacy*, *The Dance of Anger* and *The Dance of Deception*.

THE FEMALE SIDE OF JEALOUSY

What makes us jealous? As a rule, women are more likely than men to feel jealous or envious of relationships, while men are more often tormented by differences in status, income and power.

The big problem with jealousy and envy is that they distract you from the matter at hand—namely your own life. If you are preoccupied with someone else's circumstances, you might not pay sufficient or appropriate attention to enhancing your own, says Dr. Glass.

On the other hand, jealousy and envy do you some good if they motivate you to change—to improve your appearance, learn new skills or

WHEN TO SEE A DOCTOR

Uncontrolled, jealousy and envy can be so intense and so un-relenting that you need help dealing with them, says Leah J. Dick-stein, M.D., professor and associate chair for academic affairs in the Department of Psychiatry and Behavioral Sciences and associ-ate dean for faculty and student advocacy at the University of Louisville School of Medicine and past president of the American Medical Women's Association. Call your local mental health clinic, employee counseling service or therapist if:

- Jealousy or envy is interfering with important relation-ships in your life.
- You are so distracted by feelings of envy and jealousy that you can't focus on things that you want to accomplish.
- You have been dogged with jealousy and envy most of your life.
- You find yourself blaming or threatening people of whom you are jealous or envious.
- You avoid venturing out because you are afraid that you'll see things that make you envious or jealous.

work on your self-esteem, says JoAnn Magdoff, Ph.D., a psychotherapist in private practice in New York City.

Here's what experts have to say about managing jealousy.

Acknowledge your feelings. Denying your feelings is stressful, says Leah J. Dickstein, M.D., professor and associate chair for academic af-fairs in the Department of Psychiatry and Behavioral Sciences and associ-ate dean for faculty and student advocacy at the University of Louisville School of Medicine and past president of the American Medical Women's Association. Admit to yourself that you're jealous and learn from it. (In-terestingly, women seem to find it easier to acknowledge jealousy than men do, according to an Australian study.)

Ask yourself why you're jealous. If your husband, for example, ap-pears to be flirting with a co-worker, says Dr. Magdoff, you may actually be jealous of his relationship with his job, especially if it seems to offer more satisfaction than his relationship with you.

Of course, it's also possible that something may be going on with the woman at the party, says Dr. Glass. If you think so, tell him what you're feeling without making accusations.

Question your assumptions. If your friend gets a raise, don't carry on as though that precludes your getting a raise, too. "All too often, when someone else gets a raise, we act as though there's less possibility that we will receive one," says Dr. Tangney. "But that's a faulty assumption. There are actually very few situations in which that's true."

Turn envy into admiration. "If you envy someone because she has some quality, trait or skill that you don't, use that as a guide," says Dr. Glass. Take steps to cultivate the quality that you admire. If you wish that you could quote poetry, sign up for a poetry course. If you wish that you were slimmer, buy an exercise bike. If you wish that you had better business savvy, take an accounting course.

"Learn from the person who has what you want," says Dr. Dickstein. "You can ask her, 'What did you say in the interview for this job? How did you learn to do this?' Ask for her advice. You can turn someone you envy into an advisor and mentor."

Jet Lag
Cross Time Zones without Fatigue

*J*et lag can ruin the first couple of days of a trip for even the most frequent of fliers, interfering with alertness at business meetings or making you too miserable to sightsee.

What happens? You cross time zones too fast for your body clock to catch up. The result? You're in Europe (or L.A. or wherever), but your body clock is still back home. Which means that you're completely out of sync with the local day-night cycle, and you feel miserable.

"Jet lag affects everyone differently, but the most common symptoms include fatigue, sleep disturbances and insomnia, mild depression or irritability, gastrointestinal distress and headaches," says Maria Simonson, Sc.D., Ph.D., director of the Health, Weight and Stress Clinic at the Johns Hopkins Medical Institutions in Baltimore and a medical consultant to the International Cabin and Cockpit Crew Association.

Morning Light Is the Key

Suzan E. Jaffe, Ph.D.

Sleep disorder specialist Suzan E. Jaffe, Ph.D., didn't want jet lag to spoil precious moments of her Paris honeymoon. The consultant to the Veterans Administration Medical Center Sleep Disorders Center at the University of Miami in Coral Gables practiced what she preaches to many of her clients.

"The morning that my husband and I arrived, rather than climbing into bed and sleeping off jet lag, we sat in the sunshine on the hotel porch, having hot coffee and croissants and reading the paper," says Dr. Jaffe. "At first my husband thought that I was crazy, but he went along with it."

Sure enough, the bright morning sunlight helped their internal biological clocks to shift to Paris time. The newlyweds spent the afternoon strolling around the city and sight-seeing rather than sleeping. And they made it through the week without typical jet-lag symptoms like fatigue and moodiness.

Travel from east to west is usually easier to adjust to than travel from west to east. That's because you're pushing your body clock ahead instead of back. "It's much easier to rally and stay up later than it is to go to sleep earlier and get up earlier," says sleep disorder specialist Suzan E. Jaffe, Ph.D., a consultant to the Veterans Administration Medical Center Sleep Disorders Center at the University of Miami in Coral Gables. As a general rule, if your body is left to its own devices, it could take you about one day for every time zone that you crossed to adjust to the new schedule. And by that time, you could be back home again. The good news is that there are travel tricks that you can use to help reset your body clock more quickly.

CHANGE WITH THE TIMES

Photocopy these tips and tuck them in your suitcase for after-landing relief.

Get with the local motion. There's something to the old saying, "When in Rome, do as the Romans do."

"Adopt the local schedule as quickly as possible—the first day—to help your biological clock adjust to the new time zone," says Dr. Jaffe.

Eat when the locals do; wake up and go to sleep when they do. Force yourself to remain awake until at least 10:00 P.M. local time. This will help you get up on schedule the following morning, says Dr. Simonson.

Take a coffee break. If you've traveled from west to east, a single dose of caffeine (one cup of coffee, for example) at breakfast in your new location may help you stay alert, since you have essentially awakened six hours earlier than you customarily do. So suggests a small-scale study headed by Margaret L. Moline, Ph.D., director of the New York Hospital–Cornell Medical Center Sleep-Wake Disorders Center in White Plains, New York.

"Used sparingly and appropriately, caffeine can help you shift to the new time zone and get you over a hump in the day," suggests Dr. Jaffe. Don't overdo it, though. "Restrict coffee after lunchtime, or you may end up overstimulated, jittery and wide awake in the middle of the night."

Let the sun shine in. Exposure to light at the new destination helps convince your body clock that you truly are on a new time schedule, says Dr. Moline.

Research has shown that timing is important: In general, if you fly from west to east, get lots of sun early in the day, then restrict sunlight after 4:00 P.M., says Dr. Jaffe. If you fly from east to west, do the opposite. Restrict morning sunlight and get as much late-afternoon sun as you can. That doesn't mean that you should sunbathe—just go out shopping or relax at an outdoor cafe.

Snack for your stomach's sake. Your gastrointestinal system will be tender until it adapts to your new mealtimes. "You may not be able to stomach heavy meals or exotic local delicacies for a day or two. Until your gastrointestinal system has a chance to adjust, eat lightly and stick to foods that you're used to," says Dr. Jaffe.

Work it out. If it's daytime when you land, get some light outdoor exercise shortly after you arrive, like walking around the block or jogging, suggests Dr. Simonson. "The activity will help your circadian rhythms— 24-hour cycles—to biologically adjust to the time of day in the new place."

Snap up a nap. If you need to feel refreshed for an activity later in the day, take a short snooze. "You don't need a sleeping pill—just a nice quiet room," says Dr. Moline.

Limit daytime snoozes to no longer than 1½ hours and don't nap after 5:00 P.M., so you can fall asleep at bedtime, advises Dr. Simonson.

Give alcohol a rest. You may think that a cocktail will relax you, but it will actually do more harm than good. "Alcohol depresses your central nervous system and interferes with sleep patterns. It may help you fall asleep, but you'll wake up feeling lousy, because the drug effect still lingers," says Dr. Jaffe. "Don't drink in flight or on the first day after you arrive."

Knee Pain
Ice and Other Therapies

We demand a lot from our knees. We use them to go up and down stairs, bend when we pick up packages and children, run for fitness and walk properly even if we wear attractive-but-oh-so unnatural footwear like high heels.

Formed where the end of your thighbone, calf bone and kneecap meet, the knee is a complex joint: The bones are joined by ligaments, and the kneecap is attached to the bones by tendons.

Some protection is provided by two cushions, or pads (called meniscus), and by the bursae (strategically placed sacs of fluid that reduce friction.

The knee has to withstand a lot of pressure in a small space, yet "the knee wasn't constructed very well for the demands that we place on it," says Margot Putukian, M.D., team physician at Pennsylvania State University in University Park and assistant professor of orthopedic surgery and internal medicine at the Milton S. Hershey Medical Center in Hershey.

No wonder that the small, overworked joint rebels.

BE KIND TO YOUR KNEES

Women often get knee pain from kneeling to talk with or pick up kids, to garden or do filing or from running or walking a lot, says Elizabeth Arendt, M.D., associate professor of orthopedic surgery at the University of Minnesota in Minneapolis. "Housemaids knee" refers specifically to bursitis of the joint of the knee, and not to global knee pain.

331

WHEN TO SEE A DOCTOR

If your knee hurts and, despite use of home remedies, doesn't improve after a week, you should see a doctor, says Margot Putukian, M.D., team physician at Pennsylvania State University in University Park and assistant professor of orthopedic surgery and internal medicine at the Milton S. Hershey Medical Center in Hershey.

If the pain is so significant that you can't walk, it hurts to walk or your knee swells up, see a doctor immediately.

Here's what women doctors say that you can do to lighten the stress on your knees and reduce pain. (For practical ways to manage knee pain caused by arthritis or bursitis, see pages 24 and 537.)

Rest makes sense. If knee pain is triggered by gardening or other activities that you love, it's tempting to continue what you're doing, despite the pain—not a good idea.

To relieve the pressure and ease the inflammation and soreness, "get off your knees," says Letha Griffin, M.D., an orthopaedic surgeon at the Peachtree Orthopaedic Clinic in Atlanta.

Then, ice them. Apply an ice pack for no longer than 20 minutes at a time, as frostbite can occur on your skin, says Dr. Griffin. Ice your knees several times a day when they hurt or swell. Make sure that the ice is in a padded pack or wrapped in a towel so that it doesn't come in direct contact with your skin.

Wrap it and raise it. You should also compress your knee with a bandage that is secure but doesn't cut off circulation, like an Ace Bandage or a slip-on elastic knee sleeve, available at drugstores, says Dr. Griffin. Prop up your knee on some pillows to elevate it above heart level.

Kill the pain. An over-the-counter remedy containing aspirin, ibuprofen, ketoprofen (such as Orudis) or acetaminophen can help ease the pain, says Dr. Griffin.

Shed some weight. "If you're overweight and can lose weight, drop those pounds," says Dr. Arendt. "It will help relieve pressure on your kneecaps."

Wear comfortable, low-heeled shoes. High heels increase the pressure on your knees, says Dr. Griffin. "Instead, try walking around in shoes with low heels or no heels, or wear walking or running shoes."

Change positions. "Sitting for a long time can also put a lot of pressure on your kneecaps," says Dr. Arendt. Check the height of your chair to make sure that your feet are planted firmly on the ground. If they're not, get a lower chair or a stool for your feet.

Stretch your knees. From time to time during the day, bend forward and relax and straighten out your knees to make sure that they don't stiffen, says Dr. Arendt.

Break up long drives. Call it commuter's knee. "Your knees can really get stiff from being held in the same position during a long drive," Dr. Arendt says. "If you have cruise control, go for it—and stretch out your knees." If you don't, try to shift positions from time to time and try to take a break from driving once an hour.

Labor Pain

Beyond Deep Breathing

*L*ook up *labor* in a medical dictionary, and you'll see it described as "the function by which the product of conception is expelled from the uterus through the vagina to the outside world." In everyday language, labor (or childbirth) is better described as the effort used to push a baby through an opening that is usually the size of a tampon.

Labor is work—literally. And it takes not only one big push but four stages of delivery. First, the uterus (or womb, which carries the fetus) begins to contract and the cervix (the opening to the uterus at the top of the vagina) widens. In stage two the uterus continues to contract more frequently as the mother forcefully pushes the baby out through the vagina.

But wait, there's more: Next, the placenta (which attaches the fetus to the womb) is expelled or pushed out. Within hours after delivery—stage four—the uterus returns to near-normal size.

There's no way around it: Having a baby hurts, says Eileen Mur-

Medication Is Okay (and Sometimes Advisable)

If you plan to have a child naturally, great," says Eileen Murphy, M.D., clinical instructor in obstetrics and gynecology at Northwestern University Medical School in Chicago. If despite your best efforts, however, you find labor pain intolerable, allow yourself the option of pain-relief medication.

Intense pain can interfere with uterine contractions, and it can slow delivery. What's more, using medication in the early phases might help you later. "You'll need energy for the pushing phase. You shouldn't be so exhausted and depleted that by the time you're dilated ten centimeters (about four inches), you're seeing stars.

"If you're at a high level of pain for too extended a period, childbirth may no longer be the self-actualizing experience that you had hoped for. Nor is it necessarily healthy for the baby," says Dr. Murphy. So if you need medication, consider it.

phy, M.D., clinical instructor in obstetrics and gynecology at Northwestern University Medical School in Chicago. The pain, understandably, causes anxiety. And the more worked up you get, the more your body releases adrenaline, a stress hormone that interferes with the uterus's ability to contract efficiently, possibly prolonging labor and increasing discomfort, says Dr. Murphy.

So efforts to reduce labor pain can be aimed at helping you work with, not against, the delivery process. There are even some ways to speed delivery—the sooner to enjoy the product of your labors.

NOT FUN, BUT WORTHWHILE

Here's what women physicians and other health professionals trained to assist women during labor and childbirth advise for minimizing pain and maximizing the birthing experience.

Eat. First pangs of labor? Don't stop eating, says Martha Barry, R.N., adjunct clinical faculty member of the University of Illinois School of Nursing and a certified nurse midwife at Illinois Masonic Hospital, both in Chicago. You need fuel. At home have something easy to digest like soup or a sandwich. Later, during the more active phase of labor, you may not feel like eating, and the hospital or birthing center may discourage it.

Drink plenty of liquids. Labor is an athletic event of sorts: lots of huffing and puffing and sweating. As with other athletic efforts, your body requires fluid during the workout. If you become dehydrated, you might have more painful contractions, or your contractions may become irregular, says Dr. Murphy. Drinking adequate fluid improves the action of the smooth muscles of the uterus, which helps maximize the effect of contractions. Drink water, apple juice or other clear liquids liberally every hour or a sip after each contraction.

Urinate. A full bladder adds to labor pain, says Barry. Try to urinate at least once an hour.

Try different positions. "I encourage women to change positions frequently during labor to keep themselves moving with the contractions," says Mindy Smith, M.D., associate professor in family practice at the University of Michigan in Ann Arbor. This takes the focus off the pain and puts it on the process. It might even speed delivery.

For instance, switching positions may help change the alignment of the fetus and can often provide pain relief and encourage descent of the baby in preparation for childbirth, says Barry.

Warm yourself. "Hot compresses are really helpful," says Chicago-based Amy Durbin, a certified Bradley childbirth instructor with the American Academy of Husband-Coached Childbirth. A warm washcloth placed on your lower abdomen right above your pubic bone, either between contractions or during, is fine.

Step into a hot shower. When the pain gets intense, take a hot shower, suggests Barry. "A lot of women have trouble with labor when they have dilated five centimeters or so—about two inches." The warmth of the water provides comfort and relaxation and can make labor more tolerable.

Breathe. "Breathing techniques don't take away the pain, but they do keep you from tensing up," says Barry. "That tension in itself can make things more painful. It also may impede labor, because you're not relaxing your muscles to allow the baby to descend."

Breathe deeply from your diaphragm rather than shallowly from your shoulders and neck, suggests Durbin. She also suggests taking a deep breath at the beginning of a contraction and another at the end. "I found in my second labor that the contractions just would not let up. Sometimes it was a struggle, but taking a nice deep breath got me through one contraction in time for the other."

Vocalize. "Groan if you feel like it," Durbin says. "Low, slow, deep tones. Cow noises, I call them." These help keep your anxiety level down.

Visualize. You can use imagery and deep breathing to help yourself relax during labor. "Imagine that your 'in' breath is a radiant white light filling your womb with health-giving energy," suggests Julie Tupler, R.N., a certified childbirth educator and founder and director of Maternal Fitness, a program in New York City that trains women for childbirth. "See your baby floating in that light and pushing its way out." She also suggests bringing along a cassette tape with calming music to play while you visualize.

Make it a team sport. Having a partner to pay close attention to you and cheer you on—whether it's your husband or somebody else—is "exceptionally helpful," says Dr. Smith. One study showed that the presence of a trained childbirth assistant decreased women's requests for an anesthetic during childbirth. A coach can help in practical ways, too.

Ask for a back massage. While some women prefer not to be touched during labor, others love it, says Elaine Stillerman, a licensed massage therapist on the staff of the Swedish Institute of Massage in New York City and author of *Mother-Massage*.

Massage on the lower back and along the spine is often helpful. A leg massage can be nice, because your legs often get very tense during labor.

Lactose Intolerance
More Calcium, Fewer Cramps

As a child you could drink a milk shake or eat a bowl of ice cream, no problem. Now the same foods leave you as bloated as the Goodyear blimp. Or running to the nearest bathroom with diarrhea. Or crampy and uncomfortable.

What's going on?

As you grow older, your intestines begin to produce smaller-than-usual amounts of lactase, a special-purpose digestive enzyme required to break down lactose, the natural sugar found in milk and other dairy products. Symptoms—such as bloating, cramps and diarrhea—usually appear anywhere from 15 minutes to several hours afterward as your intestines react to the undigested sugars.

QUICK RELIEF

If you feel ready to explode, it's too late to put that bowl of ice cream that you just consumed back in the freezer. So for quick relief of lactose-induced discomfort, women doctors offer this fast-action advice.

Down a degassing tablet. Head for a drugstore and try Charcoal Plus or Phazyme, over-the-counter pills that can help absorb gas trapped in your colon and reduce bloating, says Jacqueline Wolf, M.D., a gastroenterologist, assistant professor of medicine at Harvard Medical School and co-director of the Inflammatory Bowel Disease Center at Brigham and Women's Hospital in Boston.

Take a short hike. If you're feeling bloated and gassy, a half-hour stroll often will calm your distress, says Melissa Palmer, M.D., a gastroenterologist in private practice in New York City.

Put your feet up. "If you have stomach cramps, sometimes the best thing that you can do is nothing at all," says Wanda Filer, M.D., a family practice physician in York, Pennsylvania. Rest, relax, take a bath, put your feet up, go to bed—whatever it takes to wait out the cramps caused by lactose intolerance.

LIMIT LACTOSE

After you're feeling better, here are some suggestions on how to find out if you can't digest dairy products.

Keep a diary. "To find out if milk and ice cream are causing your distress, write down everything that you eat, when you ate it and if you experienced any symptoms," says Wahida Karmally, R.D., director of nutrition at the Irving Center for Clinical Research at Columbia University Medical Center in New York City. If you keep careful track, you should know if you have the problem within a week or so.

Go dairy-free. Don't have time to track your symptoms? "Simply stay away from milk, cheese and ice cream for a week or two," says Dr. Wolf. If you stop feeling like a helium balloon and cramps and diarrhea subside, you probably should stay away from the dairy counter.

Track food labels for lactose code words. Foods could contain hidden lactose, says Karmally. For example, whey (used in cottage cheese) is often an ingredient of canned foods. Nonfat milk solids, sour cream, sweet cream and some breads, candies and salad dressings also contain dairy products.

Limit yourself to one glass at a time. All milk—skim, low-fat, 2 percent or whole—has the same amount of lactose, says Karmally. But even if you have severe symptoms, you may be able to maintain some dairy in your life.

A study conducted at the University of Minnesota in St. Paul found that among a group of 30 individuals thought to be lactose-intolerant, almost everyone could comfortably drink an eight-ounce glass of 2 percent milk every day.

Doctors there tested 30 people who consistently reported symptoms including gas pains after drinking less than a glass of milk and found that the symptoms were minimal when they drank a glass of milk every day at breakfast for a week.

BRIDGE THE CALCIUM GAP

If you've determined that you can eat or drink little more than a glass of milk (or its equivalent) per day, women doctors say that you still have to address your need for calcium, normally provided in dairy products.

"Calcium is essential to protect against osteoporosis and heart disease," says Barbara Frank, M.D., gastroenterologist and clinical professor of medicine at Allegheny University of the Health Sciences MCP–Hahnemann School of Medicine in Philadelphia. If lactose intolerance has forced you to cut back on milk, you need to find other ways to reach the 1,000 milligrams of calcium a day that women doctors say you need.

Switch to yogurt. Yogurt (such as Dannon) with active cultures is lower in lactose than most other dairy products, and you may be able to eat that, says Dr. Crowe. But don't try frozen yogurt—all the active cultures are eliminated in the freezing process.

Link up with lactase. If you're not manufacturing much lactase on your own, buy the enzyme in tablet or liquid form. Lactase supplements such as Lactaid or Dairy Ease are available in supermarkets and drugstores, says Karmally. "Two tablets with a glass of milk will improve your tolerance of milk," she says. The liquid form converts 70 to 90 percent of the lactose, depending on the number of drops that you add to the milk, so experiment and decide which form is most effective for you.

Or buy lactose-reduced milk, sold under the same brand names.

Drink citrus. Many juices are now fortified with calcium, says Karmally. Together with lactose-reduced dairy, calcium-enriched orange juice and other juices can help bridge the calcium gap sometimes created by lactose intolerance.

Laryngitis

Rest and Recuperation for Raspiness

*I*n old movies starring actresses like Lauren Bacall, a woman with a husky, deep-throated voice came across as alluring. But if you're beginning to sound more like Lurch from *The Addams Family* television series, or if your voice is fading away to a squeak, you have a problem, and it's called laryngitis, or a swollen, irritated voice box.

To function at its best, your larynx needs to be coated in a mucous membrane that moistens and filters air before it passes into your lungs. When you have a cold or the flu, or when you strain your voice, your vocal cords can become swollen, dry and irritated. When air passes over them as you speak, the sound becomes distorted. In severe cases, you can lose your voice altogether, although the symptom will probably pass within a few days.

COAXING YOUR VOICE BACK

Women doctors suggest these simple strategies for easing the discomfort of laryngitis (and getting your voice back).

No talking, period. People often make the mistake of turning down their volume to a whisper to protect their ailing voices, says Penelope Shar, M.D., an internist in private practice in Bangor, Maine. "Don't even whisper," she says. "That puts a bigger strain on your voice than talking."

Draw yourself a broth. Drinking lots of water, decaffeinated tea, juice and good old-fashioned chicken soup—between a half-quart and two quarts of liquid a day—will help restore liquids to your parched vocal cords and make you feel better, too, says Sally Wenzel, M.D., associate professor at the University of Colorado School of Medicine and a pulmonary specialist at the National Jewish Center for Immunology and Respiratory Medicine, both in Denver. In fact, chicken soup is believed to have anti-inflammatory properties, she says.

Season with garlic. A clove of garlic (or several cloves) can be of help when you're losing your voice, since it thins the mucus surrounding your vocal cords, says Dr. Shar. So go ahead—press away! You won't have to worry about your breath in close, intimate conversations anyway.

WHEN TO SEE A DOCTOR

Occasionally, a rough and raspy voice can signal a bacterial infection or, especially in professional singers or speakers, nodules or other harmless growths on the vocal cords. Women should be aware that doctors are seeing an increased number of cases of hoarseness that are ultimately attributed to the sexually transmitted disease chlamydia.

If your laryngitis is painful as well as annoying, and it persists for more than a few days, see a doctor. If the pain is severe, making it difficult to swallow or breathe, seek help right away.

Suck on sugarless candy. Sucking on a piece of hard candy will increase your saliva production, bathing your dehydrated voice box, says Dr. Shar. They're as good as lozenges.

Opt for acetaminophen. Dr. Shar recommends acetaminophen-containing pain relievers for laryngitis, since aspirin and ibuprofen have the potential to affect your body's clotting ability, interfering with the healing process within your vocal cords.

Banish your vices (if you have any.) Smokers and heavy drinkers are at increased risk for laryngitis, and occasionally, laryngitis can be caused by allergies, irritating fumes or the backward flow of stomach acids into the throat in cases of severe heartburn, says Dr. Shar.

In general, women doctors say that the best way to lure your voice back is to not smoke and to eliminate exposure to secondhand smoke or other irritants in the air, such as dust or fumes. Avoid alcohol (even in mouthwash) and caffeine, since they irritate and dry out your already scratchy throat, says Dr. Wenzel.

(For practical ways to manage colds, congestion and postnasal drip, which can sometimes lead to laryngitis, see pages 126, 136 and 437.)

Lip Lines
Fill, Fight or Fend Off Feathering

The unfair truth is that only women develop those tiny vertical creases that radiate above an otherwise perfect upper lip line somewhere around age 35. Men do not.

"In men the skin around the upper lip ages better, because it has all those hair follicles supporting it," explains Diana Bihova, M.D., a dermatologist in New York City and author of *Beauty from the Inside Out.* Hair follicles are the shafts out of which hair—in this case, moustache hair—grows.

But aging is not the only cause of those insidious little creases, says Dr. Bihova. Lip lines are also caused by the sun's destruction of the elastin and collagen fibers that keep skin elastic. If you smoke, pursing your lips around cigarettes causes lip lines, too. Wearing lipstick—as many women do—tends to make lip lines more noticeable, as lip color tends to creep into the tiny creases, producing what cosmetics companies call feathering.

SIX STEPS TO PRETTIER LIPS

The only sure cures for longstanding, deeply ingrained lip lines are medical procedures such as collagen injections, chemical peels and laser treatments, says Anita Cela, M.D., clinical assistant professor of dermatology at New York Hospital–Cornell Medical Center in New York City. Fortunately, more superficial lines can be minimized. So if you're just beginning to notice these vexing little creases, here's what women doctors say that you can do.

Use glycolic acid. Every morning, after you wash your face, apply a lotion containing glycolic acid around your lip area, says Dr. Bihova.

The glycolic acid will encourage your skin to slough off old cells that have formed lines and replace them with the younger, smoother cells underneath. Smooth it right up to your lip line, but not on the lip line itself or on your lips, says Dr. Bihova. Your lips are composed of mucous cells, not skin cells, which are extremely sensitive to contact with glycolic acid. If you get the lotion on your lips, it won't do any good, and it will burn.

Apply a moisturizer. About ten minutes before you plan to apply lip color, smooth a moisturizer above your upper lip to further minimize

341

lines says Dr. Bihova. Choose a moisturizer that has a built-in sun-screen—a sun protection factor, or SPF, of 15 or higher—so that you can prevent future lines and prevent existing lines from getting any deeper. Whatever moisturizing sunscreen you use on the rest of your face is fine.

Lay a foundation. To fill in existing lines and prevent lipstick from migrating into lip lines, making them more obvious, Dr. Bihova suggests applying a lip fixative such as Elizabeth Arden's Visible Difference Lip-Fix Creme. Any fixative will work, though. Sold in drugstores or at cosmetic counters everywhere, lip fixatives cause a slight swelling in the skin just above the upper lip, which fills in most lines.

"A lip fixative also works like a foundation," says Dr. Bihova. "It's a primer that will keep your lipstick in place, preventing feathering."

Powder your lips. To set the fixative and ready your lips for color, lightly dust your lips with facial powder, says Dr. Bihova.

Add an outline. Using a lip pencil, outline your lips with color, then fill them in with the same pencil or one of a very close color, says Dr. Bihova. Some pencils bleed, and some don't. The only way to tell what works best is to try several different types.

Color, then blot. Apply lip color as usual, being careful to stay in the lines. Then, to further set the color, blot your lips with a fresh tissue, says Dr. Bihova.

Low Blood Pressure
Pump Up Your B.P.—And Your Well-Being

Thirty seconds earlier, Pamela had no idea that she would find her-self lying on her back in the middle of a crowd of people waiting for a bus in the noonday heat. But there she was, prone on a hot sidewalk. A month of strenuous dieting and daily tennis matches had left her vulnerable to a sudden drop in blood pressure. And when it dropped, so did she.

In the absence of problems, blood pressure hovers around 120/80 millimeters of mercury (mmHg) or so. What makes it tumble?

WHEN TO SEE A DOCTOR

If you repeatedly feel faint and light-headed during the day, check with your doctor, says Debra R. Judelson, M.D., senior partner with the Cardiovascular Medical Group of Southern California in Beverly Hills, fellow of the American College of Cardiology and president of the American Medical Women's Association. Also see your doctor if you are actually losing consciousness upon standing or if you repeatedly feel light-headed, tired or weak along with signs of internal bleeding such as dark stools, she says. In younger women low blood pressure may be a sign of chronic fatigue syndrome, according to researchers at the Johns Hopkins University School of Medicine in Baltimore. In older women, especially, symptoms of low blood pressure may suggest the possibility of serious problems such as heart disease.

In women Pamela's age—in their forties or younger—blood pressure can drop below 90/60 mmHg during pregnancy, hot weather or crash dieting, says Debra R. Judelson, M.D., senior partner with the Cardiovascular Medical Group of Southern California in Beverly Hills, fellow of the American College of Cardiology and president of the American Medical Women's Association. If someone is on high blood pressure medication or has heart problems, the blood pressure drop can be even more significant, she says.

PUMP UP THE PRESSURE

Low blood pressure can leave you feeling light-headed, sluggish or headachy. On the other hand, you can walk around with low blood pressure and not know it or feel it unless you happen to have your blood pressure checked for some reason. If you tend to experience bothersome drops in blood pressure, says Dr. Judelson, giving it a boost is easy.

Drink lots of fluids. When you're sweating your way through a heat spell, blood pressure can plummet quickly because of dehydration, says Dr. Judelson. If you're feeling faint, reach for a sports drink or bouillon. Replace lost fluids, and your blood pressure will return to normal, relieving your symptoms, she adds. The sugar in these drinks will speed fluid into your cells, and the salt will help it stay there. Of course, plain water will also work wonders.

343

Eat. Feeling woozy? When was the last time that you ate? If it has been more than a couple of hours since your last meal or snack, says Dr. Judelson, grab a bite to eat, even if it's just half a sandwich or a piece of fruit. You'll feel better in a jiffy.

Stand up s-l-o-w-l-y. Some people feel dizzy when they first stand up after sitting or lying down, a cardinal sign of momentarily low blood pressure. This is caused by blood rushing to your legs from other areas. But your body can quickly adjust to it if you sit, jiggle your legs for a few moments, then stand slowly, says Dr. Judelson. If the light-headedness returns, simply sit or lie down again until the feeling of faintness passes. Then stand up more slowly.

Low Resistance

Reinstate Your Immune Power Now

Are you frequently under the weather? Is your body a human Internet for every cold germ or cold sore? When the bug for the new flu hits town, does it bug you first?

If so, take heart: It could be that you just need to start taking better care of yourself. If you're not well-nourished, well-rested, at least moderately well-exercised and physically prepared to control the stress that faces you every day, you might find your body battling bugs more frequently than you would like. That goes double if bad habits—smoking, drinking too much alcohol or not eating the way you should—are taxing your system.

ARM YOURSELF AGAINST GERMS

The demands of running a medical practice or attending to hospital patients and raising a family teach many women physicians firsthand what it's like to catch whatever comes along. For their collective wisdom, read on.

344

Don't share. Keep telephones, drinking vessels and eating utensils to yourself whenever possible, says Margaret Lytton, M.D., a family practitioner at Thomas Jefferson University Hospital in Philadelphia. "The problem isn't usually decreased resistance; it's increased contact with other people and their germs that causes illness."

Get your daily quota of laughter. Laughter may really be the best medicine, says psychologist Kathleen Dillon, Ph.D., professor of psychology at Western New England College in Springfield, Massachusetts. "I conducted experiments where I had people watching funny movies. After they watched, the participants had measurably higher levels of immunoglobulin A, the factor that helps your body fight infections.

"I also studied nursing mothers and their babies," she adds, "and learned that mothers with good senses of humor were less likely to have upper respiratory infections—and so were their babies."

Give stress the slip. Since it's impossible to eliminate stress, learn how to manage it before it makes you sick.

Scientific evidence points to stress as a risk factor for catching colds, and direct connections between stress and various functions of the immune system have been found. In addition, Dutch researchers found that people experiencing stress produce fewer antibodies to hepatitis B vaccinations than people who aren't undergoing stress. (For practical tips on how to manage stress, see page 521.)

Work in some exercise. Some studies indicate that moderate exercise for people who do not usually get much physical activity seem to boost levels of the body's natural disease-fighting antibodies. (Other studies indicate that high-intensity exercise—say, at the level of highly competitive athletes—may increase the production of stress hormones, which in turn have a depressing effect on the immune system. So experts don't suggest running marathons for stress reduction.)

"I advise people to acquire a higher level of physical fitness through moderate exercise," says Peggy Norwood-Keating, director of fitness at Duke University Diet and Fitness Center in Durham, North Carolina. A daily brisk walk for 20 minutes or more is an excellent health booster.

Know when to call it a day. "To improve your immune status, get the right amount of rest," says Carole Heilman, Ph.D., chief of the respiratory diseases branch at the National Institute of Allergy and Infectious Diseases, part of the National Institutes of Health in Bethesda, Maryland.

In one study people deprived of four hours of sleep on four consecutive nights had a 30 percent drop in an immune system measure called natural killer-cell activity.

To make sure that you're getting enough rest, "train yourself to set

WHEN TO SEE A DOCTOR

If, despite efforts to boost your immunity, you still seem to catch everything that comes along, see your doctor for a checkup, especially if you have frequent bouts of bacterial illnesses, such as sinus infections, bacterial pneumonia and the like, recommends Margaret Lytton, M.D., a family practitioner at Thomas Jefferson University Hospital in Philadelphia. "And if you get repeated strep throat infections, it might be a good idea to have your entire family tested to make sure that one of you isn't carrying *streptococcus* germs."

lights-out time and wake-up time," advises Anstella Robinson, M.D., a fellow at the Stanford Sleep Disorders Clinic and Research Center in Palo Alto, California. "For most women, those two times should be spaced about eight hours apart." Most women with busy schedules take whatever extra time they need for daily activities out of their sleep time. They fail to recognize that better sleep hygiene may make them more productive during the day, she adds.

IMMUNITY-BOLSTERING VITAMINS

No resistance-enhancing regimen would be complete without a look at what nutrition has to offer.

Empty the fruit bowl. "Eat at least three pieces of in-season fruit a day," says Katherine Sherif, M.D., instructor of medicine at Allegheny University of the Health Sciences and on staff at the Institute for Women's Health, both in Philadelphia. "People who eat three to six pieces of fresh fruit a day live longer and are markedly healthier than those who don't." Doctors aren't sure why, but it could be because of vitamins A and C, bioflavonoids and other substances in many fruits that act as natural antioxidants, fighting disease at the cellular level by preventing damage from pollutants and other assaults. Some but not all antioxidants can be duplicated in vitamin pills, says Dr. Sherif.

Take vitamin C. "Studies that I've done on 800 people tell me that the current Daily Value for vitamin C—60 milligrams—is not the optimal amount," says Judith Hallfrisch, Ph.D, research leader at the U.S. Department of Agriculture Metabolism and Nutrient Interactions Lab in Beltsville, Maryland. "To ensure benefits, aim for between 200 and 300 milligrams a day."

Get your zinc. "Your immune system needs an adequate amount of zinc for healthy healing functions," says Eleanore Young, R.D., Ph.D., a licensed dietitian and professor in the Department of Medicine at the University of Texas Health Science Center at San Antonio. "Women should be sure to get about 12 milligrams of zinc a day."

Take a multivitamin. In one study among a group of people over age 60, those given a daily multivitamin a day for 18 months did significantly better at tests measuring their immune levels than the group given inactive look-alike pills for the same time period.

BE KIND TO YOUR SPLEEN

No use taking all those steps to build up your immunity if you're going to undermine it by taxing the systems that you're trying to enhance. Consider these suggestions.

Think before you drink. People who consume more than four alcoholic drinks a day get more colds than nondrinkers, according to research conducted by Marlene Aldo-Benson, M.D., professor of medicine at Indiana University School of Medicine and a practicing rheumatologist at Methodist Hospital, both in Indianapolis. "My work tells me that you can suppress your immune system when you drink excessively," she says.

"Alcohol lowers immunity by affecting white blood cells in the spleen, bone marrow and liver," says Dr. Sherif. "And women are particularly susceptible to its negative effects."

The reason? Women have fewer of the enzymes needed to process alcohol, so it remains longer in a woman's system than in a man's, says Dr. Sherif. "I advise my patients to drink very lightly, if at all."

Toss the butts now. "Women who smoke are more likely to have more prolonged and more severe respiratory infections," says Dr. Lytton. "Chronic smokers are also more likely to get bacterial respiratory infections rather than just viral infections. Because of this, they are more likely to have to see their doctors and take antibiotics to get better." So if you've been thinking about quitting, why not make today the day?

Low Self-Esteem
Give Yourself a Boost

*L*ow self-esteem leaves us with the uncomfortable feeling that we're not capable or deserving enough, no matter what the evidence to the contrary. We may excel as mothers, managers, professionals, technicians, friends, spouses or the founder of a highly acclaimed magazine and still lack self-worth.

"What's relevant is that these feelings of low self-worth are not warranted," says Susan Schenkel, Ph.D., a clinical psychologist in Cambridge, Massachusetts, and author of *Giving Away Success: Why Women Get Stuck and What to Do about It.*

A STRONG SENSE OF SELF

Self-esteem begins with the responses that you get from parents, siblings, teachers and peers when you're growing up, says Eleta Greene, Ph.D., a psychotherapist and director of Creative Survival Systems in New York City.

Gender enters into the mix, too, says Dr. Greene. Back when most of us were growing up, boys got kudos for achievement—doing things—and they grew up with a sense of self based on how well they mastered tasks. Girls were applauded for pleasing others—looking pretty or being nice. So we developed a sense of self based on how well we establish and maintain relationships.

"Women were taught to maintain harmony in relationships, even if that meant sacrificing their own wants and needs to keep relationships going," says Harriet Lerner, Ph.D., a senior staff psychologist at the Menninger Clinic in Topeka, Kansas, and author of *The Dance of Anger, The Dance of Intimacy* and *The Dance of Deception.* "This isn't good for self-esteem."

The cost of low self-esteem is high. If you don't value yourself, you are less likely to take care of yourself. And you are more likely to develop self-destructive habits, like addictions to alcohol, drugs, work or relationships with people who don't treat you well, say experts. Studies suggest that you are likely to be less satisfied with life all around. You can, however, boost your self-esteem and change all this. Here's how to start.

Treat yourself right—now. Don't feel selfish—treating yourself well reinforces the idea that you are worthwhile, says Dr. Greene. Do what makes you feel good, and you'll feel better about yourself. Begin doing small things for yourself this very minute. Make an appointment to get your nails done, for example. Call the bookstore and find out when the local book club meets.

If you don't exercise, start. "Exercise is a good option—it has so many physiological and psychological benefits," says Dr. Schenkel. Exercise prompts your brain to release a natural feel-good substance called serotonin. And research suggests that women who exercise regularly feel more enthusiastic, energetic and upbeat.

Talk nicely to yourself. "I look terrible." "I can't believe I said that." "I blew it."

That kind of self-deflating commentary perpetuates low self-worth, says Dr. Greene. You would never say those things to a friend, so don't say them to yourself. Instead, support yourself the way you would compliment a friend. Say to yourself, "Good point." "Smart move." "Well-done."

Plan to improve. If there's something about yourself that you don't like, take steps to change it, says Dr. Greene.

Start small. If you want to further your education, sign up for one class at the local college, see how you like it and give yourself credit when you finish. Then try for two classes the next semester.

The same goes for losing unwanted pounds. "People say things like, 'I'm so fat. I have to lose 50 pounds,' " says Dr. Greene. "And I say, 'No, no, no. First lose 5 pounds.' "

Congratulate yourself. Breaking your goals into manageable steps and rewarding successes along the way builds confidence and self-esteem, says Dr. Greene. Unreasonable goals, on the other hand, set you up for failure and erode self-worth.

Work toward self-sufficiency. Knowing that you can fend for yourself—that you don't have to depend on another person for everything—is a great source of self-esteem, says Dr. Lerner. If you have friends, turn to them for emotional support. If you don't have marketable job skills, get training. Aim for greater independence. Your self-esteem will soar.

Lupus
Keys to Comfort

*I*f you're like most women diagnosed with lupus, the first thing that you'll do when you leave your doctor's office is find a medical dictionary and look it up. You'll discover that lupus erythematosus—the full name—is a complex autoimmune disease. Autoimmune means that your body turns on itself—and in the case of lupus, inflames the blood, kidneys, skin and joints and other tissues and organs.

The medical dictionary may or may not mention that nine out of ten people with lupus are women, and each woman who has lupus will experience the disease in a very individual way.

"For some women lupus begins with fevers and achy muscles or joints, and these symptoms are likely to persist throughout her life," says Janice Dort, R.N., who has had lupus for more than 20 years and works with the Lupus Foundation of America, an educational and support service headquartered in Rockville, Maryland. "But lupus can affect other women with more sinister problems, which include kidney, blood and brain complications."

While there is no cure for lupus, it can be managed with medication and self-care. "The most important thing for women with lupus is good medical treatment," says Susan Ward, M.D., clinical assistant professor of medicine and associate director of the Jefferson Osteoporosis Center at Thomas Jefferson University Hospital in Philadelphia.

HEALING WITH REST, WRAPS AND YOGA

Once you have been diagnosed with lupus, there are a variety of strategies that you can use to manage it and keep it under control. The best advice follows.

Brace painful joints. "Wrapping painful joints in an elasticized bandage may help keep down the swelling and relieve the discomfort," says Dr. Ward.

Jump into a whirlpool or heat up the hot tub. "Many women find that they sleep better after spending 20 to 30 minutes in a Jacuzzi or a hot tub," says Dort. "The heat and swirling water soothe joints and muscles, too." If you don't have access to a hot tub, a warm bath will do.

Try a vinegar-and-water soak. "I don't know how it works, but many of my patients insist that soaking their aching hands in a basin of warm water with a few tablespoons of white vinegar relieves pain," says Dr. Ward. "It might be from nothing more than the action of the warm water. So it's worth a try."

Alternate heat with cold. Since every woman experiences a different discomfort with lupus, the treatments to relieve that discomfort will vary, too, says Dr. Ward. "Many women like heat packs over aching joints or muscles, while others prefer cold packs, and some women get relief by alternating between hot and cold."

Learn your limits. "Each woman will have her own limits," says Dort. "Learn what triggers flare-ups and avoid those triggers." For example, women who are sensitive to the sun sometimes have flare-ups after being outside too long, says Dort. Others are prone to flare-ups under stress.

HOW DIET CAN HELP

"If you have lupus, a healthy diet, built on the principles of the Food Guide Pyramid, will strengthen the disease-fighting abilities of your immune system," says Kristine Napier, R.D., member of the education committee of the Lupus Foundation of America and author of *How Nutrition Works.*

The Food Guide Pyramid, issued by the U.S. Department of Agriculture and widely disseminated by the food industry and nutrition educators, is a nutritional plan calling for 6 to 11 servings of bread, pasta, cereal and other grain foods per day; 2 to 4 servings of fruit; 3 to 5 servings of vegetables; 2 to 3 servings of meat, fish, poultry or other protein foods; 2 servings of dairy products and a bare minimum of fats and sweets.

To help build your lupus-fighting Food Guide Pyramid, try these additional tips.

Shun fat, seek carbs. "Make sure that your diet is low in fat—no more than 20 to 30 percent of your caloric intake—and high in complex carbohydrates," says Napier. That means concentrating on bread, pasta, cereal and other grain foods, plus potatoes and starchy vegetables like carrots.

Count to ten. If you have lupus, it's easy to fall into the routine of eating a few handy foods, day in and day out. But you'll fare better if you include at least 10 to 15 different foods every day to make certain that you get a broad range of nutrients, says Napier. "Be sure to include five,

351

WHEN TO SEE A DOCTOR

Consult a doctor if you experience all or most of the following symptoms for more than a week.
- Chronic fatigue unrelieved by rest
- Unexplained chronic muscle pain or joint pain
- Dry eyes and mouth
- Fever
- Rash
- Mouth or skin ulcers
- Swollen glands

See a doctor or visit an emergency room immediately if you experience:
- Chest pain
- A seizure
- Shortness of breath

If you consult a doctor for persistent problems associated with lupus, and you're told that your symptoms are "nothing to worry about," see a rheumatologist—a physician who specializes in diagnosing inflammatory diseases—if you are still concerned.

"Lupus affects different women in different ways, making it hard to diagnose, especially in the early stages," says Susan Ward, M.D., clinical assistant professor of medicine and associate director of the Jefferson Osteoporosis Center at Thomas Jefferson University Hospital in Philadelphia.

Also, pregnancy poses special concerns for women who have lupus. So if you have lupus and want to conceive, consult your physician.

or better yet, nine fruit and vegetable servings every day," she says. They're rich sources of beta-carotene (a form of vitamin A found in plant foods) and other nutrients vital to strong immunity. Since lupus is an immune disorder, your body needs plenty of foods that help strengthen the immune system.

"This is the advice that I give the women I treat, and it makes sense," says Napier.

Lyme Disease
What to Do *after* You're Bitten

One thing is for sure: The deer tick (*Ixodes dammini*), whose bite causes Lyme disease, has a much easier time finding you than you do finding it.

This tick is so tiny that, even when engorged with the blood that it has sucked from you, it's still not much bigger than the head of a pin. And, given the little bugger's propensity for seeking hidden, hairy places (the groin, scalp and armpits are preferred), a body check may not reveal a tick's presence.

Statistically, only two or three ticks in a hundred are likely to carry the spiral-shaped bacteria (known as a spirochete) that causes Lyme disease (Latin name: *Borrelia burgdorferi*). Once thought to infest ticks in just a few northeastern states, such as Connecticut, the tick-born disease is now present in all but seven states nationwide.

The classic sign of Lyme disease is a rash resembling a red bull's-eye at the site where you were bitten or anywhere on your body. The bacteria can travel to distant sites—your heart, your joints or your brain and nervous system. Consequently, you may also develop swollen joints, all-over aches, flulike symptoms, memory lapses, heart problems or other lasting effects.

A BUG YOU WANT TO AVOID

Researchers report that Lyme disease is more often contracted in the spring and summer, when the ticks are tiny—in what is known as their nymph, or growing, stage. They are easily overlooked. By fall the ticks are full-grown adults—still capable of transmitting the disease, but far easier to spot if they hitch a ride on your body.

To decrease your chances of being bitten by a deer tick, the National Centers for Disease Control and Prevention in Atlanta offer these standard guidelines.

Avoid known tick havens. Ticks are especially prevalent in May through July. Call your local or state health department to identify tick-prone locales.

Wear light-colored clothing. Hiking or biking in the woods? Doing yard work? Ticks are easier to spot on white or khaki socks, pants and shirts.

Tuck in your clothing. To keep ticks out, tuck your shirt into your pants and your pants into your socks. Then apply duct tape where pants and socks overlap.

Use a tick repellent spray. As added protection, say experts, you should spray an insect repellent containing diethyltoluamide, or DEET, on clothing and any exposed skin except your face.

Strip, shower and check. As soon as you get home, take off your clothes, shower and check for ticks. Even if one has landed on your skin, it may not start feeding right away.

DETECT, THEN TREAT

If, despite precautions, you have developed the telltale symptoms, and your doctor says that you have Lyme disease, she will probably prescribe a course of antibiotics, perhaps in combination with anti-inflammatories or other medications. At that point, here's what women doctors tell the women they treat.

Be patient. How you respond to medication will depend on what stage Lyme disease was in when you were diagnosed, says Susan Ward, M.D., clinical assistant professor of medicine and associate director of the Jefferson Osteoporosis Center at Thomas Jefferson University Hospital in Philadelphia.

"The earlier you catch Lyme, the more likely that you'll avoid its complications," she says. "With today's medications, the progression of Lyme disease, for many women, can be halted even a couple of months after the initial infection."

"Lyme disease symptoms, however, including arthritis-like pain and fatigue, may persist for weeks or even months after the disease has been cured," according to Kathy Roye, R.N., an epidemiologist at the Hunterdon County Medical Center in Flemington, New Jersey. "It is important for women with Lyme disease to realize that they are not still infected. But they will need patience as their symptoms gradually decline."

Take your medicine even if you feel better. "The course of antibiotics that you take for Lyme disease may last for as long as a month," explains Roye. "Though you may feel completely cured in a week or less, it is vital to continue the medicine for as long as your doctor recommends."

WHEN TO SEE A DOCTOR

Consult your doctor if you have removed an engorged tick from your body, says Susan Ward, M.D., clinical assistant professor of medicine and associate director of the Jefferson Osteoporosis Center at Thomas Jefferson University Hospital in Philadelphia.

Also, see your doctor if you get the distinctive bull's-eye rash—a red, circular patch that can appear three days to one month after you've been bitten by an infected tick.

Other symptoms that may signal Lyme disease include fatigue, chills and fever, headache, muscle and joint pain and swollen lymph nodes.

Symptoms of Lyme disease that may appear months after you've been bitten include numbness, tingling, facial paralysis (Bell's palsy) or other nervous system problems; heart palpitations or other irregularities and swollen joints (especially the knees).

If you have any of these symptoms, see your doctor.

SELF-CARE CAN HELP

Even if Lyme disease has progressed to the point where you have symptoms like fatigue and arthritis-like pain, doctors say that self-care strategies can ease the discomfort.

Heat up aching joints. "The muscle pain that you feel may respond to hot, moist heat," says Eileen Hilton, M.D., director of the Lyme Disease Center at Long Island Jewish Medical Center in New York. Apply a towel wrung out in hot water and keep it on the painful area until you feel relief.

Get thee to a steam room. "The hot, moist heat of a steam room is good when your body aches all over," says Dr. Hilton.

Watch what you eat. "When you have Lyme disease, good nutrition is especially important to help your body's healing process," says Dr. Hilton. "Although we're not in a position to say that taking specific vitamins will affect the course of Lyme disease, we can say that it's smart to eat a varied low-fat diet with plenty of fruits, beans, grains and vegetables."

Join a support group. "The most important thing that a woman can do when she has Lyme disease is hook up with a support group," says Dr. Ward. "It's a good way to learn how to manage the various problems that she may encounter. This helps people regain a sense of control over their lives."/

355

Marine Bites, Stings and Cuts
How to Handle Nautical Nuisances

*I*f you love to swim, snorkel or scuba dive in the ocean, you need a little knowledge of the habits of marine life in your area and of what to do in an emergency if you should get stung, bitten or cut, says Constance Nichols, M.D., an emergency physician and associate residency director in the Department of Emergency Medicine at the University of Massachusetts Medical Center in Amherst.

"Sea stingers," such as jellyfish or sea anemones, defend themselves by discharging venom from tiny poisonous cells, called nematocysts, which are found on the ends of their tentacles or spines, explains Saralyn R. Williams, M.D., a toxicologist and emergency physician at the San Diego Regional Poison Center.

"You can get stung just by brushing against portions of tentacles that have broken off and are floating in the water," says Dr. Williams. You'll experience severe burning and pain and develop red streaks, spots or blisters where the tentacles touched your skin.

ACT, DON'T PANIC

Scary as some of these nautical encounters may be, women doctors say that if you handle them quickly and properly, you can keep pain and injury to a minimum.

Wash in saltwater. If you've been stung by a jellyfish or any other stinging creature, wash off remaining pieces of tentacles by taking a dip in the ocean, suggests Dr. Williams. Just look out for more jellyfish before entering the water.

The sooner you get the tentacles off your skin, the less damage they will do.

Stay out of the pool. Don't rinse with fresh water or jump in a swimming pool, because fresh water shocks the venom cells into discharging more venom.

Took Lifeguard's Advice

May R. Berenbaum, Ph.D.

While on vacation in Honolulu, Hawaii, May R. Berenbaum, Ph.D., head of the Department of Entomology at the University of Illinois at Urbana-Champaign, waded into the tropical blue waters off Waikiki Beach for a swim. Five minutes later, she was hit with jellyfish tentacles floating in the water. She emerged from the water in pain, a line of blistery red bumps on her skin.

The lifeguard on the beach told Dr. Berenbaum to cover the sting with a paste made from rubbing alcohol and unseasoned meat tenderizer.

"I thought that he was kidding—you know, 'Oh, here's a tourist from the mainland. Let's have a joke on her,'" she says. "But he convinced me that he was serious." So she bought the necessary ingredients at a nearby store and applied the paste to her skin. "It was amazing. Within 15 minutes, the sting didn't hurt anymore."

Later, back at the university, Dr. Berenbaum researched this remedy and found that meat tenderizer is indeed a good remedy for jellyfish stings. "An ingredient in the tenderizer—an enzyme called papain—quickly breaks down proteins in jellyfish venom, so that the sting is not as painful," she explains. The rubbing alcohol minimizes the chance of infection and helps make a paste out of the powdered meat tenderizer. "It worked for me," she says.

Vanquish the pain with vinegar. Vinegar contains acetic acid, which inactivates the stinging nematocysts on tentacles, so they stop hurting you, explains Dr. Williams. (To find vinegar in a hurry, try the nearest beachside or boardwalk french-fry stand.)

Vinegar is an effective remedy for sea urchin cuts. "If you step on or brush against a sea urchin, and its spines break off in your skin, vinegar will help dissolve the spines, so they are easier to remove," says May R. Berenbaum, Ph.D., head of the Department of Entomology at the University of Illinois at Urbana-Champaign.

Remove jellyfish tentacles. Wearing rubber surgical gloves if possible, remove any large jellyfish tentacles left in your skin with tweezers, says Dr. Nichols. If small tentacles remain in your skin, "shave" them off by applying shaving cream and scraping gently with a clean dull knife or the edge

WHEN TO SEE A DOCTOR

As with bee stings, some people can have potentially fatal allergic reactions to the venom in marine animals. If you experience an outbreak of hives, difficulty breathing, nausea or redness and swelling spreading over your body away from the sting site, you need to get to a hospital immediately.

Also seek help if you are having trouble removing tentacles from your skin, or if you can't tolerate the pain of a sting.

Stingray wounds are usually deep, jagged and contaminated with debris, not to mention extremely painful. So if you're struck by one of these winged sea creatures, you must seek medical attention, says Constance Nichols, M.D., an emergency physician and associate residency director in the Department of Emergency Medicine at the University of Massachusetts Medical Center in Amherst.

It's also a good idea to see a physician if you have a cut, wound or sting that punctures your skin. "You run the risk of getting an infection from bacteria that is in seawater, and you also risk getting tetanus," says Saralyn R. Williams, M.D., a toxicologist and emergency physician at the San Diego Regional Poison Center. You need to make sure that the wound is properly cleaned and irrigated and that all debris is removed. While you're at it, have your tetanus shot updated.

of a credit card with the direction of the tentacle, not against it, suggests Dr. Williams. Whatever you do, don't pinch, rub or squeeze the tentacle pieces in your effort to remove them. Harsh handling will cause them to discharge more venom into your skin. If you can't remove all of the tentacles, get help from a doctor.

Hold still. Lie still and rest the stung area for about an hour, so that the venom won't spread to other parts of your body, says Dr. Nichols.

Treat coral cuts with care. If you feel a stinging sensation after scraping against coral, try applying vinegar and/or meat tenderizer—although some people might find the meat tenderizer aggravating to their skin—and gently scraping away any remaining coral or debris, suggests Dr. Williams. If you're cut, gently clean away any debris and coral with soap and water and apply an antibacterial ointment to the coral cut. "These tend to get infected easily, because of organisms in the water, so they have to be well-cleaned," says Dr. Williams.

Menopause
A Kind of Midlife Puberty

*T*oday, as baby boomers move into midlife with a whole new mind-set, menopause doesn't have quite the alarming effect that it used to. Yet it remains a time of profound transformation in a woman's life, as her ovaries start shutting down and production of the female hormone estrogen plummets, signaling an end to her childbearing years.

"Menopause is a perfectly normal process that occurs over several years," points out M. Eileen Beiler, Psy.D., a psychologist in Dallas and adjunct faculty member in the Department of Psychiatry and Division of Psychology at the University of Texas Southwestern Medical Center at Dallas. She says that in a group she leads for women in transition, "Menopause is compared with puberty. Remembering the process of adapting to those earlier changes can help put current changes in a familiar perspective."

The physical and emotional changes associated with menopause vary from woman to woman, but may include hot flashes, insomnia, mood swings and memory difficulties, to name a few. And some women—up to 38 percent, according to estimates—experience no symptoms whatsoever.

ATTITUDE COUNTS

If your doctor has determined that you are going through menopause, you and she may decide on hormone replacement therapy to deal with some of the symptoms—or maybe not. (For nondrug ways to deal with other bothersome changes, read about hot flashes, insomnia and mood swings on pages 292, 317 and 374.)

Women doctors offer expert advice on ways to cope with other, more general aspects of menopause.

Acknowledge sadness. If menopause feels like a loss, allow yourself to feel sad about it, says Dr. Beiler. "But remember that the ability to have a child is only one way to define yourself as a woman. Everybody experiences menopause very differently. Some women are happy to not have to worry about birth control and periods anymore."

WHEN TO SEE A DOCTOR

Menopause isn't a disease, so you don't necessarily need to see your doctor unless you are very uncomfortable, are experiencing very early signs of menopause (before age 40) or you're just plain curious, says Liliana Gaynor, M.D., D.D.S., clinical assistant professor in the Department of Obstetrics and Gynecology at Northwestern University Medical School in Chicago. Your physician can perform a blood test measuring follicle-stimulating hormone, or FSH. This female hormone shows up if you're approaching menopause, even if you're still having periods. The higher your blood levels of FSH, the closer you are to menopause.

A woman who thinks that she may be experiencing premature menopause (before age 40) and wants to have a child should see her physician or a fertility specialist immediately, says Margory Gass, M.D., director of the University Hospital Menopause and Osteoporosis Center at the University of Cincinnati. With prompt treatment, it may still be possible to sustain a pregnancy. Donor egg programs are available at some fertility centers. This allows a woman to carry a pregnancy by an in vitro procedure when she is no longer producing eggs of her own.

Talk to your partner. Open communication with your intimate other is especially important, says Dr. Beiler, both to "normalize" menopause and to address specific issues, such as the physical changes that can make sex uncomfortable. "Share your thoughts and concerns and get closer instead of creating distance."

Lubricate your love life. The once supple tissues of the vagina that produce lubrication become thin and dry in the absence of estrogen, which normally sends messages to the genitals to prepare for intercourse, says Mary Jane Minkin, M.D., associate clinical professor at Yale University School of Medicine and co-author of *What Every Woman Needs to Know about Menopause*. If sex is uncomfortable, use a lubricant like K-Y jelly or a product called Astroglide, which Dr. Minkin says is highly recommended by many of the women she counsels.

Seek emotional support. "Connecting with other women, not isolating yourself, will help you feel better," says Dr. Beiler. Check with your doctor or local hospitals for menopause support groups in your area, she suggests, "or start your own." Get together with other women friends, reminisce about your lives and plan changes that you'd each like to make in the future.

Get enough shut-eye. Hot flashes can jolt you from your sleep, says Dr. Minkin. What's more, your pituitary gland, which normally works the night shift, can wake you if it goes into overdrive because of low estrogen levels. If you need help dozing off again, try a glass of warm milk, a hot shower or an occasional sleeping pill. (Follow package directions or use only as prescribed.)

Exercise regularly. The depression that can come with menopause may be related to low levels of serotonin and endorphins, brain chemicals that influence mood, says Liliana Gaynor, M.D., D.D.S., clinical assistant professor in the Department of Obstetrics and Gynecology at Northwestern University Medical School in Chicago. "Exercise is a form of self-medication for depression, raising the level of endorphins in the brain." Low-impact aerobic exercises like running or walking are especially helpful, two or three times a week for 30 to 60 minutes each time.

Stay away from smoke. "Smoking directly affects the production of estrogen and brings on menopause two to four years earlier," says Dr. Gaynor. And smoking while on hormone replacement therapy carries a risk of blood clots and stroke.

Menstrual Problems
Strike Out Monthly Misery

*T*he good news is that you're not pregnant. The not-so-good news is that your body lets you know with symptoms like menstrual cramps, pain in your lower back and bloating. Your uterine cleanup crew has gone into gear. Leading the effort are prostaglandins, chemicals produced by the lining of your uterus that initiate uterine contractions—what you feel as cramps—to expel tissue and fluids that had built up in the event that a fertilized egg needed to make its home there. For some women menstrual fluid loss, or flow, is so heavy that anemia can result.

Sit-Ups Helped

Mary Lang Carney, M.D.

For Mary Lang Carney, M.D., her high school memories include what she calls "hideous periods."

"I threw up and got terrible cramps," recalls this women's health expert. Now medical director of the Center for Women's Health at St. Francis Hospital in Evanston, Illinois, Dr. Carney shares her secret for putting painful periods in her distant past.

"I took aspirin, I used a heating pad and I climbed in the bathtub (sans heating pad) for a warm bath," she says. And something else: She did sit-ups before, during and after her period. "Those seemed to really make a difference for me. Maybe it was just psychological, but exercising my abdominal-wall muscles worked. Not only did they help me cope with my period, but I also developed strong muscles overall."

Dr. Carney is pleased to report that she doesn't have menstrual problems any longer—"not since I had kids." Other women doctors also report that after they had kids, menstrual cramps disappeared or lessen significantly.

TOO MUCH OF A GOOD THING

Women bothered by menstrual pain, cramps and heavy bleeding might fantasize about somehow escaping menstruation altogether. Forget it: Menstruation is your body's way of setting the stage for eventual pregnancy, even if pregnancy isn't in your plans. So it's part of the deal. In fact, absence of periods, or irregular menstruation, may signal too much exercise; thyroid, cervical or endometrial problems; infertility or the beginning of menopause. (If these are your concerns, read about infertility on page 303 and menopause on page 359.)

Otherwise, women doctors offer this advice for getting through this time of the month.

Try a painkiller. For cramps and lower-back pain, women doctors recommend either ibuprofen (the main ingredient in pain relievers such as Midol, Advil and Motrin) or aspirin.

"Ibuprofen does an excellent job of relieving cramps by interfering with the body's production of prostaglandins," says Mary Lang Carney,

M.D., medical director of the Center for Women's Health at St. Francis Hospital in Evanston, Illinois. Aspirin has the same effect, she says, but acetaminophen (such as Tylenol) doesn't.

Act early. Take medication the moment that you feel cramps coming on, says Yvonne S. Thornton, M.D., visiting associate physician at the Rockefeller University Hospital in New York City and director of the perinatal diagnostic testing center at Morristown Memorial Hospital in New Jersey. "Don't wait for the cramps to build up. If you do, prostaglandins will have already been produced, and your cramps will be worse."

These painkillers will also help relieve lower-back pain, says Dr. Carney.

Warm up. Heat does wonders to relieve painful abdominal cramps and lower-back ache, says Dr. Carney. Lie down with a hot-water bottle or heating pad on your abdomen, she suggests, or beneath your lower back. Or take a warm, relaxing bath.

Cut the salt. "A lot of women crave salt around the time of their periods, but watching salt intake will help decrease the amount of bloating," says Dr. Thornton. Try alternative seasonings in your cooking and remove the saltshaker from your dinner table.

Try a little more B_6. Making sure that you get 25 to 50 milligrams of vitamin B_6 daily during your period can help relieve bloating, says Dr. Thornton. The vitamin appears to have a mild diuretic effect, she says.

WHEN TO SEE A DOCTOR

According to women doctors, the following symptoms merit a visit to your physician.

- Menstrual cycles shorter than 21 days or more than 35 days long
- Heavy bleeding for more than a week
- Heavy soaking of tampons or pads, especially when accompanied by dizziness and fatigue (a possible indication of iron-deficiency anemia)
- Severe cramps or pain unrelieved by over-the-counter medications

By the way, passing small (the size of a quarter or smaller) clots of blood in your menstrual flow is no cause for concern. Rather, it's a sign that your body's natural coagulation system is working.

It's a water-soluble vitamin, so we lose it when we urinate, she explains. Don't exceed 100 milligrams a day, though.

Get moving. Women who exercise regularly have fewer problems with cramps, says Charenjeet Ray, M.D., an obstetrician/gynecologist and associate professor in the Department of Obstetrics and Gynecology at Rush Medical College of Rush University and attending physician at Illinois Masonic Hospital, both in Chicago. Walk, swim, play tennis—whatever you enjoy—when you feel cramps coming on.

Working up a sweat can also help relieve bloating, says Dr. Thornton.

Midlife Crisis

Survive the Trauma of Transition

*I*n Hollywood movies women reach midlife and go wild.

They get all-body liposuction, buy new wardrobes, dye their hair eggplant, take over corporations and have flings with naughty next-door neighbors played by one of the Bridges.

In real life, midlife transitions are usually a bit tamer, but significant nonetheless.

"The midlife transition—beginning around age 40 or so—is significant, because it's a time of so many physical and social changes for a woman," says Carol Goldberg, Ph.D., a clinical psychologist specializing in stress management in New York City.

Goals that you set for yourself in your twenties may no longer fit the bill, says Renana Brooks, Ph.D., a family and clinical psychologist and director of the Sommet Institute in Washington, D.C. If you reach midlife having achieved your career goals, you may wonder, 'Is this it?' If you haven't reached your goals, you may wonder if you ever will.

If you didn't have children, you may long to experience motherhood, says Dr. Goldberg. And if you had children, the kids may have grown up and moved away by now. If you put your career on hold to raise children, you may long to return to work. Your relationship with your partner may have changed considerably, too. At the same time, you may be newly responsible for ailing parents—and contemplating what lies ahead for your own health.

LOOK AHEAD AND TAKE CHARGE

In short, women at midlife find themselves nose-to-nose with the question, "What should I do with the rest of my life?"

A midlife transition can be even more tumultuous if accompanied by a traumatic change, like the death of a loved one, a job loss or a life-threatening illness, notes Dr. Goldberg. For some the transition is truly rough enough to constitute a full-blown crisis.

Yet relatively few people find themselves in the midst of a bona fide crisis in midlife, according to a study conducted at the University of British Columbia in Vancouver. Dr. Goldberg estimates that no more than 10 percent of women go through a real crisis. If it's happening to you, however, the statistics are unimportant. These changes and choices can be stressful. And for most women, a new wardrobe and a fling just don't fill the bill. Consider this advice from the experts.

Remember: You are strong. Remind yourself of other difficult transitions that you've already weathered, says Dr. Goldberg. "By the time they reach middle age, most people have a sense of self and a sense of what they can do well. They've gained wisdom. They're better able to make decisions and handle changes. They feel more confident and poised. The adjustments turn out to be very positive."

Get support. "Transition can be painful, but pain often accompanies growth," says Dr. Brooks. "Try to see the transition as an opportunity for growth."

Look at life as a series of phases. Each phase, says Dr. Brooks, presents an opportunity to concentrate on a different—and potentially satisfying—aspect of yourself.

If you spent your early adulthood staying home with the kids, savor the satisfaction that you got from that role. Decide what you'll focus on next (music? writing?) and devote yourself to it.

Hatch a plan and write it down. Find a quiet spot and write down what you want to do in the next phase of your life, suggests Dr. Brooks. Maybe you want to shift focus from your career to family life or become a parent, adoptive parent or foster parent. Maybe you want to learn a new language and travel, do community work or enter politics.

WHEN TO SEE A DOCTOR

How well you weather midlife change depends in part on how well you're coping with other physical or emotional changes that are also occurring, says Carol Goldberg, Ph.D., a clinical psychologist specializing in stress management in New York City. She advises professional guidance if:

- You feel overwhelmed by anxiety, stress or loss.
- You have trouble making decisions, especially those that will effect the next phase of your life.
- Your friends are concerned because you're not your old self, you're having trouble on the job, you never want to go out or you're not functioning well in general.

Make evolutionary—not revolutionary—changes. Don't scuttle a long relationship prematurely. Ask yourself if you're really dissatisfied with your marriage, or if it only seems that way because other parts of your life aren't fulfilling. If the problem is with the relationship, explore counseling as a solution to your trouble, says Dr. Goldberg.

The same goes for your career. If your job is unfulfilling, try to ask for new projects at your workplace, she suggests. If this doesn't pan out, a career switch may be just the thing. Or you may simply need to pursue more satisfying outside interests. In any case, avoid hasty and major changes that you may regret later; try incremental ones instead.

"Before you make a decision to change jobs, talk to people in the field that you want to go into, observe them at work for a few days if possible or do volunteer work in that field during your free time," she says.

Head to the library. Call the local college for information about training in a field that interests you, says Dr. Goldberg. Don't assume that it's too late. "All kinds of people peaked later in life—think of Grandma Moses."

Migraines and Other Headaches

Natural Relief for Real Pain

*W*hat women have suspected for years has been confirmed: Headaches really are worse for women than they are for men. What is it about women's headaches that make them feel so intense and sometimes even disabling?

The answer may be estrogen. Changes in estrogen levels that govern the ebb and flow of women's menstrual cycles can cause headaches. Headache-prone women have more of them during menstruation and ovulation; then, headaches last longer and are more intense and, worse yet, are harder to treat, harder to prevent and harder to eradicate once they've begun.

In addition to hormonal changes, headaches can be caused by triggers that are as individual as women are. Joan Miller, Ph.D., a clinical psychologist in Marietta, Georgia, and author of *Headaches: The Answer Book*, cites several common provokers. They include tension, certain foods (such as lunchmeats or aged cheese), caffeine withdrawal, skipping meals, environmental factors (pollen or pollution, for example) and certain physical causes, like problems associated with sinuses, vision, teeth, fevers or head trauma.

HEADACHES AND SUPER-HEADACHES

The two major headache syndromes that affect women are migraine and tension (or muscle contraction) headaches. What's the difference? According to Patricia Solbach, Ph.D., a headache specialist and director of the Center for Clinical Research at the Menninger Clinic in Topeka, Kansas, the pain of tension headaches is most commonly experienced as a steady, uncomfortable background pressure that doesn't disable you to the point of dysfunction. Migraines, she says, feel much worse: intense, throbbing pain sometimes accompanied by nausea, vomiting and sensitivity to light and sound. Migraines can last a few hours or even a few days.

367

Cues Herself to Relax

Patricia Solbach, Ph.D.

Headache specialist Patricia Solbach, Ph.D., had gotten only the occasional headache until she was fresh out of graduate school. Now director of the Center for Clinical Research at the Menninger Clinic in Topeka, Kansas, she recalls:

"I had just landed a great job coordinating a $250,000 research grant for—ironically enough—the study of nondrug headache treatments. I had steady headache pain daily, with tremendous pressure in my eyes and temples. It was awful. I couldn't think, much less work very well. There I was, a headache specialist, and I had to find out the hard way that too much stress could cause headache pain. So I learned how to relax, and I learned some antiheadache strategies that helped relieve the pain.

"Don't wait for a headache to build. At the very first sign of a headache, cue your body to relax by taking a break and sipping a cup of herbal tea," she says. "This works by breaking the tension that causes headaches."

Over the years Dr. Solbach's responsibilities at the Menninger Clinic increased. But happily, she reports, her headaches did not. Now, if she gets one headache a month, it's a lot.

About 5 to 10 percent of women who get migraines will experience auras, which are sensations of bright, even colorful, lights that appear before the eyes prior to the onset of a migraine headache.

ALL-PURPOSE OPTIONS

There is no shortage of headache relief medicines on the market. And painkillers have their place. "Take acetaminophen, aspirin or ibuprofen according to package directions at the first sign of a headache," says Michelle Cyr, M.D., associate professor of medicine at Brown University School of Medicine and director of the Division of General Internal Medicine at Rhode Island Hospital, both in Providence. "You can often nip it in the bud."

But then again, if headache relief were that simple, you wouldn't be reading this chapter. Or perhaps you're interested in a nondrug approach.

If you have a headache right now, the tips that follow will help you feel better fast. Some will work for tension headaches, others may help your migraines and some just might help you prevent your next headache, whichever kind it is. Women doctors agree that it's a good idea to experiment: Headache remedies work differently for different headaches, for different women, at different times.

Thumbs up, pain down. "Place your thumbs right in the center of each temple," says Dr. Solbach, who sometimes gets headaches herself. "Massage firmly using a circular motion for a minute or two, or until you feel relief. If I catch it early enough, I find that I can sometimes stop a headache."

Take a hot bath or shower. "This may further help your muscles relax," says Dr. Miller.

Visualize away your headache. "Imagine that your headache pain is caused by a rope that's knotted and wrapped tightly around your head," suggests Dr. Solbach. "Then concentrate hard on seeing it unknot, inch by inch. Watch as it slowly loosens and falls away from your head."

Try necking with a heating pad. "When you have a stiff neck, you can get a headache, because the stiff muscles hurt and cause pain that can be felt in your head," says Mary Scholz, R.N., a nurse clinician and nurse manager of Headache Associates at Faulkner Hospital in Boston. Her remedy? Apply a heating pad to the back of your neck to soothe the stiffness.

Ice a migraine. "For easing migraines, ice usually works better than heat," says Dr. Solbach, "most likely because of its action as a vaso-constrictor—it shrinks blood vessels pressing on nerve endings." A re-sealable plastic bag full of ice, wrapped in a kitchen towel, works.

Feverfew for you? For occasional headaches, Sandra McLanahan, M.D., executive medical director of the Integral Health Center in Bucking-ham, Virginia, recommends taking the herb feverfew. "Research on fever-few suggests that it can be effective as a headache remedy; I've used it with success for patients with headaches. I recommend taking two feverfew cap-sules (available at health food stores) three times a day until your headache is gone." Studies indicate that feverfew has anti-inflammatory properties, which is why it might be particularly effective for migraine headaches.

Lie down in a dark room. "If you have migraines," says Dr. Cyr, "lying down in a darkened room and napping for an hour or so can usu-ally make the headache history."

Have a snack. "You can get headaches from just being hungry," says Dr. Miller, because your blood sugar drops.

"Always be aware of when you last ate," adds Julie Buring, Sc.D., as-

WHEN TO SEE A DOCTOR

"Three hundred different medical conditions can cause headaches," says Patricia Solbach, Ph.D., a headache specialist and director of the Center for Clinical Research at the Menninger Clinic in Topeka, Kansas. "Most are tension headaches, and the rest are migraines and don't constitute emergencies."

However, she cautions, "If you're experiencing the worst headache that you ever had, see your doctor right away."

The following symptoms could signal a serious condition that needs prompt medical attention.

- Confusion
- Numbness
- Vision problems
- More-severe-than-usual headache, if you're over 50
- Chronic headaches that worsen

Also, talk to your doctor if you're on the Pill and get migraines—the estrogen in oral contraceptives can exacerbate migraines.

sociate professor of ambulatory care and prevention at Harvard Medical School and an epidemiologist at Brigham and Women's Hospital in Boston. "Try eating smaller meals, spread more frequently throughout the day."

Take a coffee break. "If you feel a migraine coming on, go someplace quiet and have a strong cup of coffee. Take aspirin or ibuprofen according to package instructions," says Dr. Solbach. Like ice, caffeine acts as a vasoconstrictor, which seems to help migraines.

Or, do the caffeine wean. The surprising thing about caffeine is that either too much or lack of it can trigger pain. According to Dr. Miller, too much caffeine can lead to headaches, because of an increase in tension or a decrease in sleep (or both). Consuming less than the usual amount of caffeine can lead to very painful withdrawal headaches. "Frequently, weekday coffee or cola drinkers may drink less on weekends, and they get fierce withdrawal headaches." Dr. Miller recommends that if you get headaches, give up caffeinated drinks slowly and gradually—by four to six ounces a day—perhaps by diluting regular brew with decaf until you're finally caffeine-free. She also suggests substituting eight cups a day of noncaffeinated liquids, such as water, juices, skim milk or herbal teas.

Keep a headache diary. "Both tension and migraine headaches can have triggers," says Dr. Cyr. "Your monthly cycle can affect headaches, too." She suggests that you log the time of day and month, the foods, activities, moods—anything that could possibly trigger a headache. After a couple of weeks, read your diary. See if anything obvious is causing your headaches and avoid the source if you possibly can.

"It's a very individual thing," says Dr. Buring. "For many, chocolate can be a migraine trigger—though it doesn't trigger my migraines—but red wine will immediately send me right around the bend."

Avoid migraine triggers. Dr. Cyr recommends avoiding the most common offenders: that is, foods that have been aged, fermented, pickled or marinated. Other reputed problem foods are those containing monosodium glutamate, or MSG (such as canned soups), nitrates or nitrites (such as lunchmeats).

ADDED HELP FOR KILLER MIGRAINES

Once a migraine takes hold, it's a bugger to relieve. So women doctors offer this additional advice for migraine sufferers in particular.

Restock your magnesium. An Italian study indicates that people with migraines are likely to have lower blood levels of magnesium than non-migraine-sufferers, and suggests that magnesium supplements for people with migraines warrant further study. Good food sources of magnesium include green leafy vegetables, legumes, seafood, nuts and whole grains.

Regulate sleep patterns. "People who work irregular shifts have trouble with their migraines," says Scholz. "Circadian rhythms seem to play a part in migraines. Try to get to sleep and wake up at the same times each day and don't sleep late on weekends." Also, avoid napping during the day, as this may change your circadian rhythms.

Give aspirin a chance. An aspirin a day may keep migraines away, suggests Dr. Buring. She conducted a study using low doses of aspirin regularly to prevent migraines. "The problem with some of the prescription drugs used to try and prevent migraines (like beta and calcium channel blockers, antidepressants and mood-regulating drugs) is that they are like hitting a little problem with an awfully big hammer," she explains. "In our study we found that taking a regular 325-milligram aspirin tablet every other day, regularly, cut repeat migraine attacks by 20 percent. It might not work for everyone, but it's definitely worth trying, because if it works, it's an easy, inexpensive and relatively safe solution."

Mononucleosis
No Longer a Forced Sabbatical

*B*ack in the Dark Ages (the 1960s and 1970s), there was something sort of sexy and vaguely attractive about mononucleosis, also known as the kissing disease. Being diagnosed with mono held special appeal—many students were sent home from college for whole semesters to recover, substituting a full schedule of watching game shows and soap operas for attending political science classes and antiwar rallies.

Triggered by the Epstein-Barr virus, mono is easily diagnosed by a blood test showing abnormally high numbers of white blood cells with a single nucleus. Typical symptoms include fever (often over 102°F) sore throat, swollen glands, an enlarged spleen and, of course, extreme fatigue.

Despite its reputation as something that you get from your sweetheart, mono can be spread by coughing, sneezing and sharing eating and drinking utensils as well as kissing. And it's less contagious than a cold or flu. You may be exposed to the virus and fight it off or experience just a touch of mono—not a full-blown debilitating episode. By midlife the odds that you'll contract mono are slim: Your teenage son or daughter is more likely to get mono than you are.

SHORTEN YOUR CONVALESCENCE

There is no drug for the virus that causes mono. But don't worry: These days, you don't have to stay home and watch game shows (unless you want to). In the event that you come down with mono, women doctors offer this advice.

Keep your spirits—and your activities—up. Jeanne F. Arnold, M.D., clinical assistant professor of medicine at Boston University School of Medicine, advises her college-age mono patients to try and maintain as much of a normal schedule as possible. "We used to tell everyone to go home and take to their beds, but now we tell them to try attending their classes if at all possible."

Rest when you're tired. That doesn't mean, says Dr. Arnold, that you shouldn't cut back your workload and get some extra rest. "Yes, limit after-school activities and, yes, rest when you're tired. But if you're

WHEN TO SEE A DOCTOR

Mononucleosis is self-limiting—in other words, the virus usually runs its course in a few weeks, says Margaret Lytton, M.D., a family practitioner at Thomas Jefferson University Hospital in Philadelphia. "You can get mono and not even know it," she says. "The symptoms can be as innocent as a mild sore throat and fatigue."

You should see your doctor if you have a severe sore throat, high fever or debilitating fatigue, says Dr. Lytton. The reasons: It's rare, but mono can sometimes carry potentially serious complications, such as an enlarged liver, hepatitis or pneumonia. Or you could have a strep or other bacterial infection requiring immediate medical attention.

so sleepy that you're napping in class, take a break for a few days and make other arrangements to get your work covered."

Doctors say that most women today can expect a convalescence of two weeks or less. "Seventy-five percent of the people who contract mono feel better after just a couple of weeks," says Dr. Arnold. "A very small percentage are still very fatigued after six months. I think that the eventual outcome is based on an individual's outlook and general state of health."

Take acetaminophen. To lower your fever and soothe aches and pains or sore throat, take Tylenol, Anacin-3 or the generic equivalent, says Katherine Sherif, M.D., instructor in medicine at the Allegheny University of the Health Sciences and on staff at the Institute for Women's Health, both in Philadelphia. Aspirin is okay for adults over age 21 only, because of the risk of Reye's syndrome (a serious neurological disease) in children and younger adults.

No roughhousing. "When you have mono, your spleen usually enlarges temporarily and is displaced from its usual position of protection under the lower rib cage," says Dr. Sherif. "So I advise patients to forgo contact sports like field hockey, skiing and any other activities where you run the risk of a spleen-rupturing injury."

Mood Swings
Help for the Highs and Lows

A good mood can have a half-life that's shockingly short.

While something more stable, like plutonium, will take a good 24,100 years to disintegrate to any noticeable degree, a good mood can dissipate in mere minutes. After whistling your way through the morning commute, you can hit the skids and slide into the blues or the jitters long before lunch hits the table.

Some of us are more vulnerable to mood swings than others, but we all have them. "Minor swings into depression or anxiety are very common," says Susan Nolen-Hoeksema, Ph.D., professor of psychology at the University of Michigan in Ann Arbor.

Women may be more vulnerable to mood swings than men, says Dr. Nolen-Hoeksema. "Our research has found that women tend to focus more on negative moods—to worry about them—and that can makes the moods worse."

Certain hormonal shifts may make women more susceptible to downward spins, says Bonnie Spring, Ph.D., professor of psychology at the University of Health Sciences/Chicago Medical School. That's why some of us find that we're particularly moody the week before our menstrual periods, after childbirth or during menopause.

STABILIZING THE PENDULUM

Even when you're feeling most vulnerable, though, you can lessen the severity of mood swings, even head some off at the pass, say doctors. Here's how.

Act, don't brood. If you feel yourself slipping into depression or anxiety, get up and do something—take a walk or clean the clutter off your desk. "One of the best ways to stop a mood from getting really severe is to do something that gives you a sense of control and accomplishment," says Dr. Nolen-Hoeksema.

Exercise for 20 minutes. "We know that exercise has an antidepressant effect," explains Dr. Spring. In a study at Texas A&M University College of Medicine in College Station, women reported significant improvements in mood after 20 or more minutes of walking.

Distract yourself. Just about any activity can help take your mind off your mood. If you can stop ruminating for a while, you can get perspective on whatever triggered the swing and think about that more clearly.

"Ponder the problem again later, when you're no longer in the throes of a mood, so you can figure out why you got upset and what you can do about it," says Dr. Nolen-Hoeksema.

Think rationally. Sometimes you're too depressed or anxious about something to take your mind off your mood, even temporarily, says Dr. Nolen-Hoeksema. In these cases you can get some perspective (and relief) by asking yourself three key questions: One, what is the evidence that what you think is going to happen will actually happen? If you're anxious about losing your job because you didn't get that promotion, consider the supporting evidence—or lack thereof. If you're doing quality work, on time, then your anxiety is probably unfounded.

Two, are there alternative ways to think about this situation? Maybe your boyfriend is suddenly quiet because he's having problems at work, not because he's thinking of breaking up with you. Talk to him about it.

And third, if the worst did happen, how would you cope? You could start looking for a new job, for example. Or, should you and your boyfriend indeed break up, it wouldn't necessarily be easy, but you could start over in a new relationship.

Get a second opinion. To help you think rationally, talk things through with a friend, says Dr. Nolen-Hoeksema.

Treat yourself. If you're dropping into a depressed or anxious mood, pampering yourself may help, says Dr. Spring. Take a bubble bath, buy yourself some flowers and put them on your desk or listen to music by your favorite composer, for instance. Plan for "down" days by making a list of mood-lifting treats.

Grab some mood food. Certain foods or food combinations set off a series of chemical reactions in your brain that help determine whether you feel content, on one hand, or anxious or depressed on the other, says Elizabeth Somer, R.D., author of *Food and Mood* and *Nutrition for Women*.

If you're spiraling into a depression, Somer suggests eating a snack that combines protein with carbohydrates—like half a turkey sandwich. "The combination helps turn on neurotransmitters—naturally invigorating brain chemicals."

Reach for a bagel. If you're free-falling into anxiety, an all-carbohydrate snack like a cinnamon-raisin bagel with jam might help, Somer says. That combination turns on calming neurotransmitters (though it might also make you sleepy).

Skip the alcohol. Essentially, alcohol is a depressant. If you're already blue, it will make you feel worse, says Somer. So if your mood is floundering, don't take solace in a drink.

Watch the caffeine. Caffeine—a stimulant—will make you feel more anxious if your nerves are fraying, Somer says. If you're jittery, cut back on the java, tea, cola and chocolate.

Get enough sleep. You're especially vulnerable to mood swings when you're sleep-deprived, says Dr. Spring. Get enough sleep, particularly when you know that swings are more probable, like during the week before your period. If you have insomnia, try different remedies until you find what works for you.

Morning Sickness
Beat the Queasies

Some women say that they enjoy being pregnant. They're usually the ones who don't experience morning sickness. The Centers for Disease Control and Prevention in Atlanta doesn't track morning sickness, but women doctors estimate that 30 to 90 percent of pregnant women experience nausea and vomiting, usually between the seventh and fourteenth week of pregnancy. What's more, morning sickness can occur at any time of the day. An unlucky few get morning sickness throughout pregnancy.

While not all women get the queasies during pregnancy, for those who do, it's often the biggest problem of the first trimester, says Helen Greco, M.D., an obstetrician/gynecologist at Long Island Jewish Medical Center in Hyde Park, New York.

MOTION SICKNESS WITHOUT THE MOTION

Being too queasy to stomach food—or keep it down—can leave you hungry and tired, says Mindy Smith, M.D., associate professor in family practice at the University of Michigan in Ann Arbor. Short of hi-

Eat and Sleep

Mindy Smith, M.D.

Women doctors aren't immune to morning sickness. That includes Mindy Smith, M.D., associate professor in family practice at the University of Michigan in Ann Arbor.

"I have a queasy stomach to begin with, and my mother threw up every day during her first two pregnancies," Dr. Smith says. "So when I became pregnant, I was pretty sure that I was also going to be sick."

Early in her pregnancy, Dr. Smith took a leave from work—a move that she credits with preventing morning sickness.

"I ended up not having a single episode of vomiting. But I did nothing but eat and sleep. Most women are working or taking care of kids, and they feel like they can't tend to what their bodies need."

bernating until the daily bouts of nausea subside, experts offer these tips for relief.

Keep crackers handy. The best way to beat morning sickness is to keep saltine-type crackers at your bedside and eat a few before you even get out of bed in the morning, says Jennifer Niebyl, M.D., professor and head of obstetrics and gynecology at the Hospitals and Clinics at the University of Iowa in Iowa City.

Wash them down with juice. Next to the crackers, keep a chilled container of juice or water, says Dr. Niebyl. Fluids keep you from becoming dehydrated, which can make matters worse.

Try watermelon. If you can't keep juice or water down, eat a few chunks of ice-cold watermelon, suggests Miriam Erick, R.D., senior perinatal nutritionist at Brigham and Women's Hospital in Boston, where she works with women hospitalized for severe morning sickness, and author of *Take Two Crackers and Call Me in the Morning! A Real Life Guide for Surviving Morning Sickness.* Erick calls this type of food a solid liquid.

Eat small, frequent meals. It's easier for your stomach to digest just a few bites at a time, and you'll be less likely to get nauseated, says Dr. Greco.

Make sure you don't overeat. Eat just enough to satisfy your

WHEN TO SEE A DOCTOR

If you experience routine bouts of morning sickness during pregnancy, it won't hurt to mention it to your physician during your regular prenatal visits. If you can tolerate little or no food or liquids, are not gaining weight or are losing weight, however, call your doctor *immediately*, says Mindy Smith, M.D., associate professor in family practice at the University of Michigan in Ann Arbor. Severe morning sickness may require hospitalization.

hunger, because more could just make you feel worse.

Save part of your lunch for the middle of the afternoon and part of dinner for a bedtime snack, says Dr. Niebyl.

And take snacks along when you're away from home, adds Dr. Smith.

Act on your cravings. "Ask yourself what you would have if you could eat anything in the world," suggests Erick. What appeals to you? Something salty? Sweet? Soft and chewy? Crisp and crunchy? Then eat whatever food satisfies your craving. Potato chips? Spaghetti? Jell-O? If you want it, eat it, because in 30 minutes you could want something different.

Chew on anise. Herbalists have found that the volatile oils in anise seeds calm the stomach and relieve nausea, says Mary Bove, a naturopathic physician with the Brattleboro Naturopathic Clinic in Vermont and a licensed midwife. Ask your obstetrician if it's okay to chew a few.

Ask your OB about B_6. Taking 25 milligrams of vitamin B_6 helps some women, says Dr. Smith.

In fact, Dr. Niebyl conducted one of two studies in which women who took 25 milligrams of vitamin B_6 three times a day (a total of 75 milligrams per day) for three days reduced nausea and vomiting associated with pregnancy.

Vitamin B_6 is available in supermarkets and drugstores in 50-milligram doses, so you need to break the pills in half, says Dr. Niebyl. Use caution, though: The Daily Value for vitamin B_6 is 2 milligrams a day, and very high doses—more than 100 milligrams a day—can be toxic. So, as with other vitamins, if you're pregnant, don't take B_6 without medical approval.

Press your point. An acupressure point in your wrist can help relieve nausea, according to both Dr. Smith and Elaine Stillerman, a licensed massage therapist on the staff of the Swedish Institute of Massage in New York City and author of *Mother-Massage*. The point is on the underside of your forearm, about 1½ inches away from your wrist, dead center between the ligaments. Press it with the pad of your thumb and hold for a slow count of ten. Breathe normally and repeat three to five times or until the nausea subsides.

Apply seasickness bands. Developed for motion sickness and available at drugstores, Sea-Bands apply constant pressure to acupressure points for nausea, say both Dr. Smith and Stillerman. Or you can try Stillerman's do-it-yourself-version: Affix a dried bean like a kidney bean over the point with an adhesive bandage and wear it overnight.

Motion Sickness
End Nausea and Cold Sweats

Any woman who has ever been on a boat in rough seas or braved a turbulent airplane ride is probably all too familiar with the dreaded symptoms of motion sickness: that queasy feeling that makes your skin turn pale and clammy, your head feel heavy and your stomach start to churn. Other symptoms include dizziness, fatigue, sweating, faintness, difficulty breathing, even blackouts. "The most perturbing symptom is the stomach distress—queasiness, nausea and even vomiting," says Susan Herdman, Ph.D., associate professor of otolaryngology at the University of Miami in Coral Gables.

THE CONFUSED BRAIN

Motion sickness occurs when your brain receives conflicting signals about the movement affecting your body. Your eyes may tell you one thing, but your inner ear system and your legs tell you another. Say you're inside the cabin of a boat where you can't see the choppy waves outside. Everything looks perfectly still. But your legs and inner ear system sense

379

WHEN TO SEE A DOCTOR

If you're pregnant, you may be more susceptible to motion sickness, says Glenda Lindseth, R.D., R.N., Ph.D., associate professor of nursing at the College of Nursing of the University of North Dakota in Grand Forks. If you've been traveling and have three to five severe episodes of vomiting, see a physician to make sure that you're not dehydrated, and that you and your fetus are okay.

that you're bobbing around like a lobster buoy atop the waves. When your brain receives these signals that don't match, it gets confused—and you get sick, says Dr. Herdman.

Motion sickness can strike even when you're riding in a car or train. So if you're a busy woman who needs to travel, repeat attacks could seriously derail your lifestyle.

Certain situations may make some women especially vulnerable to motion sickness. If you're pregnant and you're prone to morning sickness, your stomach is already irritable, and you'll be even more likely to get green around the gills if you step onto a rocking boat, for example. "The increase in certain hormones during pregnancy may change your body's tolerance to motion sickness, it seems," says Glenda Lindseth, R.D., R.N., Ph.D., associate professor of nursing at the College of Nursing of the University of North Dakota in Grand Forks.

Likewise, women who are on the Pill or taking hormone replacement therapy for menopause may be more susceptible to nausea while traveling, because the medications boost levels of certain hormones and may make their stomachs more sensitive, says Dr. Lindseth. In fact, in a small study of airsickness in pilots, Dr. Lindseth found that all of the female pilots who were using contraceptive pills became significantly more airsick than other pilots.

A MIND-BODY APPROACH

The cure for motion sickness is to get back on solid ground; you should feel better once you stop moving. But that's not always an option. Short of bailing out of a moving vehicle (not a wise move), here's what women doctors say that you can do to soothe your stomach and get a smoother ride.

Choose a good seat. "The best thing that you can do is sit where you reduce conflicting sensory signals," says Dr. Herdman. If you're on a boat, get out of the cabin and sit on deck, where you can see the movement of the water. If you're in a car, sit up front, where you can see the road.

Watch where you're going. "When you can see where you're going, the visual cues from your eyes match more closely what your inner ear system says, and you're less likely to get sick," says Dr. Herdman. So focus on something outside the vehicle. And don't read; it confuses your senses.

Snack smart before you depart. A study of the diets of pilots on the day of travel revealed that those who ate a light meal within two to three hours before flight were less likely to get airsick than those who flew on an empty stomach. "It's best to opt for light servings of pasta, bread, grain (like cooked oatmeal) or fresh fruits and vegetables," advises Dr. Lindseth, lead author of the study.

Eat light on traveling day. Dr. Lindseth's study also showed that pilots who ate fatty, high-calorie foods before flight were more likely to report airsickness than those who ate light. "Avoid foods packed with fat or protein for two to three hours before your trip and during travel," she recommends. Dairy and meat products such as ice cream, cheeses, lunch-meats, bacon and ham are among the worst culprits.

Munch low-salt snacks. If you're going to be traveling, and you're prone to motion sickness, low-sodium, low-fat crackers are ideal. But beware of salty, sodium-packed treats like potato chips or corn chips, which tend to make stomachs more queasy en route, says Dr. Lindseth. Extra sodium causes the body to retain water, which seems to affect the fluid balance in and around cells, and therefore may contribute to motion sickness sensations, she says.

Calm down! "If you're prone to motion sickness, the more anxious you get while traveling, the more sick you will probably feel," says Dr. Lindseth. In fact, worrying about motion sickness may actually bring on the symptoms. So sit down, relax and stay calm. Try not to get upset or exert yourself.

Breathe in, breathe out. One of the best ways to calm your mind and body is to control your breathing, says Patricia Cowings, Ph.D., a psychologist at NASA in Moffett Field, California, who developed a six-hour biofeedback training program to teach astronauts (women as well as men) how to overcome feelings of motion sickness in space.

"As part of our program, we recommend breathing at the constant rate of two seconds in, two seconds out," says Dr. Cowings. "Also try to keep the volume constant—not too deep, not too shallow." When you control your breathing, other stress responses will calm down too—your heart rate will slow, your muscles will relax and your blood pressure will come down—so you'll be less anxious and less likely to get sick, she explains.

Snap up some ginger. "Ginger actually settles the stomach, so it's very likely to help," says Dr. Herdman. In a study of sailors on a ship in open seas, those who received one gram of powdered ginger root (the equivalent of one capsule bought in a health food store) experienced less vomiting and cold sweating while traveling through heavy waves than sailors who received a placebo.

Taking one or two powdered ginger capsules bought in a health food store, three times a day on travel days, will help soothe the stomach, says Tori Hudson, N.D., a naturopathic physician and professor at the National College of Naturopathic Medicine in Portland, Oregon.

Take medications with care. As a last resort, if you have a history of motion sickness but absolutely can't avoid travel and nothing else works, you can head off queasiness by taking an over-the-counter medication about 30 to 60 minutes before you depart. "If you wait until the motion sickness starts, it's too late. You'll be even sicker by the time the medicine kicks in," says Dr. Lindseth.

The drawback of these off-the-shelf medications is that they do have side effects. The active ingredients in many of these drugs, including dimenhydrinate (Dramamine) and meclizine (Bonine), work by making you drowsy—so you'll make it through the ride, but you'll be out of commission. Other side effects include dry mouth and, rarely, blurred vision, says Dr. Herdman. Read the warning labels. You may want to try them out ahead of time, so you know how they will affect your body while you're traveling.

Size 6? Take half the amount. If you're petite, take the lowest dosage recommended on the label. "The amount recommended on the label is usually safe and effective for most adults, but a very petite woman who weighs only 100 pounds or so may want to cut back on the dosage even more, because her smaller body may not metabolize the drug as well," suggests Jean L. Fourcroy, M.D., Ph.D., past president of the American Medical Women's Association and the National Council of Women's Health.

Muscle Aches and Pains

Soothe Next-Day Soreness

Every January 2, health clubs are jammed with women resolved to get back in shape once and for all—or lose their holiday weight gain. And every January 3, millions of women wake up with sore muscles.

New exercise recruits are not the only ones who experience muscle pain. The same thing can happen when you clean out your flower beds in spring or finally get around to washing the windows.

According to women doctors, overuse—doing too much too fast—is the most common cause of simple muscle aches and pains.

After not using your muscles for months or years, suddenly forcing them all to jerk into high gear may well inspire rebellion from tiny tears that develop within the muscle tissues. You can't see them, but you sure can feel them.

"You'll feel achy and sore," says Debra Zillmer, M.D., an orthopedic surgeon and medical director of the Gundersen Lutheran Sports Medicine Clinic in La Crosse, Wisconsin.

HELP YOUR MUSCLES HEAL

Whether it's your first sore muscle or an achiness that you've felt before, relax. The pain isn't permanent, and it probably won't last long. Meanwhile, women doctors offer these suggestions to help ease the pain more quickly.

Take a 24-hour sabbatical. "The very first step to heal an overuse injury is to rest the muscles that are hurting," says Margot Putukian, M.D., team physician at Pennsylvania State University in University Park and assistant professor of orthopedic surgery and internal medicine at the Milton S. Hershey Medical Center in Hershey. Give your muscles a 24-hour layoff after they start to ache, she says.

Ice it. To speed the healing process, Dr. Zillmer advises using ice. It reduces swelling and soreness, slows bleeding from tears and soothes bruises.

383

Place a wrapped ice pack or even a bag of frozen vegetables on your aching muscles for up to 20 minutes out of every hour until the pain subsides, says Dr. Putukian. (Don't eat the vegetables.)

Distract yourself. Sitting around whining about how much you hurt will only make aches worse. So do something to get your mind off the hurt. "Watch the dog dig up a bone, listen to a relaxation tape or soothing music or do anything that lifts your spirits," says Kathleen Lewis, R.N., a nurse in Decatur, Georgia, and author of *Successful Living with Chronic Illness.*

"Studies have shown that when you focus on the pain, your muscles actually tense up more," she says.

Shake a leg. Don't run out and exercise when your muscles hurt, but when the discomfort eases, get out there and play to your level of fitness. Your body will tell you how much to do or not do, says Lewis.

"If you use your muscles every day, they're likely to be more limber and a lot less prone to the strains and pains of overuse," she says. Try low-impact aerobic exercise—exercise that gets your heart pumping—such as walking or swimming for half an hour at least three times a week.

For repeat aches, try heat. "Women with chronic muscle pain often do better with heat than with cold, because it increases circulation and muscle flexibility," says Dr. Zillmer. Try a heating pad, a warm bath or even just a warm towel on the affected area for no more than 20 minutes at a time.

Muscle Cramps
Freedom from Kinks and Knots

Say you're playing tennis—and doing pretty well. One minute you're fine, then suddenly, for no apparent reason, your calf muscle knots up and you can't move.

What's happened is that your muscle has tightened and shortened, causing sudden, severe pain, explains Debra Zillmer, M.D., orthopedic surgeon and medical director of the Gundersen Lutheran Sports Medicine Clinic in La Crosse, Wisconsin. In active, healthy women, muscle cramps generally result from overexertion and dehydration—like spending five hours playing tennis in hot, summer heat and forgetting to take sips from your water bottle.

"When you don't have enough fluid in your system, it leads to an electrolyte imbalance that causes your muscles to cramp up," says Dr. Zillmer.

Electrolytes are chemicals in the body—sodium, magnesium, calcium and potassium—that help the cells function normally. An imbalance occurs when we have too much or too little of one or more electrolytes in our system. The main electrolytes affecting muscle cramping are potassium, sodium and calcium.

Other cramps, not related to fluid intake, occur after inactivity—like sitting too long in one place without moving a muscle. Sometimes you can even get a cramp when you're just lying in bed, though no one is sure why.

TAKING THE CRIMP OUT OF CRAMPS

Though people most often get cramps in their calves, you can also get them in your thighs or feet—or just about any muscle. But women doctors say that wherever the knotting up and whatever the cause, most cramps can be eased by a few simple measures.

Massage gently. To relax the tightened area, Dr. Zillmer suggests gently massaging the area that's cramped—whether it's a crick in your calf from overexercising or a spasm in your feet from wearing high heels all day.

S-t-r-e-t-c-h. "Next, stretch the muscle out slowly and gently, as long as you don't feel pain," says Dr. Zillmer.

For calf cramps, do a wall stretch. Stand about three feet away from the wall, with your knees straight and your heels on the floor. Lean into the wall, supporting yourself with your hands. You will feel the stretch of your calf muscles. Hold for 60 seconds and repeat three times, says Dr. Zillmer.

Slurp fluids. "If you get muscle cramps after golf or other forms of exertion, drink water or a sports drink or juice to rehydrate and restore your electrolyte balance," says Dr. Zillmer. Most of the time water will be sufficient to rehydrate you. The exception is if you have spent several hours exercising in extreme heat. You are then better off choosing a sports drink containing electrolytes, she adds.

WHEN TO SEE A DOCTOR

Muscle cramps usually go away on their own, even if you do nothing, says Margot Putukian, M.D., team physician at Pennsylvania State University in University Park and assistant professor of orthopedic surgery and internal medicine at the Milton S. Hershey Medical Center in Hershey. But if you're drinking plenty of fluids and eating a balanced diet (plenty of grains, cereals, beans, fruits and vegetables and few sources of animal fat or sugar) and keep getting cramps, see a doctor. Frequent, intense muscle cramping may be a sign of a more serious condition, such as a blood clot or electrolyte problems.

Focus on calcium, potassium and general hydration. The electrolyte imbalance that causes muscle cramps can also be caused by deficiencies of calcium and potassium in the diet, says Margot Putukian, M.D., team physician at Pennsylvania State University in University Park and assistant professor of orthopedic surgery and internal medicine at the Milton S. Hershey Medical Center in Hershey. To beef up your calcium levels, she suggests low-fat dairy products such as yogurt and skim milk. For potassium, focus on sweet potatoes, turkey, bananas and orange juice.

Undo a cramp with ice. "Ice is both a pain reliever and an anti-inflammatory," says Judith C. Stern, a physical therapist in private practice in Westchester, New York. Stern suggests you keep a paper cup of ice in the freezer for just such emergencies, then massage the area on and around your cramp as needed. "Tear down the edge of the cup and, holding the paper end, rub the ice over the cramped muscle. This way, it won't be too cold to hold," says Stern.

Massage the area with ice for no more than ten minutes or until the area is bright red, which indicates that blood cells have returned to heat the cramped muscle. Or use an ice pack or if nothing else is handy a bag of frozen vegetables.

Heat is another option. Heat improves superficial blood circulation and makes muscles more flexible, so some people find that heat is more soothing for muscle cramps than ice, says Stern. Try a heating pad for 20 minutes at a time, or even a warm shower or bath. Massage the muscle with your hands following ice or heat.

Move around. "Inactivity also is a cause of cramps," says Valery Lanyi, M.D., physiatrist at Rusk Institute of Rehabilitation Medicine at New York University Medical Center in New York City. So if you've been on the road for an hour, get out and walk around for five minutes.

Nail Biting
Unlearn a Bad Habit

Women doctors say that nail biting is a familiar—albeit unhealthy—reaction to stress.

"We're all under stress, and we all have to do something with it," says Loretta Davis, M.D., associate professor of dermatology at the Medical College of Georgia School of Medicine in Augusta. "Some women take up jogging to control stress, and some women bite their nails."

Some woman want to quit once and for all, so that their hands look beautiful for their wedding or some other special occasion, says skin-care specialist Lia Schorr, owner of Lia Schorr Skin Care Salon in New York City. Others are motivated by other reasons. For one thing, think of all the germs that you're putting in your mouth.

AVERSION THERAPY

Trying to stop biting your nails is a lot like trying to quit smoking or avoid overeating—success depends partly on behavioral changes and partly on analyzing why you continue the habit.

For simple nail biting, women should start with the easiest remedies first, says Frances Willson, Ph.D., a clinical psychologist in Sherman Oaks, California, and chair of the Health Psychology Committee of the Los Angeles County Psychological Association.

Make them taste bad. Dr. Willson suggests nail paint, available at drugstores, to make your nails taste objectionable. Standard advice says that it takes seven to ten days to break a habit. So give it some time.

When not in public, wear cotton gloves. That way, you can't get at your nails, says Dr. Willson.

Or buy a box of adhesive strips. Wearing an adhesive bandage around the tip of each finger can also act as a deterrent to nail biting, says Dr. Willson.

Carry worry beads. Trisha Webster, a hand model with the well-known Wilhelmina Modeling Agency in New York City, suggests wearing something like worry beads and fingering those when the urge to chew strikes. "The important thing is to find something to do with your hands," she says.

Encourage yourself. "When it comes to breaking this habit, I believe that encouragement works better than punishment," says Dr. Willson. For many women who bite their nails, a manicure is very encouraging.

Shorter is better. Well-manicured nails leave you little nail to bite. If necessary, file your nails between manicures so that you won't bite them in order to trim them, says Dr. Willson.

Nail Discoloration
Get Rid of Yellow Stains

*N*ail polish is one of the accessories that many women take for granted, changing colors every few days to coordinate the color of their nails with their wardrobes. Or maybe sticking with a classic shade of dragon red, touching up nicks and chips between manicures as their nails grow out. After a few weeks, they remove all the polish, only to discover that their nails have a decidedly yellowish tint.

If your nails are discolored, it may be caused by nail polish, especially if you favor red polish, says Phoebe Rich, M.D., clinical assistant professor of dermatology at Oregon Health Sciences Center in Portland.

"Discoloration is often caused by the yellow dye that's in many of the red polishes," says Dr. Rich. If you don't wear red polish, other products may discolor your nails.

WHAT YOU CAN DO

If your nails are discolored, don't try to aggressively scrape away the stains, warns Dr. Rich. You'll damage your nails. Instead, she offers this advice.

Let your nails grow out, sans polish. "It's best to let the staining disappear, which it will do on its own," says Dr. Rich. In four to six months—the time that it takes a nail to grow out—the stains will be gone.

Use a base coat. "I find that if you apply a base coat and then add a high-quality polish, you can use bright red with less chance of staining," says skin-care specialist Lia Schorr, owner of Lia Schorr Skin Care Salon in New York City.

A coat of clear nail polish works well too, says Dr. Rich.

Avoid formaldehyde. If you want stain-free nails, read labels closely and avoid nail products that contain formaldehyde, says Marianne O'Donoghue, M.D., associate professor of dermatology at Rush-Presbyterian–St. Luke's Medical Center in Chicago.

Smoke less (if at all). Red polish isn't the only reason why nails turn yellow, says Loretta Davis, M.D., associate professor of dermatology at the Medical College of Georgia School of Medicine in Augusta. The nicotine in cigarettes leaves powerful stains. "Patients of mine who smoke cigarettes to the very end are quite likely to have stained nails. The stains remain until the nail grows out and only disappear if they don't continue to smoke."

Wear protective gloves. Hair stylists, nurses and other health care workers who work with dyes or chemical solutions may end up with stained nails, say women dermatologists. If you work with strong chemicals, always wear protective gloves.

WHEN TO SEE A DOCTOR

If you've quit smoking and stopped coloring your nails, and they're still discolored, consider seeing a doctor.

Some medications can cause changes in nail pigmentation. Rarely, discoloration is caused by what doctors call yellow nail syndrome—a slow thickening of the nails that may occur in people with pulmonary (lung) disease or other conditions.

Nail Fungus
A Side Effect of Artificial Nails

A fungal infection of any kind is upsetting, especially if it occurs on your nails, so visible to you and everyone else. Yet nail fungus is quite common, say women doctors.

Fungus of the nails can be stubborn and "may produce dramatic changes in the nail," says Elizabeth Whitmore, M.D., assistant professor of dermatology at Johns Hopkins University School of Medicine in Baltimore. "Typically, the nails thicken and turn white or yellow. They can also be scaly and crumbly and begin to split. Sometimes the nails may even shed."

Ironically, one of the chief causes of nail fungus can be traced to a practice adopted to enhance women's beauty: wearing artificial nails.

Artificial nails are glued on, and if separated from the natural nails, moisture can get under the tip, creating a cozy place for fungus to grow. When fungal infection occurs, it may cause no symptoms. However, if an associated secondary bacterial infection occurs, pain, swelling and throbbing may be the result. Typically, antibiotics are needed to clear the secondary bacterial infection.

"I make my living with my hands, but I make it a policy to not wear false nails," reports Trisha Webster, a hand model with the well-known Wilhelmina Modeling Agency in New York City. "Women get so used to them that they forget to give their own nails a rest."

Many women are allergic to the glue or acrylic used to cement the nails in place, says Elizabeth Abel, M.D., clinical associate professor of dermatology at Stanford University School of Medicine. Some women are also allergic to the formalin in nail polish. Symptoms include redness, scaling, swelling and pain in the nail folds or adjacent tissue. Complications include bacterial infections and such bothersome reactions as oozing and drainage from around the nail.

If you don't wear artificial nails and develop a nail fungus anyway—say, on your toenails—the problem could be caused by yeasts, molds or other members of the fungi family. Fungi can travel back and forth between hands and feet.

"Yeast infections of the nails can pose a problem for people who have their hands in water a great deal," says Loretta Davis, M.D, associ-

WHEN TO SEE A DOCTOR

Typical signs of a nail bacterial or fungal infection include:
- Painful swelling around your nail folds and debris under your nail causing separation
- Yellow, white, green or brown discoloration

If you think that you have a nail infection, consult a dermatologist for an accurate diagnosis and proper medical treatment.

ate professor of dermatology at the Medical College of Georgia School of Medicine in Augusta. "Usually, what happens is that people develop a break in their cuticles, and that's the entering point."

PREVENTION WORKS BEST

Women doctors say that nail fungus is easier to avoid than to treat. Here's what they advise.

Avoid artificial nails. Since wearing artificial nails is the most common cause of nail fungus in women, you can save yourself a lot of grief by not wearing them.

Keep hands and nails dry. After you wash your hands, dry them well. "If you must keep your hands in water for any length of time, wear cotton-lined latex gloves," advises Dr. Davis.

Moisturize. Dry, cracked cuticles, nails and skin can be an entry point for infection, according to Dr. Davis. She recommends keeping your hands well-moisturized at all times.

Nausea

Stop the Heaving

What do bus fumes, pregnancy and week-old tuna noodle casserole have in common? All three can make you nauseous. So can a rocky ride on a rolling boat, too much cognac, and some powerful medicines.

One way to deal with nausea is to end it all—by throwing up. Sometimes you feel better, and sometimes you don't.

STILL THY STOMACH

Nausea is somewhat individualistic—no single cure is guaranteed to work for everyone, every time. So women doctors offer the following remedies that may work for you.

Put your feet up. "Sometimes the best thing you can do is nothing," says Wanda Filer, M.D., a family practice physician in York, Pennsylvania. Put your feet up, sit still, don't move around. It will give your stomach a chance to calm down, she says.

Starve your stomach. If you're vomiting or feel like you're about to, don't eat or drink anything for a couple of hours, in order to give your stomach time to settle down, says Dr. Filer.

Then sip a bit. When your stomach stops heaving, sip some flat soda, water, Gatorade-type fluid replacement drink or chicken broth once or twice every five minutes. "But sip, don't gulp, so that the liquid has a chance to settle down," she says.

Have a small snack. If you're queasy, food may be the last thing you want to think about. But once your stomach starts to feel a little less shaky, it can help to eat something.

"Your stomach often will feel less queasy if you eat a little bit of plain food, like crackers," says Sheila Crowe, M.D., gastroenterologist and assistant professor of medicine in the Department of Internal Medicine in the Division of Gastroenterology at the University of Texas Medical Branch at Galveston. But be sure not to overdo.

"As long as you're nauseated, stick with small amounts of low-fat foods," Dr. Crowe says.

WHEN TO SEE A DOCTOR

If you're nauseous for a day or two and can link your discomfort to something you ate, pregnancy or other probable cause, it's probably not serious enough to warrant medical attention. But if you're sick for more than three days or you frequently feel nauseous for no obvious reason, see a doctor. This is particularly true if you're also vomiting, experiencing abdominal pain or losing weight unintentionally. Your doctor needs to find out what's going on and get the problem under control.

Shy away from rich, highly seasoned dishes. Spicy, fatty foods like chili and pizza are hard to digest when you're nauseated, says Dr. Crowe.

For now, forgo milk. Milk and dairy products like cottage cheese contain protein and fats that are hard to digest and make the digestive system work extra, says Dr. Crowe. So until your nausea subsides, stick with clear fluids such as water and broth and avoid dairy in all forms.

Take a shot of bismuth compound or antacid. Over-the-counter products such as Pepto-Bismol and Mylanta often soothe squeamish stomachs, says Dr. Crowe.

Go for the ginger. "Ginger combats the nausea associated with pregnancy, seasickness, carsickness and just about everything else except the nausea associated with chemotherapy," says Tori Hudson, a naturopathic physician and professor at the National College of Naturopathic Medicine in Portland, Oregon.

Ginger in capsule form—available in health food stores—is the strongest, so it has the greatest medicinal effect, Dr. Hudson says. "Take one or two capsules three times a day as long as you feel nauseous," she says.

If you prefer to drink your ginger, go to the produce section of your supermarket and buy some fresh ginger root, Dr. Hudson says. When you get home, cut off a slice about as long as your index finger and simmer it in about 16 ounces of hot water for 15 minutes. "That will make about two cups of soothing ginger tea," says Dr. Hudson.

Or try crackers and ginger. If you need help getting the ginger tea down, Dr. Hudson suggests eating a bland food, like a cracker, with it.

Mix up a ginger juice cocktail. If ginger tea doesn't soothe your nausea, try tincture of ginger, available at health food stores, says Dr. Hudson. Dunk 30 drops into a few ounces of water or juice and drink it

393

down three or four times a day until you're no longer nauseous.

Or, sip ginger ale. Dr. Hudson says you might also want to try some ginger ale—yes, the same thing your mother gave you when you stayed home from school, she says. There isn't much ginger in it, but there's enough to settle your stomach in a mild case.

(For details on dealing with nausea associated with pregnancy, read about morning sickness on page 376. For details on nausea caused by travel and transportation, read about motion sickness on page 379.)

Neck Pain
Surprising Causes, Easy Solutions

*I*f your neck had the flexibility of a crane or a swan, trying to parallel park would be no problem. Neither would sitting at a keyboard for hours as you input data into a computer, read e-mail or write reports. And it certainly would make watching fireworks or craning your neck to watch a play or musical from the back rows easier.

In reality, our necks don't have much flexibility. And if you keep your neck in an unusual position too long—jutting forward, for example, or sleeping in an awkward position—you risk an irksome episode of neck pain.

"The neck is like a pole on which a 14-pound bowling ball sits," says Annie Pivarski, ergonomics and injury prevention program supervisor at Saint Francis Memorial Hospital in San Francisco. "It's subject to a lot of stresses."

Though both men and women suffer from neck pain, it's particularly prevalent among women tied to desk jobs.

"Neck pain is especially prevalent in women in clerical positions, because they lean over their desks or computers for long periods of time, which strains the upper back or neck," says Mary Ann Keenan, M.D., chairman of the Department of Orthopedic Surgery at the Albert Einstein Medical Center in Philadelphia.

SIMPLE STEPS TO RELIEF

Okay, so for whatever reason, your neck hurts. Relax. Women doctors say that you may be able to get rid of the pain in your neck posthaste by trying these simple home remedies.

Head for the freezer. Applying an ice pack or ice wrapped in a washcloth can ease the acute pain and stiffness, says Pivarski. Try it for 15 or 20 minutes.

Or try heat. Some women feel that heat works better than ice, says Dr. Keenan. Try a warm shower, letting the water run over your neck, or a heating pad at a comfortable setting—low or medium, not hot—for no more than 20 minutes at a time, she says.

Stretch those muscles. "These stretches don't take much time, but they ease neck stiffness. And you can do them at home or at work," says Sheila Reid, P.T., coordinator of rehabilitation services at The Spine Institute of New England in Williston, Vermont.

One example: Turn your head all the way to one side, then back to the center so you're facing straight ahead, and then all the way to the other side. Look down at the floor, bring your head back to a straight-ahead position, next look up at the ceiling, then bring your head back. Repeat a few times a day, as needed.

IS IT YOUR SHOES? OR YOUR CHAIR?

When it comes to preventing repeat episodes of neck pain, women doctors suggest a few tactics that may come as a surprise. Here's what they suggest.

Save high heels for special occasions. Few women make a connection between footwear and neck pain. "High heels knock your spine out of alignment, which also makes your neck jut forward," says Pivarski. Try to save high heels for special occasions, and wear low-heeled shoes or flats most of the time.

Take a load off your shoulder. "A heavy purse on one shoulder strains your neck as well as your back and shoulders," says Dr. Keenan. Switch to a fanny pack or backpack or carry your purse across your chest. Load heavier belongings into a suitcase on wheels, as do many flight attendants and travelers. Or buy the wheels and a couple of bungee cords from a discount store and roll your luggage along.

Tilt your chair back. Often, neck pain is caused by jutting your head forward. The solution? Bring your reading material to you.

When you read or watch television, recline your chair so that your

WHEN TO SEE A DOCTOR

If you try home remedies but your neck continues to hurt after a few days, see a doctor, says Mary Ann Keenan, M.D., chairman of the Department of Orthopedic Surgery at the Albert Einstein Medical Center in Philadelphia.

See a doctor immediately if your pain radiates to your shoulder, arm or wrist, says Dr. Keenan. It could signal a heart problem, and it's better to be on the safe side than to ignore the symptom.

head is supported by the back of the chair or a wall, Dr. Keenan says.

"It's okay to sit on a couch or an easy chair, as long as you change positions frequently (say, once an hour), so that your neck doesn't get stiff," says Margot Putukian, M.D., team physician at Pennsylvania State University in University Park and assistant professor of orthopedic surgery and internal medicine at the Milton S. Hershey Medical Center in Hershey.

Adjust your PC monitor. "If you work at a computer, make sure you don't have to crane your neck to look at your monitor," Dr. Keenan says. Adjust your monitor so it's at eye level.

Get a copy holder. "You can easily strain your neck from looking back and forth from the computer to copy off to the side and lower than the screen," says Pivarski. A copy holder attached to the monitor at eye level will allow you to read documents without straining your neck.

Wear a headset. Do you cradle the phone receiver between your ear and shoulder while taking notes or writing on a computer? "Consider switching to a headset and saving your neck stiffness and pain," says Pivarski.

Trade up to a down pillow. To keep from waking up with a stiff neck, choose a pillow made of down or other pliant material or one of the orthopedic pillows instead of solid foam rubber, says Reid. "A good pillow follows the contours of your neck instead of leaving your neck unsupported," says Reid. And sleep on your side or back, not your stomach.

Nicotine Dependency
Quit Smoking Once and for All

*W*hen it comes to incentives to quit smoking, scare tactics don't work. Women know that smoking causes lung cancer. They know that it raises their risk of stroke and heart attack—a whopping tenfold if you also take birth control pills.

Smokers and nonsmokers alike are also now learning that smoking contributes to osteoporosis and cancer of the mouth, larynx, esophagus, cervix and pancreas. What's more, it can lead to early menopause, fertility problems and miscarriage.

Chances are, if you smoke, you've tried to quit—several times—but just couldn't kick the habit. In a survey by the Centers for Disease Control and Prevention in Atlanta, 73 percent of the 22 million American women who were smoking in one year said that they wanted to quit. But 80 percent of those who had tried to quit said that they couldn't even manage to cut back. More than a third reported significant withdrawal symptoms: irritability, anxiety, hunger, fatigue, dry mouth, headaches, insomnia, constipation and, of course, cigarette cravings.

TRY, TRY AGAIN

The truth is, cigarettes are just as addictive as cocaine or even heroin—and equally hard to ditch.

"Studies show that it's very difficult for people to stop using products containing nicotine," says Anne Geller, M.D., neurologist and chief of the Smithers Alcoholism Treatment and Training Center at St. Luke's-Roosevelt Hospital Center in New York City and past president of the American Society of Addiction Medicine. Also, fear of weight gain—a common occurrence among ex-smokers—also keeps many women from quitting.

But it's worth trying to quit again. Smoking can cause permanent damage. Nicotine withdrawal, by contrast, is only temporary.

Here's what you can do to minimize withdrawal symptoms and avoid weight gain.

Switch brands first. A few weeks before you plan to quit, try switching to a brand that's lower in nicotine than what you currently smoke, suggests Nancy Rigotti, M.D., assistant professor of medicine at

WHAT WOMEN DOCTORS DO

Reward Yourself along the Way

Anne Geller, M.D.

No doubt about it—giving up cigarettes can be rough. Just ask Anne Geller, M.D., neurologist and chief of the Smithers Alcoholism Treatment and Training Center at St. Luke's-Roosevelt Hospital Center in New York City and past president of the American Society of Addiction Medicine. Dr. Geller experienced nicotine withdrawal firsthand when she quit a 17-year cigarette habit in 1980 (and learned some withdrawal-coping strategies in the process.)

When she was quitting, Dr. Geller soaked away the irritability and anxiety in a nightly hot bath. "I also found that exercise was another wonderful antidote to the irritability and anxiety.

"After I quit I was more interested in dessert than I had been," she adds. "While I was smoking, my after-dinner cigarette had always been my 'goodie.'" So that she wouldn't be tempted, she stopped making desserts.

And once a week, Dr. Geller says that she would take the money that she saved on cigarettes and spend it on a record or some other small treat. "If you're quitting smoking, try to build some pleasurable activities—little purchases, movies—into your schedule, so that you don't feel so deprived."

Harvard Medical School and director of Quit Smoking Services at Massachusetts General Hospital in Boston. Just make sure that you don't smoke more cigarettes than usual or inhale more deeply, since that defeats the purpose.

Have half a cigarette. If you can quit cold turkey, consider yourself lucky. More than likely, you'll need to cut back gradually to ease withdrawal symptoms, says Dr. Rigotti. She suggests smoking only half of each cigarette. Or allowing yourself to smoke only during certain times of the day. Or putting a progressively lower limit on the number of smokes that you're allowed daily. Once you're down to five or six, quit altogether.

Ice dry mouth. If you've just quit, and your mouth feels dry and cottony, or if your throat, gums or tongue hurts, try sipping ice-cold water or fruit juice, suggests the National Cancer Institute.

Snack sensibly. Make sure that you have lots of low-calorie snacks on hand—fruit, cut-up raw vegetables, small packages of flat bread, skim milk or sugarless gum. By taking the low-cal route, you can eat more without gaining more. But don't automatically reach for food when you think that you're hungry. Try having a no-cal drink—preferably water—first. Drink through a straw, if that helps. You may think that you're hungry, but you really need a drink, or you simply want something in your hand or mouth, says Dr. Geller.

Exercise more, smoke less. Women doctors say that exercise relieves irritability and anxiety, and it helps you avoid adding extra pounds when you quit.

"Increasing the amount of aerobic exercise that you do is one of the best ways to control your weight," says Dr. Rigotti. If you walk for 20 minutes three times a week, make it 30 minutes a stretch, or do 20 minutes four times a week.

Heal the headache. Aspirin and other pain relievers can soothe a nicotine-withdrawal headache, says Dr. Geller. A warm bath or shower may also do the trick.

Draw a warm bath. Relaxing in a hot tub of bathwater can also help ease anxiety and irritability, says Dr. Geller. If there's no bath in sight, try visualizing yourself in a soothing, pleasant place. Or relax with some deep breathing: Take a long, deep breath, count to ten and release. Repeat five times.

Hang in there. Most relapses happen the first week after you quit, when withdrawal symptoms are the strongest, says Dr. Rigotti. Make quitting easier by avoiding things that you associate with cigarettes—like alcohol or other smokers.

"Most people make four or five attempts before they succeed in quitting," notes Dr. Geller. "Just remember: One cigarette doesn't have to lead to a pack, and a relapse doesn't mean that you're never going to quit."

Nosebleeds

Dam the Red-Nose River—Fast

*A*ll you did was sneeze, and suddenly, there seems to be an awful lot of bright red blood dripping down your face. Yikes! You have a nosebleed.

"It's easy to get a bloody nose, because inside the nose, blood vessels are close to the surface, where they can easily rupture," says Karin Pacheco, M.D., staff physician in the Division of Allergy and Immunology at the National Jewish Center for Immunology and Respiratory Medicine in Denver.

STAY CALM

"It's important not to panic," says Dr. Pacheco. "Ninety-nine times out of 100, you can stop your own nosebleed without medical intervention, as long as you remember what to do."

Give it a pinch. "Use your thumb and forefinger to pinch your nostrils shut," says Susan Fuchs, M.D., associate professor of pediatrics at

WHEN TO SEE A DOCTOR

Seek emergency treatment for your bloody nose if you experience any of these problems.

• If you can't breathe through either nostril after a blow to your nose, your nose may be broken. Apply ice and pressure and see a doctor or go to an emergency room for evaluation.

• If you're swallowing lots of blood, you may have a nosebleed from deep within your nose. (This is typical in people who have been struck in the face.)

It's also a good idea to consult your doctor if you frequently get nosebleeds for no obvious reason.

the University of Pittsburgh School of Medicine and attending physician in the emergency room at Children's Hospital of Pittsburgh.

"If your nose still bleeds after five minutes, pinch your nostrils shut again and don't let go for fifteen minutes," says Dr. Fuchs. If bleeding continues after you apply 15 minutes of pressure, it's time to see a doctor.

Apply ice. "If you were hit in the nose, apply ice and pressure," says Dr. Fuchs. "The ice will help reduce swelling and slow the bleeding." Lying down with a bag full of ice cubes—wrapped in a towel—pressed on your nose should do it.

Don't blow your way into another bleed. "If you've successfully stopped a nosebleed by pinching it shut, don't blow your nose," says Dr. Pacheco. "You'll dislodge the clot that has formed, and your nose will start bleeding again."

No cotton, please. "Don't stuff your nose with cotton in an attempt to quell a nosebleed. The cotton will adhere to the scab that forms inside, and you'll rip it away when you remove the cotton, causing another nosebleed," says Dr. Fuchs.

Oily Hair

Shine without Grease

You start out every morning with clean, shiny hair. But by bedtime, your hair looks greasy, lame and lank.

The problem?

"An overproduction of oil," says Patricia Farris Walters, M.D., clinical assistant professor of dermatology at Tulane University School of Medicine in New Orleans and a spokesperson for the American Academy of Dermatology. In other words, the sebaceous (oil-producing) glands that are attached to the hair follicles pump out so much goop that the cells along each shaft are slickly coated. Since hormones control the production of oil in your scalp, there is really no way to change the amount of oil produced.

SECRET WEAPONS AGAINST OIL

Here's what women doctors advise to combat oily hair.

Shampoo frequently. Wash your hair more often, and make sure that you get it clean when you do. With oily hair, wash once, then rinse and wash again. Leave the shampoo on for several minutes to give the detergent time to remove the dirt and oils, says Dr. Walters.

Try a dandruff shampoo. "Most people with oily hair also have dandruff, since the same hormones can stimulate both conditions," says Dr. Walters. Shampoo your hair with a dandruff shampoo that contains coal tar derivatives, even if you don't have dandruff. Dandruff shampoos tend to dry out even the oiliest hair.

As an added bonus, coal tar has a natural conditioning effect, which adds softness and shine without adding the oils contained in man-made conditioning products. This eliminates the need for adding any conditioners to detangle or add shine, says Wendy Resin, hair-care manager at the Neutrogena Corporation in Los Angeles. Neutrogena T/Gel shampoo contains coal tar and can be purchased at drugstores.

Cut down on conditioners. Most conditioners and styling products tend to contain oils and other ingredients like emollients and resins that can weigh the hair down—the last thing that you need if your hair is oily, says Yohini Appa, Ph.D., director of product efficacy at Neutrogena.

Alternate with a clarifying shampoo. Every other shampoo, use a shampoo that's high in cleaning agents such as sodium lauryl sulfate and low in any kind of conditioners such as lanolin, says Dr. Walters. These clarifying shampoos, as the cosmetics industry sometimes calls them, actually strip oil from the scalp as well as the hair shaft, says Resin. She suggests Neutrogena's Anti-Residue Shampoo.

You might also want to try Pantene's Pro-Vitamin Clarifying Shampoo.

Oily Skin

On-the-Spot Control

*O*ily skin isn't all bad. Sure, oily skin leaves your nose shiny or creates a small puddle in the middle of your forehead. Yet oil also makes our skin soft and supple.

The key is to strike a balance, to somehow regulate oiliness for maximum benefit with minimum mess.

AN OIL-REDUCTION PLAN

"Oily skin tends to be hereditary. It's an overproduction of sebum (oil) from the sebaceous (oil) glands," says Karen S. Harkaway, M.D., clinical instructor of dermatology at the University of Pennsylvania School of Medicine and a dermatologist at Pennsylvania Hospital, both in Philadelphia.

If your oil glands seem to be working overtime, give these tips a try.

Swab the decks, matey. Skin-care companies have come up with nifty foil-wrapped packets of alcohol-saturated wipes for oily skin. They're similar to the larger wipes that women with children often carry for tidying up kids away from home. The smaller facial wipes are easy to tuck into your handbag or briefcase. Then, when you notice that your nose is shiny with oil, you can peel a packet apart in a bathroom and wipe the oil from your face. The alcohol cuts through the oil and dries up your skin. "They smell nice and refreshing and they're very convenient," says Dr. Harkaway. Look for Tyrosum wipes, among other brands, in major drugstores, or ask your pharmacist to order them.

Wash with care. If you have oily skin, you may be tempted to scrub that oil away every chance you get. But washing your face too much—more than three times a day—may stimulate your skin to produce *more* oil. "Every skin pore is a little oil factory," says Mary Lupo, M.D., associate clinical professor of dermatology at Tulane University School of Medicine in New Orleans, "and your skin knows how much is produced—as if it had a little dipstick. So if you constantly remove that oil, your skin says, 'Oops! Not enough oil. Better make some more.'"

Hard scrubbing and rubbing stirs up the oil glands, too, so be gen-

tle. And if you have oily skin, avoid superfatted soaps (intended to moisturize as they clean) like Dove and Tone—your skin doesn't need any
added oil. "Antibacterial soaps (like Dial and antibacterial Lever 2000)
are helpful," says Susan C. Taylor, M.D., assistant clinical professor of
medicine in the Department of Dermatology at the University of Pennsylvania School of Medicine in Philadelphia. That's because oily skin has a
tendency to clog the pores and foster bacterial growth.

Rely on witch hazel. Among dermatologists witch hazel is a popular astringent. Don't let the name fool you. "Witch hazel is mild and
doesn't have a lot of added ingredients," says Mary Ruth Buchness,
M.D., chief of dermatology at St. Vincent's Hospital and Medical Center
in New York City. It's always best to keep skin-care products as simple as
possible—use the purest products. And be wary of natural products containing essential oils (extracts of herbs used in aromatherapy and massage)—some people are allergic to them.

Go powder your nose. Talcum powder, whether it's formulated for
the body or if it's loose face powder, is oil-free. What's more, talc blots
the oil on your skin. "People with oily skin need a little powder after they
bathe and when they apply makeup," says Dr. Lupo.

Apply loose face powder after applying foundation, says Dr. Buchness. Pressed powder is not recommended, because it contains some oil
and may make acne worse in susceptible women.

Orgasm Problems
Peak Pleasure Can Be Yours

*I*f sex were a banquet, orgasm would be dessert. If it were a European
journey, it would be Paris. If it were a romance novel, the part where
the star-crossed lovers sigh and finally find one another.

Just as it would be a mistake to rush through the appetizer and entrée, give short shrift to Florence or skip those tantalizing scenes where he

casts her longing glances and she casts them back, it would be a mistake to overlook the pleasure of foreplay—and all that follows—by focusing too narrowly on orgasm.

"If a woman is bent on achieving orgasm, she can end up missing out on the pleasure of everything else—and missing out on orgasm," says Sharon Nathan, Ph.D., a sex therapist and clinical assistant professor of psychology in psychiatry at Cornell University Medical College in New York City. "However, if she's bent simply on achieving pleasure, she's not going to end up that far from orgasm."

The truth is, most women don't achieve orgasm every time, but they do enjoy sex tremendously. According to one nationwide survey, 29 percent of women say that they always have orgasm, while 40 percent say that they're extremely pleased with their sex lives. Do the math: Lots of women enjoy sex whether they have an orgasm or not.

That's not to say that orgasm isn't particularly pleasant. It's the wonderful release of delightful tension that builds during sex. When you're aroused, extra blood flows to your genitals, creating this tension. In the moment of release, your vaginal muscles contract and release rapidly in spasms of extreme pleasure, says Dr. Nathan.

SECRETS OF A SATISFYING CLIMAX

Assuming that your doctor has ruled out medical reasons for an orgasm problem, says Barbara Bartlik, M.D., a psychiatrist and sex therapist with the Human Sexuality Program at New York Hospital–Cornell Medical Center in New York City, there is really nothing holding you back from a good orgasm—or several.

The obstacles that most often stand in the way—inhibitions, communication problems, inexperience, fear of letting go, stress and depression—can be overcome, says Barbara Keesling, Ph.D., a sex therapist in Orange, California, and author of *Sexual Pleasure* and *Talk Sexy to the One You Love*. Here's what you can do.

Talk yourself into it. "The most common reason why women have difficulty achieving orgasm is that they don't give themselves permission," Dr. Keesling says. "And this stems from being taught that 'nice girls don't.'"

The trick in giving yourself permission is challenging beliefs about sex that you've held since childhood. If you do challenge them, you'll probably find that many of them don't hold up. Ask yourself: Do the sex rules that your parents taught you still make sense now that you're a grown-up? Why shouldn't you enjoy sex now?

Know thyself. You have to be sufficiently aroused to reach orgasm, and to get sufficiently aroused, you need to know what makes you feel good. The best way to find out, says Dr. Bartlik, is to explore your body.

To start, set aside 20 minutes when you know that you won't be interrupted.

"First, do something relaxing, like taking a hot bath," explains Dr. Bartlik. "Then, look at your genitals in a mirror. Put some lubricant on your finger and touch them. Touch your vaginal lips, your clitoris and your vagina. Find out which areas are most sensitive and what kind of touch feels good. Sometimes using a vibrator can help, though you may not feel comfortable doing that right away."

Practice touching yourself in ways that heighten your arousal to the point of orgasm. When you have an orgasm, you'll feel your vaginal muscles contract around your inserted finger about once every second, explains Merle S. Kroop, M.D., a psychiatrist and sex therapist in New York City.

Speak up. When you find what you like, tell your partner about it, says Dr. Nathan.

While you're at it, get in the habit of talking about all facets of your relationship with one another. Unresolved conflicts can put the damper on sex, and orgasm, adds Dr. Bartlik.

Try new positions. If you're like most women, you'll need clitoral stimulation to achieve orgasm, says Dr. Bartlik. The surest way to climax, then, is to have your partner fondle your clitoris with his fingers or tongue or to stroke your clitoris yourself. (It may be easier to achieve the right kind of clitoral stimulation during intercourse if you're on top.)

Some women have an extra-sensitive spot on the wall of the vagina, about two inches inside the vaginal opening. Stimulating this spot, called the G spot, can also lead to orgasm. The G spot gets a lot of friction during rear-entry intercourse, so if your vaginal wall is responsive, give that position a try, suggests Dr. Keesling.

By trying a lot of different positions, you'll find the ones most likely to lead to orgasm, says Dr. Keesling.

Osteoporosis
Prevent "Little Old Lady Syndrome"

*I*f you're 45 years old or younger and think that it's too early (or too late) to start worrying about osteoporosis, think again: The earlier you think about it, the better, says Susan Allen, M.D., Ph.D., associate professor of internal medicine in the Department of Internal Medicine at the University of Missouri Hospital and Clinic in Columbia. According to top women doctors who specialize in osteoporosis, this disease could easily become yesterday's news if, starting now, you eat calcium-rich foods and engage in regular weight-bearing exercise.

"Osteoporosis is 100 percent preventable," says Susan Ward, M.D., clinical assistant professor of medicine and associate director of the Jefferson Osteoporosis Center at Thomas Jefferson University Hospital in Philadelphia. According to Dr. Ward, women's bodies were originally designed to not last much past menopause, when estrogen production slows and finally ceases. The lack of estrogen triggers an increase in bone resorption—in other words, bone loss.

BANK BONE NOW

The good news is that the time to lessen your osteoporosis risk is right now. Women doctors offer these proactive measures to prevent or slow the progression of the disease.

Bone up on calcium. Premenopausal women need at least 1,000 milligrams of calcium a day, says Doris Gorka Bartuska, M.D., director of endocrinology, diabetes and metabolism clinical services at Allegheny University of the Health Sciences in Philadelphia. Once past menopause, women should be getting 1,200 to 1,500 milligrams a day, she says.

The best sources of calcium? Low-fat dairy products. Nonfat yogurt (onc cup has 452 milligrams), skim milk (one cup has 302 milligrams) and part-skim mozzarella cheese (1 ounce has 181 milligrams) top the list. Of course, taking calcium carbonate, calcium gluconate or other forms of calcium supplements is the easist way to ensure that you get what you need each and every day of the week.

Stay (or get) active. "Incorporate activity into your lifestyle now,"

407

WHEN TO SEE A DOCTOR

Since there is no pain associated with early osteoporosis, it's important to be aware of the risk factors, so that you can head off the disease by taking precautions now. A simple 15-minute test called the DEXA scan (dual energy x-ray absorptiometry) measures your bone density and tells whether you're at risk for osteoporosis. Ask your doctor about having a DEXA scan if you:

- Are thin and small-boned
- Have irregular menstrual periods or fewer than ten cycles a year
- Have a history of eating disorders
- Have a family history of osteoporosis
- Take corticosteroids, anticonvulsants like phenytoin (Dilantin), thyroid medication or blood thinners
- Have generalized bone pain and tenderness
- Experience frequent fractures

says Susan A. Bloomfield, M.D., assistant professor of kinesiology at Texas A&M University in College Station. "The most important thing is to do something active every day." Dr. Bloomfield advises women to alter sedentary routines—for example, she says, "Never sit when you can stand, or ride when you can walk. Any exercise is better than no exercise at all."

Take a walk. "Every woman should have a program that includes weight-bearing exercise," says Dr. Allen. "And one of the very best and easiest is walking."

"Schedule yourself for a daily 20-minute walk," suggests Dr. Ward.

Join a smoking-cessation program. "Smoking cigarettes can lower estrogen levels," says Dr. Bartuska, "and it has a negative impact on bone density."

A study on female twins suggested that a woman who smokes a pack of cigarettes a day may experience a 5 to 10 percent reduction in bone density at the time of menopause, a deficit that could increase the risk of fracture.

Skip coffee and alcohol. "Put both alcohol and caffeine on your no-no list," says Dr. Bartuska. "Both are diuretics that leech calcium from your bones."

In addition, alcohol may be toxic to bone-forming cells and may interfere with intestinal absorption of calcium, say experts. Plus, drinking affects your balance and, as you get older, increases the chances that you'll fall and break a bone.

Overweight
A Passport to Slenderness

Women all over the United States are struggling with weight gain. Women doctors are no exception.

"I lost weight not just for cosmetic reasons but for its health implications," says Jan McBarron, M.D., a weight-control specialist and director of Georgia Bariatrics in Columbus, Georgia.

If you're even 20 percent overweight (say, you should weigh 120 pounds, but tip the scale at 144 pounds), health risks soar for high blood pressure and cholesterol, diabetes and other diseases, says Dr. McBarron.

According to the Harvard University Nurses' Health Study, an ongoing study of about 115,000 women, even gaining 15 or 20 pounds more than you weighed at age 18 increases your risk of heart disease or other serious illnesses.

LEAVE EXCESS POUNDS IN THE DUST

The news is not all bad. Luckily, dropping even ten excess pounds can lower your cholesterol by five to ten points and your blood pressure as much as six points, says Dr. McBarron. Here is some help with slimming down forever.

Watch less TV, get more exercise. The only way to lose weight and keep it off is to exercise, even if it's something as simple as turning off the TV and going for a walk around the block, says Susan Zelitch Yanovski, M.D., director of the Obesity and Eating Disorders Program at the National Institute of Diabetes and Digestive and Kidney Diseases at the National Institutes of Health in Bethesda, Maryland.

"Physical activity is crucial—for health and weight loss," says Dr.

Now Wears a Size 7

Jan McBarron, M.D.

As a weight-control specialist and director of Georgia Bariatrics in Columbus, Georgia, Jan McBarron, M.D., has lived the counsel that she gives.

"At one point I wore a size 22 and weighed 200 pounds," says Dr. McBarron, who now wears a size 7. "I had tried every diet craze that came along. I would lose weight, then it would all come back *plus* 10 pounds.

"When I reached 200 pounds, I thought, 'I can't diet anymore. I'm going to look at my thin friends and see what they do, then do what they do.'

"My thin friends ate breakfast, lunch, dinner and occasionally, dessert," she says. "But they also took the stairs, parked farther away from the door at the mall and were more active in general. So I did the same.

"I lost about ten pounds a month, and my weight has been stable for the past nine years," she says. And she has never missed her large-lady wardrobe.

Yanovski. You become overweight when you take in more calories than you burn up, she says, and nothing burns up calories and fat like exercise.

To get the maximum benefit, you should do aerobic exercise—that means exercise that increases your respiration and heart rate—such as walking, running or bicycling, for 30 minutes most days of the week, says Dr. Yanovski.

Walk a little now and a little later. "If exercise seems overwhelming at first, start small and work up to it," says Dr. Yanovski. "Walk for 15 minutes at lunch and another 15 minutes when you get home from work, or walk for 10 minutes, with a goal of gradually increasing your exercise time."

AND BY ALL MEANS, EAT

Exercise works faster if you also take in fewer calories. But you don't have to crash diet. Here is what women doctors tell women who want to lose excess pounds.

Trim 600 calories a day from your present diet. The simplest way to do this is to eat less, says Dr. McBarron. You can easily do this by switching from whole milk to skim, ordering foods like fish and potatoes—baked instead of fried—switching to fat-free mayo and salad dressing and taking similar small calorie-saving steps.

Eat half as much. Do you usually fill your plate or, if you're at a restaurant, eat everything that you're served? "Try eating half as much," says Maria Simonson, Sc.D., Ph.D., director of the Health, Weight and Stress Clinic at the Johns Hopkins Medical Institutions in Baltimore. Chances are, you'll be able to meet your need for nutrition without feeling deprived.

Chew the fat less. You don't have to leave out fat entirely, but you should keep it to 20 percent (240 calories if you eat 1,200 calories a day) of your diet: That includes butter, fat in meat or nuts and, yes, the occasional sweet treat, Dr. McBarron says.

Her Secret is Tabasco

Maria Simonson, Sc.D., Ph.D.

One of the nation's most widely quoted weight-loss counselors, Maria Simonson, Sc.D., Ph.D., director of the Health, Weight and Stress Clinic at the Johns Hopkins Medical Institutions in Baltimore, also used to have a substantial weight problem. She ate everything—fries, steaks and ice cream—until health problems forced her to reconsider.

At five feet six inches, Dr. Simonson has kept her weight constant at 165 pounds for 15 years. Here's what she does to keep the pounds from coming back.

"When I order a meal at a family restaurant, I'll ask for a carry-out box. When my food is served, I immediately put half in the box," she says.

"I try not to eat foods that are fattening or cooked with fat, but I don't count every calorie. I eat very slowly and drink water before meals," she says. "And I eat small portions. At this point, if I sat down to a full meal at a restaurant, I would lose my appetite.

"I love spicy foods. It's impossible to overeat on spicy foods, because they fill you up so quickly. Whenever I travel, particularly abroad, I carry a bottle of Tabasco sauce. I use it on everything but ice cream."

WHAT WOMEN DOCTORS DO

WHEN TO SEE A DOCTOR

If you have a chronic health problem such as diabetes or high blood pressure, see a doctor before embarking on a weight-loss program.

If you're more than 20 pounds overweight, your risk of developing certain serious health conditions is higher than average, so see your doctor for periodic checkups.

Break your nightly fast. "Breakfast is the day's most important meal, because it's your body's signal that it's time to fight fat," says Dr. McBarron. While you sleep, your body stores food as fat so that you won't starve to death. Eating lets your fat-burning enzymes know that it's time to get up and go to work. If you don't eat, your body will continue to store food as fat.

"Strange as it may sound, you're likely to lose weight if you start eating breakfast, even if you don't cut calories the rest of the day," Dr. McBarron says.

Flip lunch and dinner. Exercise burns up calories, which means that your body will burn up food better while you're active, so eat your main meal at midday and eat something light (like salad with fat-free dressing) for dinner, says Dr. McBarron.

Chew your food—a lot. "Chew each morsel 10 to 15 times slowly," says Dr. Simonson. You'll enjoy it more and digest it better, and the effort of chewing each bite thoroughly will make you less inclined to overeat.

Drink up. Water slows your appetite and keeps food moving quickly through your digestive tract, Dr. Simonson says. "Drink a large glass of water ten minutes before meals. It'll fill you up, so you'll get full faster."

Eat with a fork. Finger food is a no-no, Dr. Simonson says, because we just naturally eat more when it's easier to get to. Don't eat straight from the bag or the box. Your mother was right: You should eat sitting at the table, with your food on a plate or in a bowl, and use the proper utensil.

Ditch the low-fat snacks. Low-fat desserts are deceptive, Dr. McBarron says. They are full of sugar and often contain as many or more calories as high-fat desserts. Worse, excess sugar converts to fat when your body digests it. Instead, eat a piece of fresh fruit, she suggests.

Stay away from alcohol. Alcoholic beverages—as well as alcohol-free drinks—are very high in calories, Dr. Simonson says. A piña colada, for example, has 262 calories—more than a slice of pepperoni pizza.

What's more, "people who drink eat more and eat worse," says Marion Nestle, Ph.D., professor and chairperson of the Department of Nutrition and Food Studies at New York University in New York City.

Painful Intercourse
Turn "Owww" into "Ahhh"

As intensely pleasurable as sex can be, it can be downright painful now and then.

All sorts of things can make intercourse hurt. Vaginal infections, injuries, allergic reactions and insufficient lubrication can do it, says Barbara Bartlik, M.D., a psychiatrist and sex therapist with the Human Sexuality Program at New York Hospital–Cornell Medical Center in New York City. Sexually transmitted diseases, improperly healed adbominal surgical scars, bladder conditions, chronic constipation and reproductive organ disorders like endometriosis and fibroids can also lead to pain during or after sex. So can psychological conflicts.

MAKING LOVE, COMFORTABLY

If sex is painful, and your doctor has ruled out an underlying medical cause, you can get comfortable again by following these simple strategies.

Check your cabinets. Vaginal irritation can make sex agonizing, says Sharon Nathan, Ph.D., a sex therapist and clinical assistant professor of psychology in psychiatry at Cornell University Medical College in New York City. Common irritants include latex condoms and ingredients in laundry detergents, bubble baths, douches, contraceptive creams and spermicides. Try eliminating potential culprits for a week or so and see if the pain or irritation clears up, suggests Dr. Nathan. Bathe without bubbles. Use a different contraceptive cream. Try one of the new, nonlatex condoms.

But don't switch to lambskin condoms, unless you're absolutely sure

WHEN TO SEE A DOCTOR

If pain during intercourse is severe, see your gynecologist for an exam right away. If the pain is mild, try self-help strategies for a few days. If that doesn't do the trick, see your doctor, advises Barbara Bartlik, M.D., a psychiatrist and sex therapist with the Human Sexuality Program at New York Hospital–Cornell Medical Center in New York City.

that your partner is HIV-negative and monogamous. Lambskin condoms block sperm but won't block transmission of the human immunodeficiency virus, says Gretchen Lentz, M.D., assistant professor of obstetrics and gynecology at the University of Washington Medical Center in Seattle.

Extend foreplay. To give yourself more time to get aroused and lubricated, prolong the cuddling, stroking, caressing and kissing before intercourse, Dr. Bartlik says. Having sex when you're not fully lubricated can cause both irritation and pain.

If you always feel pain, you and your partner might try stimulating one another with your mouths or hands and saving intercourse until the very end, suggests Dr. Bartlik. In the event that penetration is still painful, skip intercourse and bring one another to climax orally or manually.

Assume a new position or two. Some positions make sex more comfortable than others. Experiment until you find the ones that work best for you, advises Dr. Bartlik.

Try an over-the-counter lubricant. Hormonal changes that occur during breastfeeding and menopause can make vaginal tissues drier and thinner and make sex painful, says Dr. Bartlik. Certain medications, like antihistamines, can also cause vaginal dryness.

Whatever the cause, applying over-the-counter water-soluble lubricants (like K-Y jelly, Replens or Gyne-Moistrin) before intercourse can help, says Dr. Bartlik. In fact, a New York University study that compared over-the-counter lubricants with prescription ones found that the former did an equally good job. Follow package directions.

Get comfortable. A combination of psychological and physical factors can contribute to a condition called vaginismus, in which the muscles around the vaginal entrance spasm involuntarily, making intercourse extremely painful, even impossible, explains Merle S. Kroop, M.D., a psychiatrist and sex therapist in New York City.

Often, women who experience vaginismus feel great anxiety about insertion or penetration. Some were raised in households where sex was considered bad or degrading. Others have had traumatic sexual experiences, says Dr. Kroop.

The following exercise, designed to dispel fear of sexual penetration and restore a sense of control during sex, may help, says Dr. Nathan.

Set aside some time when you can be alone and relax. Undress and lie in a comfortable position with your legs bent at your knees and your feet flat. Put a dollop of lubricant on your finger and insert just the tip into your vagina, pushing down as if you were trying to defecate. (This procedure relaxes the muscles at the entrace to the vagina without any risk of a bowel accident.) Leave your finger in your vagina for a minute until you get used to the feeling. Then move it further in, up to the first knuckle. Now practice tightening and relaxing your vaginal muscles around your finger. To tighten, contract the same muscles that you use to stop the flow of urine while on the toilet.

Continue practicing the technique, each time inserting your finger a little further, then tightening and relaxing your muscles around it. With practice, you should feel progressively more confident about your ability to control your muscles and more relaxed about having something in your vagina.

When one finger is easy, try inserting two. When that's comfortable, ask your partner to insert one, then two of his fingers. Eventually, he should be able to insert his penis, says Dr. Nathan.

Panic Attacks
Calming Techniques That Work *Fast*

*H*eart galloping, hands trembling, sweat running down her face, Alison had her first panic attack in her early thirties. She never figured out why. A wave of intense and terrifying anxiety washed over her, then dissipated in the space of an hour.

Several years later, panic returned—first one attack, then another, to the point where Alison dreaded going to work. As a high-level executive at a major multinational corporation, Alison (not her real name) was afraid that she'd have an attack in front of her staff.

"Alison called in sick so often that she lost her job," says Irene S. Vogel, Ph.D., a psychologist and director of Vogel Psychology Associates in the Washington, D.C., metropolitan area who later successfully treated Alison's panic.

As debilitating as they are unpredictable, panic attacks are relatively common. They happen to perfectly reasonable people, like you.

"A large number of adults have had panic attacks at some time in their lives," says Dr. Vogel. "Some never have more than one or two and don't even know that they had one." They may blame their symptoms on something else, such as drinking too much coffee.

We're all more likely to have panic attacks during periods of stress. But some of us seem to inherit a vulnerability to attacks, say researchers, since the attacks appear to run in families. For reasons that scientists don't completely understand, panic attacks are more common in women than men.

MORE THAN JUST A CASE OF NERVES

The symptoms of a panic attack vary from person to person, but they usually include a combination of the following: difficulty breathing, sweating, chest pain or discomfort, loss of balance, feelings of unreality, trembling, tingling or numbness in the extremities, nausea, palpitations, smothering sensations and hot or cold flashes. There is always an overwhelming anxiety. Most attacks last just minutes, and few go on for more than an hour.

WHEN TO SEE A DOCTOR

If you think that you're having panic attacks, but you aren't sure, see your doctor. Certain medical conditions or medications can cause similar symptoms.

If indeed the problem is panic, experts recommend immediate professional help, because treatment gets more difficult the more entrenched the problem becomes. Recurring panic attacks may lead to agoraphobia, characterized by irrational fears and avoidance of places or situations in which the panic occurs.

In addition to self-help coping techniques, professional treatment may involve a variety of approaches, from behavioral therapy to medication (at least temporarily).

People who experience panic worry that they're having heart attacks or dying or going crazy, explains Dr. Heitler. That explanation compounds the anxiety and perpetuates the symptoms—the pounding heart, the sweating, the shallow breathing—further convincing people that they really are having a heart attack, dying or going crazy.

What's more, worrying that you'll have a panic attack increases the odds that one will indeed occur, says Dr. Vogel.

SCIENTIFICALLY PROVEN PANIC BUSTERS

Panic attacks can be beat. If your doctor has confirmed that what you are experiencing is bona fide panic and not something else, you can learn to cope with the symptoms—calmly. Here's how.

Talk yourself out of it. "Tell yourself, 'Okay, I'm having a panic attack. I know that I'm not having a heart attack or dying or going crazy. This won't last long. It will pass. I'll get through it,'" says Dr. Vogel. This self-talk—part of an approach called cognitive behavioral therapy—should take the edge off the anxiety, and your symptoms should start to fade.

What's more, practicing self-talk should also take the edge off your fear of future panic attacks and lower your general anxiety level so that further attacks are less likely. Researchers in Sweden reported remarkable success after teaching the technique to people prone to panic attacks. After treatment all but a few were panic-free.

Relax, one muscle at a time. While you're reminding yourself that you're going to be fine, try deep breathing or some other relaxation technique, like progressive relaxation, says Dr. Vogel. Relaxation helps diminish symptoms, end attacks and lower the odds of future attacks.

To give progressive relaxation a try, sit in a comfortable chair, close your eyes and follow these instructions from Martha Davis, Ph.D., a psychologist at Kaiser Permanente Medical Center in Santa Clara, California, and co-author of *The Relaxation and Stress Reduction Workbook*.

To start, clench your right fist. Keep it tightly clenched for about ten seconds, then release and let it go limp. Repeat with your left hand, then both hands simultaneously. Next, bend both your elbows and tense your arms. Then relax them and let them hang at your sides. To continue, tense then relax both your shoulders and your neck; wrinkle then relax your forehead and brows; squeeze your eyes shut and clench your jaw, then relax. Moving on, tense and relax your stomach, lower back, both thighs, buttocks, both calves and both feet. The whole process should take about ten minutes. Try to do these exercises about twice a day.

Paper Cuts
When Stationery Cuts Like a Knife

We've all done it: Hurrying to open an envelope or sheaf of paper, you slide your finger under the flap and instantly feel the paper slice your finger.

A paper cut is deceptively tiny but deep. It throbs and stings so badly that you feel like every nerve ending in your body is centered in your fingertip.

Because they are superficial, paper cuts heal fast, says Wilma Bergfeld, M.D., head of clinical research in the Department of Dermatology at the Cleveland Clinic Foundation. But they can be very uncomfortable for a few days—especially if you need to use your fingertips for typing, dialing or other tasks. "Every time you move your fingertip, the cut opens again," says Dr. Bergfeld.

Women tend to get paper cuts more frequently in the winter, when

WHEN TO SEE A DOCTOR

Women doctors say that most paper cuts heal well with home treatments and don't require medical care. However, you may want to see a physician if your paper cut becomes red, swollen, inflamed, crusty or sore.

dry air and heat sap away skin's natural moisture. "Skin on the hands, especially, becomes dry and rigid—meaning that it's more vulnerable to the paper's sharp edge," says Dr. Bergfeld.

HELP FOR THE SLICED AND SLIVERED

Fortunately, paper cut relief is right at your fingertips, say women doctors. Here's what they recommend you do to reduce the pain and help heal the cut.

Clean it. "Gently run warm water over your fingertip for a minute or so until it is totally clean, so that it doesn't become infected," says dermatologist Karen E. Burke, M.D., Ph.D., an attending physician at Cabrini Medical Center in New York City and at Greensboro Specialty Surgical Center in North Carolina.

Soothe with salve. After cleaning the cut, apply a dab of antibacterial ointment, such as Bacitracin, recommends Dr. Burke. The ointment will help kill germs, and it also moisturizes the cut so it heals faster.

Cross it off. To close the gaping cut, gently push both edges together and apply a small strip of surgical tape—which sticks better than an adhesive bandage, according to Dr. Burke. "Position the tape perpendicular to the paper cut, so that the cut and the tape form an X. Then pull it tight across the cut, so that the skin will stay together and heal."

Glue it together. It sounds crazy, but you might want to hold the cut together with Krazy Glue. "It stings when you first put it on, but it is not harmful," says Sheryl Clark, M.D., assistant clinical professor of dermatology at Cornell Medical Center and an assistant attending physician in medicine at the New York Hospital, both in in New York City. "Just a little dab will do it. It helps seal out air, so that the paper cut is not painful while it heals."

One caution, though. "It's rare, but some people are allergic to Krazy Glue," says Dr. Bergfeld. "So if your skin becomes red, inflamed, swollen or sore, discontinue it and see a doctor."

Coat it with zinc oxide. You know that white stuff that lifeguards put on the sides of their noses to protect them from the sun? It works for paper cuts, too, and you can buy it inexpensively in drugstores. "Zinc oxide is a thick paste that seals out air and makes the cut more comfortable. And the zinc itself helps wounds heal more quickly," says Dr. Clark.

Do the night shift. "Nighttime is the perfect time to apply treatment to a paper cut, because you don't have to use your hands while you sleep," says Dr. Bergfeld. "At night you can really gob up the cut with an antibacterial ointment, like Bacitracin, and then cover it with a bandage."

Work smart. And next time, says Dr. Bergfeld, use the letter opener.

Performance Anxiety
Say Good-Bye to On-Stage Jitters

It has been called the performer's plague. In mild cases the voice wavers and the knees knock. A case of uncontrolled jitters can reduce the most skilled actor or singer to a quivering wreck.

Of course, you don't have to be a performer to get performance anxiety. "Anyone and everyone experiences it," says Dianne Chambless, Ph.D., professor of psychology at the University of North Carolina at Chapel Hill. If you've been through an important job interview, a final exam, a key performance review or a public speech, odds are that you're familiar with the classic signs of performance anxiety: galloping heartbeat, shaky knees, trembling voice and a turbulent stomach.

Understandably, perfectionists are more likely to experience performance anxiety; they put a lot of stock in others' opinions, says Sandra Loucks, Ph.D., professor of psychology at the University of Tennessee in Knoxville and the University of Tennessee Medical Center. So does anyone who is running short on self-esteem.

To be fair, performance anxiety can have its up side. In moderate doses it can energize us and motivate us to prepare and excel, says Lenora Yuen, Ph.D., a psychologist in Palo Alto, California.

"There is a very important relationship between anxiety and performance," explains Dr. Yuen. "If there is no anxiety—or very little—performance tends to be lower. As anxiety increases, performance improves—to a point. After a while, anxiety gets too high, and it interferes with performance."

PERFORMANCE POINTERS

The secret, then, is keeping performance anxiety under control. Here are some suggestions.

Envision success. If you have just minutes to go before delivering a speech or taking an exam, breathe deeply and relax with some soothing imagery.

"Imagine yourself performing the task well, and imagine yourself and your family celebrating the outcome afterward," suggests Dr. Loucks.

Make it vivid. Envision yourself as you would appear if you were seeing yourself in a movie, suggests Dr. Chambless. Watch yourself as you deliver that rousing oratory or zip through those test questions with ease. Then watch as you toast your success with your loved ones. This will not only put you in a positive frame of mind, but also boost your confidence and calm you.

Or try another channel. As an alternative, see yourself in a completely different and serene setting, like a thatched hut in Fiji, suggests Dr. Yuen. "Some people find this technique helpful. If you love the ocean, see yourself at the shore. Or envision yourself in a hammock under a tree—any safe, calming place." You'll feel calmer.

Say to yourself, "It's normal to be nervous." If you're about do something unnerving, like making a speech in front of a roomful of people, realize that most women would be unnerved in your situation. Don't knock yourself. "Take into account that this is something that most people are anxious about," says Dr. Chambless. "Realize that it's okay to be a little nervous."

Expect improvement momentarily. Once you get started, performance anxiety usually subsides. If the first sentence out of your mouth during your yearly review with your boss has a tremolo, don't sweat it. "That will settle down," says Dr. Chambless.

Think through potential mistakes. If you have some time on your hands, try to figure out exactly what you are afraid of, Dr. Loucks suggests. Is it the failure or the success? What consequences in particular? Then figure out what you would do if those consequences came your way and then envision yourself doing just that. Visualizing yourself handling even the worst-case scenario will help you to get the anxiety under control.

"Let's say, for instance, that you imagine yourself forgetting what you're going to say in the middle of a speech," says Dr. Yuen. "You could then imagine reminding yourself, the way a soothing parent would, that no one is perfect, that you don't have to be perfect. Then envision yourself picking up the next phrase of the speech and going on."

Be prepared. "There is no substitute for being prepared," says Dr. Loucks. "Rehearse—no, *over*rehearse—your performance until it's so natural, so automatic, that later, you don't have to spend a lot of time or energy trying to remember it under more stressful circumstances."

Perm Problems and Disasters
Salvation Is Simple

Grown women still have nightmares about home perms administered by their mothers back in the 1950s—usually, right before school pictures were taken. Instead of darling curls like those gracing the little girl pictured on the box, they usually ended up with a dreaded case of the frizzies. And the smell!

Luckily, perms have come a long way since then. For one thing, they smell better. Nevertheless, an occasional disaster does strike. In fact, *Modern Salon* magazine reports that frizzies are still the number one perm complaint.

Perm mistakes are generally hard to correct, because permanents are, logically enough, intended to make permanent changes in your hair shaft, says Rebecca Caserio, M.D., clinical associate professor of dermatology at the University of Pittsburgh, who has had more than a few perms herself.

WHEN TO SEE A DOCTOR

If a perm leaves your scalp red and tender, check with your doctor, suggests Diana Bihova, M.D., a dermatologist in New York City and author of *Beauty from the Inside Out*. The chemicals in the perm solution may have left your scalp irritated. If so, applying an over-the-counter hydrocortisone lotion, liquid or spray can reduce the irritation and prevent scarring, which can lead to hair loss.

RESCUE TECHNIQUES

Most of the time, perms turn out just the way you plan, especially if you've had your hair permed by a professional hair stylist, says Liz Cunnane, a consultant trichologist (a hair-care specialist) at Philip Kingsley Trichological Centre in New York City. But if your perm leaves your hair too curly, too loose, too frizzy or otherwise flawed, here's what experts suggest.

Stay calm. When you realize that you have a disaster on your hands, don't let the adrenaline surging through your body cause you to panic, says Cunnane. "People panic and do things like try to put more perm solution on their hair or redo the perm. They end up making it worse than it was to begin with." Perming over just-permed hair can cause extensive hair breakage.

Pick up the phone. If you've used a home permanent kit, call the toll-free number listed on the package, says Cunnane. It's sort of a 911 for perm emergencies. An expert who is familiar with the particular product that you used will be on the phone in seconds—ready to talk you through any corrective action that can be taken.

In the event that you've had your perm professionally done, and there's a problem, phone the shop and ask them what they might be able to do to correct it. Since they know exactly what chemicals were used and how your hair was processed, they're the ones most likely to be able to get you out of any difficulty.

Condition a too-tight curl. To loosen a too-tight curl, buy a heavy-duty conditioner and work it through your hair, says Cunnane. Rinse and style, then follow up by using your regular shampoo and conditioner every day for the next two weeks—substituting a deep conditioner for your regular one once each week.

Style a too-loose wave. If your perm doesn't seem to have locked in the amount of curl or wave that you expected, just comb it into the best style that you can and leave it alone, says Cunnane. Deep-condition your hair twice within the following week. Then, if your hair still refuses to curl the way it was supposed to, redo the perm. And this time, pay close attention to the perm's instructions. When a perm doesn't take, says Cunnane, it's usually because the neutralizer—the chemical that creates the new bonds that dictate your hair's new shape—was not correctly applied.

Pessimism
Find the Sunny Side

At times it makes sense to expect something bad to happen—if your broker flees the country, for instance, or if Mike Wallace shows up to interview the head of your company.

Some of us, however, sweat it even when the Fates have spun smooth stretches in the threads of our lives. If you're a pessimist, you see threats where optimists see challenges. Optimists expect things to work out, figure that they'll be able to handle whatever comes down the pike and attribute unexpected disasters to things that they can change.

Naive, you say?

While optimism can sometimes foster false expectations, it's a more reasonable outlook overall, says Susan Jeffers, Ph.D., a psychotherapist in Los Angeles and author of *Feel the Fear and Do It Anyway*. "Probably 95 percent of what we worry about never happens."

Pessimism is a self-fulfilling prophecy. Even in somewhat limited doses, hard-core pessimism can rob you of enjoyment, make you unpleasant company, discourage you from trying new things and, having tried them, keep you from persevering.

"On the other hand, if people expect a good outcome, they'll keep working toward that outcome," says Lisa Aspinwall, Ph.D., assistant professor of psychology at the University of Maryland College Park. And, along with depression, entrenched pessimism may undermine your immunity and heart health.

LESS POUTING, MORE PROBLEM-SOLVING

If gloomy predictions are casting too long a shadow over your life, you can cultivate a more optimistic outlook, says Dr. Jeffers. Here's how.

Plan for the worst. Not all pessimists are blanket doom-and-gloomers, says Julie K. Norem, Ph.D., associate professor of psychology at Wellesley College in Wellesley, Massachusetts. "They're anxious about particular situations—public speaking, for instance." So they plan for disaster: They imagine the worst-case outcome of whatever they dread—forgetting what they're going to say, for instance—then hatch a plan to avoid it. In this case they rehearse until the speech comes effortlessly.

This strategy works, because it dissipates their anxiety. And since high anxiety interferes with performance, they perform better. Dr. Norem says that the strategy is particularly good for turning situation-specific pessimism into something constructive.

Empower yourself with affirmations. All-around pessimism assumes powerlessness: "There's nothing I can do to stop these lousy things from happening." You're less likely to wait for the other shoe to drop if you feel more effective, says Dr. Jeffers. She suggests using affirmations—positive statements that you make about yourself to yourself. Telling yourself, "Whatever happens, I'll handle it" will make you feel more in control, and that will make you feel more confident about the future.

Learn coping skills. When you find yourself in the inevitable tough spots, a few key coping tactics can help, says Margaret Chesney, Ph.D., professor of medicine at the University of California, San Francisco, School of Medicine. Start by sorting out what you can change and what you can't. Simply analyzing the event makes you feel more in control. Once you figure out what you can change, you can turn to problem-solving and making the change happen.

Let's say that everyone in your department gets laid off, says Dr. Chesney. You can't do anything about that. But you can affect your odds of landing a new job: Update your resume, network, attend career-change seminars and consider this an opportunity to try new things.

Hang out with the upbeat. Pessimism, like optimism, is infectious, says Dr. Jeffers. So spend your time with optimistic types.

Shake it off with exercise. Studies indicate that optimists are more likely to exercise regularly than pessimists. Researchers aren't sure if exercise makes people optimistic, or if they start out as optimists and keep exercising because they expect to live longer. There is, however, ample evidence that exercise improves mood, says Dr. Aspinwall.

Hey—it's worth a try, right?

Phlebitis
Day and Night Relief for Inflamed Veins

Simply translated, phlebitis means that the veins in your legs—those closest to the surface—are inflamed. A variation—deep-vein phlebitis—is more serious, says Lenise Banse, M.D., a dermatologist and vein expert at the Northeast Family Dermatology Center in Clinton Township, Michigan. Deep-vein phlebitis affects veins buried deeper and is usually caused by a clot in the affected veins. With thrombophlebitis—inflammation with clotting—matters can get tricky.

"If a clot breaks loose, it could find its way to the lungs or heart with fatal consequences," says Dr. Banse.

What puts you at risk for phlebitis, be it mild or serious?

"Genetics, smoking and varicose veins," says Toby Shaw, M.D., associate professor of dermatology at Allegheny University of the Health Sciences MCP–Hahnemann School of Medicine in Philadelphia. "Also, if phlebitis runs in your family, birth control pills add to your risk, since they can promote blood coagulation, and a clot is coagulated blood."

FOR MILD EPISODES

Thrombophlebitis is usually treated in a hospital with clot-busting medication, says Dr. Banse. If you've been told that you have superficial phlebitis, self-care can help alleviate the redness, itching, pain and swelling that results from inflammation.

Cool it. For immediate relief, Dr. Shaw recommends cool compresses made with Domeboro Astringent Solution, sold at drug stores. Empty one packet of powder into a basin filled with cool water, mix, then soak a clean washcloth in the solution. Wring out the washcloth and apply it to the inflamed area, she says.

Super-moisturize. To relieve itchiness, moisturize with Lac-Hydrin Five, an over-the-counter lotion found at drugstores, says Dr. Shaw.

Try medicated cream. If using a moisturizer isn't 100 percent effective, Dr. Shaw recommends you also apply an over-the-counter cortisone cream such as Cortaid with aloe. Topical antibiotic ointments such as Polysporin can also speed healing.

WHEN TO SEE A DOCTOR

Anyone who has phlebitis runs the risk that a clot will form in a deep vein, says Toby Shaw, M.D., associate professor of dermatology at Allegheny University of the Health Sciences MCP–Hahnemann School of Medicine in Philadelphia. Pay attention to warning signs—notably, severe pain and swelling, says Dr. Shaw. If the pain or swelling in your leg increases, do not hesitate to check with your doctor.

With the help of a friend, you can also check for what's called Homans' sign, says Dr. Shaw. Ask someone to put their hand on the back of your leg over your calf as you're seated and then use their other hand to flex your toes forward toward your knee.

"If flexing the foot in that way triggers considerable pain, you may have a clot," says Dr. Shaw. If so, go to a hospital. Doctors can dissolve blood vessel clots with heparin, a blood-thinning drug.

Elevate your leg. To relieve pain and swelling, says Dr. Shaw, sit in a chair with your foot propped three to six inches higher than your hips until the inflammation subsides.

Cushion your feet. At night, sleep with one pillow under your head and two pillows under your feet to elevate them properly, says Dr. Shaw.

Wear support hose. During the day, wear a good pair of support panty hose or medical support hose prescribed by your doctor, says Dr. Banse. Do not wear knee-high stockings—they interfere with circulation and aggravate the very problems you're trying to alleviate.

Move it. Once the initial pain and redness has disappeared, get moving, says Dr. Banse. Frequent walking—say, for a few minutes every hour or so—will aid circulation and prevent flare-ups. (Don't wear doctor-prescribed support hose for exercise, though—if worn while walking, medical hose can interfere with circulation, thus counteracting what you're trying to do.)

Pinkeye

When Your Eyes "Have a Cold"

*P*inkeye is the commonly used term for an eye infection known as conjunctivitis. It's sometimes called red-eye, because the infection renders the eyeball (or eyeballs) either pink or bloodshot red. If you have pinkeye, your eyelids may be irritated and itchy, and your eyes may leak a watery discharge, just like your nose does when you have a cold.

Pinkeye may be caused by a virus and may accompany a chest cold or sore throat. But it may also be caused by bacteria or irritations such as dry eyes, pollution or allergies, says Dickie McMullan, M.D., an ophthalmologist in private practice in Atlanta.

Chances are, if you get pinkeye in one eye, it will spread to your other eye, no matter how careful you are, says Jody Piltz, M.D., assistant professor of ophthalmology at the University of Pennsylvania School of Medicine in Philadelphia.

SUPREME RELIEF

The good news is that, left untreated, viral pinkeye almost always goes away by itself within a matter of weeks, says Dr. McMullan. And there are a number of ways to ease the discomfort—and control the contagion until your eyes get back to normal.

Keep your hands away from your eyes. "If you rub your eyes, they'll turn twice as red and feel more irritated," says Silvia Orengo-Nania, M.D., assistant clinical professor of ophthalmology at Baylor College of Medicine in Houston. And rubbing your eyes is likely to spread the infection from one eye to the other.

Apply a cold compress. Place a cool washcloth or wet paper towel over your eyes to soothe the irritation, says Dr. Orengo-Nania. Repeat for ten minutes at a time, as often as you feel the need.

Wear glasses, not contacts. "If you have pinkeye, wearing contacts feels like a splinter," says Charlotte Saxby, M.D., an ophthalmologist with the Group Health Cooperative of Puget Sound in Seattle. "Plus, the contact holds the germ right against your eyeball." If you wear glasses instead of contact lenses while your eye is infected, your eye is likely to heal a lot faster.

WHEN TO SEE A DOCTOR

Pinkeye that lingers for longer than a week may signal a more serious problem, says Silvia Orengo-Nania, M.D., assistant clinical professor of ophthalmology at Baylor College of Medicine in Houston. See your doctor if you experience:

- Puslike discharge from one or both eyes
- Loss of vision
- Dull, strong pain or sharp pain in one or both eyes

Don sunglasses when you go out. Sunlight irritates pinkeye, says Dr. Orengo-Nania. Sunglasses with ultraviolet protection will help reduce the glare and make you less self-conscious about baring your red or pink eye to the world.

Drop in artificial tears. Available over the counter, artificial tear drops will flush out and soothe your eye, says Dr. Saxby. Use them as frequently as you need to.

Or try special eyedrops. Other over-the-counter eyedrops, such as Naphcon-A, combine a decongestant and antihistamine (to help stop the itching), says Kathleen Lamping, M.D., associate clinical professor of ophthalmology at Case Western Reserve University in Cleveland.

But don't use them for more than two weeks without a break, cautions Dr. Orengo-Nania. Eyes easily become habituated to vasoconstrictors—substances that shrink blood vessels—so if you overuse these drops, your eyes will start looking red even after your pinkeye clears.

Throw out your eye makeup. If you wear makeup while you have pinkeye, you'll contaminate your makeup wand or liner and may spread the pinkeye to your other eye, says Dr. Orengo-Nania.

Wash away discharge twice a day. Lay a warm, wet cloth or towel over your eyelids for a minute or two and then wipe gently away toward the corner of your eye, says Dr. Saxby. To make sure that you don't spread pinkeye to other family members, it's best to launder the towel after each use.

Plantar Warts

Painful Blemishes on Your Sole

*I*f it feels like you have a pebble in your shoe every time you step down and put weight on your foot, you may have plantar warts.

Check your shoe. If, instead of a pebble, you find an ugly growth on the sole of your foot, look it over. Is the growth hard and flat? Does it hurt when you try to move it from side to side? Can you see tiny, pinpoint dots of blood in it?

If yes, then it's most likely a plantar wart, not a callus, says Suzanne M. Levine, D.P.M., clinical assistant podiatrist at Cornell Medical Center in New York City.

A plantar wart is just like any other wart, except that it's found on your sole. (Plantar is the medical term for the bottom surface of the foot.) The red dots are the ends of capillaries that are trapped in the wart, she explains. The wart is a noncancerous growth caused by the human papillomavirus, or wart virus. It's contagious and can be spread from person to person.

The wart virus thrives in moist places, and people typically pick up plantar warts by walking barefoot at swimming pools and health clubs or in locker rooms or public showers, says D'Anne Kleinsmith, M.D., a staff dermatologist at William Beaumont Hospital in Royal Oak, Michigan. You're also more susceptible if your feet sweat more than average or if your immunity is low, she says.

Plantar warts can be small, or large enough to cover the entire heel or ball of your foot. The larger they are, the more painful they get, says Dr. Levine.

ACT QUICKLY

Women doctors say that plantar warts sometimes disappear on their own. But don't count on it. Other times, they linger for years if not treated.

Take a footbath. Dunk your feet in a basinful of water mixed with a special drying preparation, such as Domeboro, which comes in little packets or tablets. "This is a solution of aluminum salts that dries out and toughens the skin," says Dr. Kleinsmith. "Mix it into the water and soak your feet in it for about 15 minutes."

WHEN TO SEE A DOCTOR

Although some plantar warts will disappear on their own or with home treatments, many stubbornly remain. See a doctor if:
- You don't see an improvement within a month or two.
- Your warts are getting thicker or more painful, or they're spreading.

Keep your feet dry. "Eliminating moisture is key to drying out a foot wart," says Dr. Levine. Use towels to dry off your feet after showering (and then launder those towels separately so that you don't spread the virus to others). Then apply foot powders containing cornstarch or talc to dry your skin, she recommends.

Hoof it to the drugstore. Dr. Levine suggests trying an over-the-counter wart medicine like Compound W, Duofilm, Duoplant, Occlusal and Dr. Scholl's preparations, available at drugstores. Many of the products contain salicylic acid, which dries out warts. The acid will eat away the wart. "The problem is, they can eat away at good skin, too," she adds. "To reduce the chance of irritating healthy skin, read the directions and follow them carefully."

Stick with it. Over-the-counter wart medicines work if you are religious about using them, but they can require six to eight weeks of treatment, says Karen K. Deasey, M.D., chief of dermatology at Bryn Mawr Hospital in Pennsylvania. So be patient. (The larger or deeper the wart is, the less effective these home remedies will be, says Dr. Levine.)

Patch them up. Some wart preparations come in little patches, usually containing salicylic acid. "You stick the patch on overnight. In the morning, you take it off and use an emery board to file down the wart and make it as thin as possible, so that the medicine will soak in better. The next night, you apply a new patch," explains Dr. Kleinsmith.

"These medicated patches come in boxes of 24, and I usually tell my patients that they may have to go through two boxes until the wart goes away," says Dr. Deasey.

Polish off a wart. Some preparations come in a nail-polish base that you paint onto the wart. "Every couple of days, you peel off the polish, and a little bit of the wart comes off with it," explains Dr. Deasey.

Put your warts in film. A few heavy-duty wart preparations, such as Viranol gel and Duofilm, come in the form of a plastic film, which you stick right onto the wart, says Dr. Deasey. "Most of these don't require covering, because when they dry, they form their own covers. They won't stick to your socks or shoes."

Cushion the blow. Callus pads can help take the pressure off a painful wart, says Dr. Deasey.

Adopt a hands-off policy. Try to avoid touching or fiddling with your plantar wart, because you may spread the wart to your fingers, says Dr. Deasey. "You may need to use your hands to apply treatment, but be sure to wash them thoroughly immediately afterward, so that the wart virus won't spread."

Poison Ivy and Poison Oak

Minimize the Misery

Why is it that some women break out in poison ivy after just looking at the stuff, while others can practically swim in it and emerge unscathed?

Some people are allergic and others are not allergic to the thick, oily substance, called urushiol, in the resin emitted by poison ivy or poison oak, says Susan C. Taylor, M.D., assistant clinical professor of medicine in the Department of Dermatology at the University of Pennsylvania School of Medicine in Philadelphia. "If you're allergic to one, you're probably allergic to the other." But if you've never had poison ivy, that doesn't mean that you're immune. "This allergy can develop at different stages in life. You may get an outbreak at some time in the future," she says.

ACE THOSE SNEAK ATTACKS

If you have already come in contact with a nasty three-leaved plant—either from direct contact, carrying contaminated clothing or pet-

WHEN TO SEE A DOCTOR

You don't necessarily need to see a doctor for poison ivy or poison oak, says Mary Ruth Buchness, M.D., chief of dermatology at St. Vincent's Hospital and Medical Center in New York City. But if the rash lingers despite treatment with over-the-counter preparations, or if it's severe, you don't have to suffer on your own. A trip to the doctor may shorten the course of the outbreak, she says.

Women doctors suggest that you see your doctor for poison ivy or poison oak if:

- Itching and swelling is severe or keeps you up at night.
- The rash covers a large area of your body.
- Fluid weeping out of the blisters is turning honey-colored (you may have an infection).
- The rash occurs on your face.
- The rash occurs near your eyes, or your eyes are swollen shut.

"If you're taking any medications, check with your doctor before taking an antihistamine for the itching of poison ivy, to make sure that it won't interact with other medications," adds Amy Newburger, M.D., assistant clinical professor of dermatology at Columbia University College of Physicians and Surgeons in New York City and a dermatologist in Scarsdale, New York. "And don't take an antihistamine without consulting your doctor if you are pregnant or have high blood pressure," she cautions.

ting your exposed dog or cat—women doctors offer these practical strategies to minimize itching and discomfort.

Head straight for the laundry room. The resin can stick to your clothing and gloves, so you need to take everything off and wash your clothing in hot, soapy water. "As soon as you come inside, go right to the laundry room, take your clothes off and dump them into the washer," recommends Mary Ruth Buchness, M.D., chief of dermatology at St. Vincent's Hospital and Medical Center in New York City.

Also, thoroughly rinse off your shoes. "Otherwise, the next time that you touch the clothes—even a week later—you could pick up the resin and get poison ivy," says Amy Newburger, M.D., assistant clinical professor of dermatology at Columbia University College of Physicians and Surgeons in New York City and a dermatologist in Scarsdale, New York.

Rinse off the resin. Next, head straight for the shower and rinse, rinse, rinse your skin with warm water and soap to remove the irritating substance. "If you can cleanse the resin off your skin in the first two hours, you may be able to remove it and prevent the rash—or at least minimize it," says Dr. Newburger.

"The longer you leave the resin on your skin, the more intense and widespread the rash will be, says Dr. Buchness.

Ice the itch. For lingering itchiness, "run ice water over the rash or hold an ice cube against your skin for a few minutes," recommends Dr. Buchness. "Cool things are comforting to itchy skin."

Milk it. Soak a washcloth or a piece of gauze in cold milk and hold the compress on your skin. "This old-time remedy really works," says Dr. Buchness. "If someone calls us on the weekend with an emergency outbreak of poison ivy, and all the pharmacies are closed, this is what we recommend." Presumably, something about the fats or proteins of the milk is soothing to the skin, although there is no real scientific explanation.

Soak in oatmeal. Add a powdered colloidal oatmeal preparation (available at drugstores) to a tub full of water and soak in it for about 15 minutes. "Oatmeal baths are very soothing to the skin," says Dr. Buchness.

Apply a menthol cream. When you're feeling better, go to the drugstore and scan the shelves for poison ivy preparations containing ingredients such as menthol and camphor (which soothe skin), and pramoxine (a topical anesthetic that relieves pain and itching), suggests Dr. Buchness.

Use calamine early. If you don't mind its pink color, calamine lotion can help dry out poison ivy blisters. You don't want to use calamine after the blisters have crusted over, because at that point it overdries skin and enhances the itch, says Dr. Newburger.

Visit with the good witch. Witch hazel, a clear lotion that you can get in drugstores, is soothing and cooling to itchy, rashy skin, says Dr. Newburger. Dab a witch hazel–soaked cotton ball on the rash for relief.

Poor Concentration
Focusing Strategies for the Easily Distracted

*I*f you can't concentrate, it's hard to get anything done. It's hard to get your work in on time, with all the details straight, so that your boss doesn't give you The Look. It's hard to enjoy books, not to mention plays, movies, concerts and ballets. And it's hard to learn new subjects, languages, sports, crafts and hobbies or simply remember people's names or follow instructions.

When your attention takes a detour, the culprit may be one type of distraction or another—worry, stress, hunger—or the cat scratching at the screen door.

Lack of sleep can also sap your powers of concentration, says Irene Colsky, Ed.D., adjunct professor of psychology and education at Miami-Dade Community College and president of the Colsky Associates, a firm offering learning and memory seminars. Some women find that they have a particularly hard time paying attention in the last months of pregnancy or during menopause, when insomnia is a common problem.

And of course, a lack of interest in the subject at hand is sure to scatter your attention, says clinical psychologist Miriam Ehrenberg, Ph.D., adjunct clinical associate professor of psychology at the City College of the City University of New York in New York City and co-author of *Optimum Brain Power*.

FOCUS, FOCUS, FOCUS

You can improve your powers of concentration, say doctors. "Everyone can be focused; it's not a gift given to just a lucky few," says Dr. Ehrenberg.

Here's how.

Block out distractions. Shut the door, turn off the TV and take the phone off the hook, and you'll cut out a lot of distractions, says Dr. Ehrenberg. If necessary, tell the people that you share space with that you'd rather not be disturbed.

Do one thing at a time. It's difficult to focus on any one task if you're working on several simultaneously, says Dr. Ehrenberg. You're

435

WHEN TO SEE A DOCTOR

If as a child you found it difficult to concentrate on school-work, and as an adult you still have a hard time concentrating, you may have attention deficit hyperactivity disorder, also known as attention deficit disorder (ADD). Trademark symptoms include impulsiveness, inattention and hyperactivity, which can cause trouble at work and in relationships.

Check with your primary care physician. If you have ADD, it can be treated with behavior modification, medication or both.

Other possible causes of poor concentration include depression, drug reactions or an underlying health problem, which all need to be ruled out or treated.

bound to take longer or make more mistakes, because your mind simply can't be in two places at once. Instead, block out time for each task or project and tackle each in turn.

Take a deep breath. Anxiety can cloud your concentration, says Dr. Ehrenberg. Deep breathing can help quiet the nagging inner voice that says, "Am I going to be able to finish this? Will it be good enough?" Take a deep breath and hold it for five seconds while pressing your hands and fingers together, palm to palm. Then slowly exhale through your lips while letting your hands relax. Do this five or six times until you relax.

Surprise your brain. Activities that give your brain a workout—reading books on subjects new to you, solving puzzles, learning new languages or instruments—translate to sharper thinking, studies find.

Experiment with background music. Some people work best in total silence, while others do better with musical accompaniment, says Dr. Ehrenberg. Research suggests that baroque music—J. S. Bach in particular—is conducive to learning. Go with whatever works for you.

After an hour, take a break. Getting focused is one thing; staying focused is another. After a while your brain (and the rest of your body) needs a break, says Dr. Ehrenberg. To refresh and refocus, take a quick walk around the block.

Concentrate on exercise. A regular exercise program—steady workouts of 45 minutes each—can also hone your power of concentration. When researchers at the University of Pittsburgh School of Medicine put women on treadmills and had them walk until they burned 350 calories, the women reported feeling more clearheaded afterward. This amounts to walking three miles in about 45 minutes, a rate of four miles per hour.

Exercise seems to improve the vital flow of oxygen to the brain, Dr. Ehrenberg says. It can also help alleviate distracting anxiety and depression.

Have a snack. Concentration wavers when your blood sugar levels fall, and frequent small meals keep levels steadiest, says Dr. Colsky. So if you're about to tackle a task that demands concentration, have a bite to eat—half a tuna sandwich, for example, or some other combination of protein and carbohydrate. Research suggests that a protein-carb combination keeps you more alert than protein or carbohydrate alone.

Remember mineral-rich foods. Studies have also linked diets deficient in boron (found in fruits, especially prunes, dates and raisins), iron and zinc (found in red meat) to difficulty concentrating. So if you don't get these minerals regularly in foods, a multivitamin with iron may help, says Gail Mattox, M.D., associate professor of psychiatry at Morehouse School of Medicine in Atlanta.

Postnasal Drip
Give Phlegm the Slip

*Y*ou know the sound: The disgusting hacking, snorting, hawking, sucking attempt that other people sometimes make to clear their throats of the steady mucus flow called postnasal drip. Admit it: Maybe you've even made the sound when you thought no one was listening. Not exactly ladylike—or effective. Hack 'til you're blue in the face; the annoying drip is still there.

What is this scourge known as postnasal drip? The by-product of a cold or sinus problem, postnasal drip occurs when the mucus that normally flows unnoticed from the nose via the back of the throat increases in volume or becomes thick or sticky. And if it's caused by a chronic sinus problem, it's likely that your postnasal drip problem will be chronic, too.

WHEN TO SEE A DOCTOR

"If your mucus is foul-smelling, greenish or yellow, you probably have a sinus infection," says Barbara P. Yawn, M.D., associate professor of clinical family medicine and community health at the University of Minnesota in Minneapolis and director of research at the Olmsted Medical Center in Rochester, Minnesota. "You need to see your doctor for antibiotic treatment."

OUT WITH THE BAD

Clearing up the cold, allergy or sinus trouble is the best solution to postnasal drip. In the meantime, women doctors offer these quick-fix postnasal drip remedies.

Flush your gullet. "The goal is to thin the mucus so that its flow down the back of your throat isn't so noticeable," says Barbara P. Yawn, M.D., associate professor of clinical family medicine and community health at the University of Minnesota in Minneapolis and director of research at the Olmsted Medical Center in Rochester, Minnesota. "Drinking plenty of fluids, particularly in the winter when indoor air is dry, keeps the mucus thin and watery."

Sip soup or tea. "Hot liquids, like tea and soup, are especially effective at loosening and thinning the secretions," says Dr. Yawn. "They should provide fairly instant relief."

Close your mouth. "Breathing through your mouth will dry and thicken the secretions, so breathe through your nose," says Dr. Yawn.

Warm the air you breath. "By the same token, cold, dry air will dry and thicken your nasal secretions," says Dr. Yawn, "So in the winter, use a scarf to cover your nose and mouth."

Give your nose a bath. "A nasal wash can alleviate a postnasal drip," says Karin Pacheco, M.D., staff physician in the Division of Allergy and Immunology at the National Jewish Center for Immunology and Respiratory Medicine in Denver. "Use a plain over-the-counter saline spray or make your own: one cup of water, a half-teaspoon of salt and a pinch of baking soda in a child-size bulb syringe. Spray several squirts into your nose, then blow, several times a day."

Give your face a steam bath. Try using a facial steamer for alleviating postnasal drip, suggests Dr. Yawn. "Raising the temperature of the nose and mouth with moist steam will thin the postnasal drip secretions."

Postpartum Problems
Cures for Soreness and Discomfort

Somewhere along the line, women have gotten the notion that within six weeks after childbirth, they should be fully recovered and feeling back to normal, says Mindy Smith, M.D., associate professor in family practice at the University of Michigan in Ann Arbor and herself a relatively new mom. "But that's unrealistic—six weeks is way too soon for someone trying to incorporate a brand-new human being into her life while trying to recover physically."

A REPAIR KIT FOR THE NEW MOM

Give yourself six to eight *months*, says Dr. Smith. Meanwhile, here's how she and other experts suggest you take care of your most immediate postpartum discomforts.

Focus on the three R's. That's rest, rest and rest. "For the first week at least, make your home in bed," says Martha Barry, R.N., adjunct clinical faculty member of the University of Illinois School of Nursing and a certified nurse midwife at Illinois Masonic Hospital, both in Chicago. "Get up and do whatever you want, but no more."

Ask for help. Enlist the aid of your spouse or partner, a relative or friend to help take care of the baby, do chores and keep visitors at bay, advises Barry.

Eat, drink and be nourished. "Get a good meal at least three times a day," says Barry. Foods high in protein (like lean chicken and fish) and vitamin C (like grapefruit and oranges) hasten the healing process, she says. And have a glass of water or another beverage at least once an hour, especially if you're nursing.

Drink herbal tea. Minor bleeding from the uterus or from an episiotomy (an incision in the birth opening) or laceration during childbirth is quite normal. Drinking shepherd's purse tea for the first two days, then switching to tea brewed with equal parts of raspberry leaves, nettle, yarrow flowers and squaw vine can help you heal, says Mary Bove, a naturopathic physician with the Brattleboro Naturopathic Clinic in Vermont and a licensed midwife.

WHEN TO SEE A DOCTOR

Visit your obstetrician for a general checkup six weeks after having your baby, says Mindy Smith, M.D., associate professor in family practice at the University of Michigan in Ann Arbor. Call before then if:

- Vaginal discharge increases substantially. (Normally, bleeding tapers off and lightens in color over a period of three to six weeks.)
- Your uterus feels tender or your breasts feel sore and warm (especially if accompanied by a fever). You could have an infection.

Take vitamin E. Daily doses of 800 international units of vitamin E, taken for two to three weeks, will help slow bleeding, too, says Dr. Bove. Vitamin E improves the health of the small blood vessels in the uterine wall. Be sure to get your doctor's okay before taking such high doses of this or any vitamin.

Apply cold and heat. Apply an ice pack (wrapped in a towel) off and on for a few hours to reduce pain and swelling around the vagina, says Barry. Then switch to a warm washcloth to increase circulation and hasten healing.

Wear sanitary pads. To absorb the pale, menstrual-like fluid normally discharged after childbirth, women doctors advise wearing menstrual pads, not tampons. The reason? Mostly because of soreness, but also because there is a higher risk of infection while the cervical opening is still wider than usual, explains Dr. Smith.

Water yourself. If urination is painful, Barry suggests you use a plastic water bottle and squeeze water over the urethra as you void, which dilutes the acidic urine.

Counter incontinence. You can get your vaginal canal back in shape and regain control over urination by doing Kegel exercises, says Julie Tupler, R.N., a certified childbirth educator and founder and director of Maternal Fitness, a program in New York City that trains women for childbirth. Kegels work the muscles that you use to stop and start the flow of urine. While sitting, squeeze those muscles and count to ten. Release and repeat 20 times. Do five sets a day. "A good time to do it is while feeding the baby," suggests Tupler.

Shrink hemorrhoids. Soak four- by four-inch gauze pads in witch hazel, an astringent. Layer them in wax paper and freeze them, then place them directly on hemorrhoids for 10 to 20 minutes two or three times a day, says Dr. Bove.

Take an over-the-counter painkiller. Sometimes uterine cramps and other postpartum pains are best treated by taking acetaminophen or ibuprofen, says Dr. Smith, neither of which will adversely affect a breast-feeding baby.

Sleep on your stomach. You can help your uterus shrink back to its normal size by sleeping on your stomach, says Barry.

Breastfeed. The uterus of a woman who breastfeeds will shrink back into shape more quickly than that of a woman who doesn't, says Yvonne S. Thornton, M.D., visiting associate physician at the Rockefeller University Hospital in New York City and director of the perinatal diagnostic testing center at Morristown Memorial Hospital in New Jersey.

Massage your uterus. To help your uterus contract further, massage your abdomen in a clockwise circular direction every four hours, says Elaine Stillerman, a licensed massage therapist on the staff of the Swedish Institute of Massage in New York City and author of *Mother-Massage*. Continue for up to two weeks or until the color of any discharge is pale pink.

Air a C-section. If you've delivered by cesarean section, you have a major abdominal incision. If your incision is moist from heat or sweat, help it heal by drying it several times a day with a heat lamp or a hair dryer set on low, suggests Dr. Smith. In the process, be sure to push folds of slack abdominal skin away from the incision.

Posture

Sit and Stand Tall and Straight

For many women, posture problems begin in junior high school. Perhaps you developed early and got into the habit of slouching to hide your breasts. Or maybe you were a head or so taller than most of your girlfriends *and* half the guys at school, so you slouched to minimize your height. Or maybe you were short, and years of wearing high heels to compensate pushed your hips forward into a "swayback."

Whatever the reason, poor posture can lead to back pain, one of the most common reasons women seek medical help. As you get older, poor posture can result from osteoporosis—a degenerative spinal condition that can cause spinal changes leading to a slumped-over, shoulders-caved-in stance (also called kyphosis or dowager's hump) in little old ladies.

"The hump is formed when your spine collapses on top," Irene Von Estorff, M.D., physiatrist and assistant professor of rehabilitation medicine at Cornell Medical Center in New York City. The result: Your shoulders get rounded and slumped.

More than appearance is at stake.

"Poor posture is a major concern," says Shirley Sahrmann, Ph.D., associate professor of physical therapy at Washington University School of Medicine in St. Louis. "Women develop osteoporosis and get a kyphotic posture. But if you already have kyphosis, it can be even worse."

STAND TALL FOR HEALTH AND BEAUTY

Women doctors say that it's never too late to learn to stand tall and improve your posture. In fact, the sooner you start, the higher the odds that you'll avoid the little old lady stance associated with osteoporosis. Try these suggestions.

Take the string test. "The first step toward learning good posture is becoming aware of what yours looks like," says Dr. Von Estorff. So stand in front of a mirror and notice your stance. Face the mirror and see if your shoulders are even, she says. Then view your posture from the side.

"If your shoulders are slumped forward and your head is down, imagine that you have a string in the middle of the ceiling pulling you up from the crown of your head so that you can stand tall again," says

Rebecca Gorrell, education director of the Canyon Ranch wellness program in Tucson, Arizona.

Your weight should be distributed evenly on both feet, and your chest should be lifted and open, with your adbominals slightly contracted to support your lower back. Lifting and pressing your breastbone slightly forward will cause your shoulders to relax down, says Gorrell.

Lean against a wall. Good posture isn't standing in a rigid military stance, ready to salute your commanding officer. It means standing straight, but at ease, while tightening your abdominal muscles by pulling your tummy in and up, says Dr. Sahrmann.

How can you tell if you have it right? "Stand with your back against the wall and your heels three inches away," Dr. Sahrmann says. "You should be able to put your hand between the wall and your back at your waistline, with your head and shoulders close to, if not touching, the wall.

"Make sure that your knees are straight. If your knees are properly aligned, it's really hard not to stand straight," says Dr. Sahrmann.

Or try this as an exercise, she says: Stand with your back against the wall, tighten your abdominal muscles and raise your arms above your head without letting your back pull away from the wall.

Lift a leg. "If you're standing for long periods of time, place one foot on a rail or a stool to relieve back pain and maintain good posture," says Gorrell.

Don't sway with baby. To ease back pain and maintain good posture, any load should be carried squarely in front of you, using two hands. That includes your baby. "Holding your baby on one hip can lead to a permanent change in back and hip alignment," says Dr. Sahrmann.

Sit well. "To maintain good posture and avoid back pain, it's important to sit in a well-supported office chair," says Dr. Sahrmann. That means a chair in which your arms are supported so that your shoulders don't slope downward, your thighs are parallel to the floor, your knees are slightly higher than your hips and your feet touch the ground. If your feet don't touch, use a footstool.

Install a good chair in your home office. If, like millions of others, you find yourself seduced into spending hours online at your home computer, women doctors say that you also need a posture-friendly chair in your home office. So don't just pull over any old chair. Make sure that you're sitting on a chair with good back support.

Rotate with your chair. If your work arrangements require rotating your body, use a chair that rotates, too. "It is most important not to twist or rotate your body through large ranges of motion while sitting," says Dr. Sahrmann.

443

Keep moving. Don't stay in any one position at your desk for too long, says Dr. Von Estorff. "We lean forward to work at our desks," she says, and it's important to get up and stretch or even stretch in the chair.

Use a small pillow. When you're driving or flying or even sitting in an office chair for a long time, a small airline-size pillow or cushion or even a rolled-up towel placed behind the small of your back will help promote good posture by maintaining the natural curve in your spine, says Gorrell.

Relax your shoulders. "There's no special reason, but women have a tendency to hunch their shoulders when they're sitting at their desks or just concentrating," says Dr. Von Estorff. If that's a habit of yours, try to be aware of it, and relax your shoulders as soon as you notice the hunch.

Square off. One simple exercise to counteract the slump: Stand and try to bring your shoulder blades together in the back by pulling back your shoulders. Hold for ten seconds and release. Repeat at least three or four times. It will help strengthen your back muscles and prevent shoulder slump, says Dr. Von Estorff.

Shrug your shoulders. Dr. Von Estorff also suggests shoulder shrugs: Hunch up your shoulders toward your ears, then lower. Repeat two or three times.

Buy a correctly engineered bra. If you're big-breasted, wearing the wrong bra can pull your shoulders down, contributing to poor posture, says Dr. Sahrmann. She suggests wearing an underwire bra or a bra with straps that cross in the back to keep your chest high and your upper body posture firm.

Spare the heels. High heels put a strain on your lower back, often causing swayback, says Dr. Von Estorff. They throw your body off balance, thrusting out your pelvis when it should be tucked in. "Save your high heels for special occasions and wear shoes that keep you firmly planted on the ground the rest of the time," says Dr. Von Estorff.

Arch your back like a cat. Strong abdominal muscles are key to correcting swayback and achieving good posture, says Dr. Von Estorff. Try an exercise called the cat back: Get on all fours and arch your back, holding your tummy in for a count of 12. Do this three or four times a day at first, gradually getting to twice that.

Tone your trunk. "For good posture, you also need strong back muscles," says Debra Zillmer, M.D., orthopedic surgeon and medical director of the Gundersen Lutheran Sports Medicine Clinic in La Crosse, Wisconsin.

"Strengthening exercises help preserve the spine, ensuring good posture and lessening the possibility of lower-back pain," says Dr.

Zillmer. She suggests push-ups or weightlifting using free weights or machines. "These exercises should be done using proper mechanics, so that maximum benefit can be obtained. See a certified athletic trainer or a physical therapist for proper instruction."

Move your whole body. Dr. Von Estorff says that regular exercise will help your posture.

"Athletes always have good posture," says Gorrell. Have you ever seen someone dunk a basket while her shoulders were rounded and slumped?

The optimum is a combination of aerobic exercises such as swimming or walking alternating with strength training such as weight lifting using free weights, machines or resistance bands, says Gorrell. Strength training should be done two or three times a week every other day or so, giving the body time to recuperate between workouts. Aerobic exercise should be done for at least 30 minutes at a time, a minimum of three times a week.

Sleep right. "If you sleep on your stomach, it will exaggerate the curve of your lower back," says Gorrell. Instead, either sleep on your side, with a pillow under your head and between your knees to keep your thighs and hips aligned, or on your back, with a pillow under your knees to relieve pressure in the lower-back area. And choose a pillow made of natural fibers (like down) that will mold to your body shape instead of a stiff synthetic that may arch your neck and head unnaturally.

(For other practical ways to prevent osteoporosis, see page 407.)

Premenstrual Syndrome
Help for Hell Week

*I*t happens every month. Everything is fine and then—wham!—a week or two before your menstrual period, you become moody, irritable, depressed, tense, headachy, bloated or tired and find it difficult to concentrate. (Or maybe you're blessed with all of the above.)

Only 1 to 5 percent of women experience serious symptoms of premenstrual syndrome, or PMS, severe enough to interfere with their work and social lives or at least get noticed by others. (Even men's magazines are reporting on PMS.) But plenty of women experience symptoms of PMS to a lesser degree, according to Karen J. Carlson, M.D., an instructor at Harvard Medical School and director of Women's Health Associates at Massachusetts General Hospital in Boston.

A PROBLEM YOU CAN LIVE WITHOUT

Rest assured, say women doctors, if you have PMS, it doesn't mean that you're neurotic (or psychotic). Nor are you necessarily suffering from deranged hormone levels. Researchers' best guess is that PMS is triggered by subtle changes in the brain's levels of serotonin, a substance that influences moods—or something similar.

Until science comes up with some kind of explanation, women doctors suggest these remedies for PMS.

Switch to decaf. Coffee—or anything with caffeine—can exacerbate the irritability and tension associated with PMS, says Yvonne S. Thornton, M.D., visiting associate physician at the Rockefeller University Hospital in New York City and director of the perinatal diagnostic testing center at Morristown Memorial Hospital in New Jersey. "Caffeine can also make you sleep less well, which makes you more cranky." So when you feel PMS coming on, Dr. Thornton suggests that you replace caffeine with decaf or herb tea.

Manage your sweet tooth. Many women crave sweets premenstrually, but eating cookies, cake or candy will probably just add to the jitters

No Rash Decisions

Ann Honebrink, M.D.

The co-director of the Center for Women's Health at Allegheny University of the Health Sciences MCP–Hahnemann School of Medicine in Philadelphia doesn't pay too much attention to her own premenstrual syndrome (PMS) symptoms. But Anne Honebrink, M.D., says that hearing about the experiences of the women she counsels, coupled with increased self-awareness, have made her more alert to the existence of PMS. When she does notice premenstrual symptoms like irritability and fatigue, she deals with them by trying to keep them in perspective.

"I really do think it helps to just step back and try to recognize PMS for what it is," she says. "You might feel like divorcing your husband or quitting your job. When that happens, I tell myself that maybe I should think about this next week."

"It helps to be able to say, 'Okay, I know I'm feeling this way now, but it will go away when my period comes.' It doesn't make PMS go away," she says. "But it can make it easier to deal with."

by dramatically raising your blood sugar levels, says Dr. Thornton. So when the urge strikes, bite into an apple instead of a candy bar.

Eat small, eat often. Smaller, more frequent meals keep your blood sugar levels steady, says Ellen Freeman, Ph.D., director of the University of Pennsylvania Medical Center PMS Program in Philadelphia. This keeps you calmer and also helps cut your craving for sweets.

Have some spaghetti. A PMS diet—heavy on complex carbohydrates such as spaghetti and whole-wheat bread—may help relieve food cravings and mood swings, says Dr. Freeman. Complex carbs play a part in increased levels of the brain chemical tryptophan, necessary for the production of serotonin, the brain chemical that is involved in mood.

Mind your minerals. A daily supplement of 200 milligrams of magnesium premenstrually may also improve your symptoms, says Dr. Carlson.

And a daily 1,200 milligrams of calcium helps relieve menstrually related headaches and other PMS symptoms, according to a study by Susan Thys-Jacobs, M.D., a physician in the Division of General Internal Medicine at Mount Sinai Medical Center in New York City.

WHEN TO SEE A DOCTOR

Premenstrual syndrome (PMS) is usually considered a minor annoyance—unless it interferes with your on-the-job performance or keeps you from getting to work in the first place. The same goes if you can't manage your children during that time of the month, or if you have blowups with your spouse. If this sounds familiar, see a physician.

If you're practicing a form of birth control other than oral contraceptives, your doctor may suggest that you switch to the Pill. Birth control pills suppress the normal cyclic fluctuations in hormone levels and, in some women, can help alleviate symptoms of PMS.

Take your vitamins. Research shows that taking 50 to 100 milligrams a day of vitamin B_6 during PMS can alleviate depression, irritability and other symptoms, say women doctors— perhaps because it plays a part in serotonin metabolism, says Dr. Carlson.

Taking 150 to 200 international units of vitamin E premenstrually also seems to help, says Dr. Carlson, though the exact mechanism is not understood.

Season sans salt. A low-salt diet can relieve premenstrual bloating, says Dr. Thornton. It may also help alleviate headaches and improve mental concentration, because women with PMS may have a degree of edema, or swelling, in their brains.

Exercise for endorphins. Aerobic exercise offers a heightened sense of well-being, because it stimulates your brain's production of the natural feel-good substances called endorphins. Exercising regularly is more important than exercising intensely, says Dr. Freeman. "You don't have to train like an Olympic athlete," she says. "Get out there three or four times a week for a half-hour walk or run."

Increasing your regular exercise levels during PMS can relieve many symptoms, says Dr. Thornton. If you normally walk for 30 minutes three times per week, do so for longer or add extra days when you're feeling premenstrual.

Brighten your mood with bright light. PMS depression may be alleviated by bright lights, according to a study at the Department of Psychiatry at the University of California, San Diego, School of Medicine. Researchers Gabrielle M. Cerda, M.D., and Barbara L. Parry, M.D., asked women who get PMS to sit three feet away from an arrangement of bright lights, gazing at the lights occasionally, between the hours of 6:30 and 8:30 in the morning or 7:00 to 9:00 in the evening seven to ten days before their periods. A significant number of the women reported feeling less depressed after the bright-light sessions. Altered circadian (day-to-day) body rhythms, which appear to be related to mood disorders, or the enhanced production of certain hormones known to have antidepressant effects, may account for the women's improved moods, say the researchers.

Procrastination
Tackle Your Obligations—Pronto!

Think over the last week or so. Chances are, you put off doing something on your to-do list: stopping at the post office to buy stamps, phoning the friend who moved out of state, dropping off the dry cleaning that's been sitting in the backseat of your car for two weeks. Minor stuff.

Everyone procrastinates now and then, says Jane Burka, Ph.D., a psychologist in Berkeley, California, and co-author of *Procrastination*. It's only natural to put off things that we find tedious (like doing our taxes) or that leave us frustrated (like returning a phone that doesn't work to the electronics store).

But ours is not a culture that takes kindly to serious procrastinators. Habitual procrastinators pay all sorts of penalties for shilly-shallying: after-school detentions, failing grades, bad performance reviews, lost jobs, irate friends, towed cars and library fines. Then there are the intangible tolls that we pay: anxiety over missed deadlines, feelings of incompetence, depression and lowered self-esteem, notes Dr. Burka.

Some procrastinators claim that they do their best work under pressure. That's true for some people, but not everyone, says Dr. Burka. "If you do your work at the last minute, and everyone thinks that you're brilliant, that's one thing," she says. "If your work is a disappointment, you have to question the premise."

DO IT NOW

If you're a procrastinator—and most people who are know it—consider this advice.

Make your motto "Get it over with." "When you procrastinate, you punish yourself by lengthening the period of time in which you dread the task ahead," says Sandra Loucks, Ph.D., professor of psychology at the University of Tennessee in Knoxville and the University of Tennessee Medical Center. Remind yourself that the sooner you get started, the sooner you'll finish.

Divide and conquer. Let's say that you have something that's due ASAP, and you haven't even started it yet. First, break the project down into several individual tasks. Then, list them.

If you break a task into its component parts, the job won't seem so overwhelming, says Dr. Burka. Plus, you can tackle each part in a relatively short period of time. "You can do a small part any time that you have a few minutes free," she adds. "Procrastinators often tell themselves that they won't start a job until they have enough time to get the entire thing done at once. But most of us don't have days that are so uninterrupted."

Give yourself mini-deadlines. Estimate how much time that you'll need for each task and give yourself interim deadlines. Then stick to your schedule. "Set a timer or an alarm clock, if necessary," says Dr. Loucks.

Punt perfectionism. Not surprisingly, perfectionists—who see anything short of faultless as failure—are often serious procrastinators, says Dr. Burka. If you're a perfectionist, try to recognize that no one, not even you, can do anything perfectly.

"This doesn't mean that you shouldn't expect yourself to do well," says Lenora Yuen, Ph.D., a psychologist in Palo Alto, California, and co-author of *Procrastination*. "A lot of people think that if they don't expect perfection, they're settling for mediocrity. But there's a big range between perfection and mediocrity."

If your work pleases others—your boss is satisfied, but you're not—you're probably setting your standards too high, writes Frieda Porat, Ph.D., a psychotherapist in Menlo Park, California, and author of *Creative Procrastination*.

Psoriasis
Relief for Achy, Flaky Skin

*W*omen don't refer to it as the heartbreak of psoriasis for nothing. This serious skin condition can be so bothersome that you probably wish you could unzip your skin and climb out of it. The hallmark symptoms of psoriasis are not pretty: the dry, red, cracking skin; the silvery scales that shed everywhere you don't want them to and the round, raised, itchy plaques. They can affect your scalp, elbows or knees, even your stomach, groin or your entire body.

MAKE IT BETTER

Why is your skin acting up, and what can you do to soothe it?

"With psoriasis, the skin cells experience a too-rapid turnover, so they build up on the skin's surface. Instead of shedding off in fine little particles, the skin cells tend to clump together and come off in big chunks. The result is thick, inflamed patches of skin along with redness and silvery scales," says Kristin Leiferman, M.D., professor of dermatology at the Mayo Medical School in Rochester, Minnesota.

Psoriasis isn't contagious, but no one knows what causes it, says D'Anne Kleinsmith, M.D., a staff dermatologist at William Beaumont Hospital in Royal Oak, Michigan. "It tends to come and go. So even though today it may look bad, it can fade again for a month or two," she says. It frequently flares up in the winter months and improves in the summer.

"Some women notice that it's worse just before their menstrual periods," says Karen K. Deasey, M.D., chief of dermatology at Bryn Mawr Hospital in Pennsylvania.

STUBBORN BUT TREATABLE

Here's what women dermatologists recommend you do to mend your cracking, flaking skin.

Target your skin with tar. Check out your drugstore skin-care shelf for bath oils, cream preparations and lotions containing ingredients made from coal tar, which can soothe psoriasis. "People might find relief from

451

WHEN TO SEE A DOCTOR

Women dermatologists say that you should consult your doctor if:

- You have severe psoriasis on your palms and soles, or if it covers a lot of your body.
- You see blistering or pus-filled blisters or little whiteheads that burst easily.
- Your skin develops any sign of infection: yellow crusting, pus or honeycomb-shaped blotches of redness.

You should see a doctor quickly if you develop a rapidly spreading rash that covers most or all of your body. You may have a streptococcus infection or other serious condition.

taking a coal-tar bath or rubbing a coal-tar cream or lotion into their psoriasis patches," says Dr. Deasey. She and Dr. Kleinsmith recommend Psorigel, Fototar and Balnetar. Ask your pharmacist to order them for you. Follow product instructions and do not apply to blistered, oozing, infected or raw skin.

"Try different products until you find what works for you," says Dr. Deasey.

They're messy but effective, says Dr. Kleinsmith. Always read instructions carefully before using.

Soak, then moisturize. Soaking in a bath can help hydrate skin, says Dr. Leiferman. But hold off on the bath oil; if you add it at the beginning of your soak, it may actually do more harm than good. "Bath oils tend to coat your skin and block out water. And if water can't penetrate your skin, it can't hydrate your cells," she says. "Soak for ten minutes to allow your skin to absorb water first, and then add oil for the last five minutes of your bath to seal in the water," she recommends. "Bath oils make the tub slippery, so step out carefully."

Moisturize right after bathing. "It's important to apply moisturizer right after you get out of the bath or shower, to seal in the water that your skin has just absorbed," says Dr. Leiferman. Moisturizing keeps your skin hydrated so that it's less likely to crack. "For best results go for a heavier cream or ointment moisturizer, which really coats the skin. Lotions evaporate too quickly to really benefit super-dry skin," she says.

Coat your skin with cortisone cream. Over-the-counter 1 percent hydrocortisone creams, such as Cortaid, can help quell itching and swelling, says Dr. Kleinsmith. But use them only when you really need them. Prolonged regular use of hydrocortisone cream can thin skin and even cause stretch marks.

Try special shampoos. "Psoriasis is particularly stubborn in the scalp. You can't get rid of it, but you can get it to calm down for a while with the use of special shampoos," says Dr. Deasey. "Check drugstores for shampoos containing either coal tars or salicylic acid, or even for everyday dandruff shampoos."

Switch shampoos frequently. "A number of doctors I have talked with recommend rotating shampoo products to produce better results," says Dr. Leiferman. "It seems that the skin on your scalp gets tolerant of one set of ingredients, so they become less effective. But if you switch off to something different, you'll see results again."

When you finish one bottle, switch to a different brand. "Go try a whole bunch of shampoos. Find four or five that you like and then just rotate them on and off," Dr. Leiferman recommends.

Take a short cut. "A long or elaborate hairstyle makes it difficult to apply daily scalp treatments," says Dr. Leiferman. She recommends short, carefree styles for women with psoriasis.

Spend a few minutes in the sun. Since psoriasis seems to improve with exposure to ultraviolet light, some dermatologists think this is one skin condition that merits a soak in the sun. "In the summer I tell women with psoriasis to go out in the sun and stay out just long enough to get the benefit of the ultraviolet light, but not long enough to burn—no more than 15 minutes or so," says Dr. Deasey.

"I do caution people to wear sunscreen on their faces and in areas where they don't have psoriasis, to protect their skin," says Dr. Kleinsmith.

Puffy Eyes
A Fast-Action Plan for Morning Pouches

For once the popular perception is correct. Crying does cause puffy eyes. So can lack of sleep, says Marianne O'Donoghue, M.D., associate professor of dermatology at Rush-Presbyterian–St. Luke's Medical Center in Chicago.

WHEN TO SEE A DOCTOR

If you wake up and one eyelid has swollen to three times the size of the other, call your doctor. It may be a sign of hives, or an allergic reaction to an insect bite, says Marianne O'Donoghue, M.D., associate professor of dermatology at Rush-Presbyterian–St. Luke's Medical Center in Chicago.

Also, see your doctor if your lids don't close all the way over your eyeballs (a possible sign of thyroid disease).

Crying and lack of sleep aren't the most common cause, though. "Sleeping on your face is probably the easiest way to get puffy eyes," says Dr. O'Donoghue. You're also more likely to wake up with puffy sacks if you're menstruating or pregnant and retaining fluid, say doctors. Ditto if you eat salty foods or drink anything—even fresh filtered water—less than two hours before you go to bed.

The fluid simply has to go somewhere, and sometimes it ends up in temporary pouches under your eyes, says Dr. O'Donoghue.

DO'S AND DON'TS FOR IMMEDIATE RELIEF

If you want to erase puffiness before you start your day, say doctors, here's what you can do.

Don't rub. If you do, says Dr. O'Donoghue, your eyes will get irritated and red—and stay puffy.

Employ a cold compress. Dunk a washcloth in cool water (or wrap ice cubes in a washcloth) and place it on your closed eyes, suggests Dr. O'Donoghue. When the cloth gets warm, wring it out and repeat. Do this three or four times. "This takes just a few minutes, but it will help drain the puffs under your eyes," she says.

Apply a cold tea bag wrapped in tissue. Tea contains tannin, a natural astringent. "The tannin in the tea may help pull the skin taut and reduce puffiness," says Dr. O'Donoghue. Five minutes should be all you need.

It is a good idea to wrap the tea bag in tissue. Otherwise, the tea will stain your skin, creating a raccoon effect. And tannic acid (a derivative of tannin) can sting, explains Dr. O'Donoghue. So keep your eyes shut.

NO MORE PUFFINESS, EVER

So much for deflating puffy eyes today. To prevent future episodes:

Raise your head with pillows. Two or three pillows will help keep fluids from pooling under your eyes, says Monica L. Monica, M.D., Ph.D., an ophthalmologist in New Orleans and spokesperson for the American Academy of Ophthalmology. But it takes hours.

Avoid salty foods and alcohol. Increasing the amount of salty foods (like chips and pickles) that you eat and drinking alcohol make you retain fluids that can collect in the eye area (and elsewhere), says Dr. O'Donoghue.

Pump Bumps
When Your Heels Take the Lumps

Pumps are minimalist footwear. They're low-cut dress shoes that stay on by gripping your feet at your toes and heels. Because the back of the shoe is contoured to fit tightly, it can bite into your Achilles tendon, the thick cord that connects your calf muscles to your heel. Wear pumps long enough, and you can develop a painful lump across the back of your heel—appropriately called a pump bump.

What's causing the pain is a combination of inflammation, calcium deposits and thickened and irritated skin, says Kathleen Stone, D.P.M., a podiatrist in private practice in Glendale, Arizona.

SENSIBLE WAYS TO EASE THE HURT

A particularly large, ugly pump bump can be removed surgically. But women doctors offer easier ways to relieve pain and reduce swelling. Here's what foot specialists recommend.

Shed shoes and apply ice. If your heel is red and swollen, chances are that the problem is an inflammation of the bursae, fluid-filled sacs right at the spot where your Achilles tendon meets your heel bone, says Dr. Stone.

WHEN TO SEE A DOCTOR

If you've tried to remedy a pump bump by switching shoes or using heel lifts, and your heel still hurts after a week or so, you could have an inflamed Achilles tendon, says Theresa G. Conroy, D.P.M., a podiatrist in private practice in Philadelphia. If not treated promptly, a temporarily inflamed Achilles tendon can become a chronic problem. So don't ignore the pain—get medical advice.

For immediate relief, half-fill a resealable plastic bag with water and crushed ice, wrap it in a damp cloth and then wrap the bag around your heel, recommends Marika Molnar, P.T., director of West Side Dance Physical Therapy in New York City. Apply the ice pack for 10 to 15 minutes, remove it for a few minutes so that your foot doesn't get over-chilled, then reapply. Repeat as needed.

Get a lift. If you favor pumps, say foot specialists, you don't have to trade in your entire footwear wardrobe for sensible shoes. Instead, use a thin foam heel insert to lift your heel, so that the back of the shoe no longer hits the sore area, suggests Theresa G. Conroy, D.P.M., a podiatrist in private practice in Philadelphia. "This is all that most women need to do." Put inserts in both shoes, even if only one foot hurts.

If you have an infection (like a sore) present, however, forget about trying to work pumps into your wardrobe and get to a podiatrist, pronto.

Give 'em some room. Squeezing your feet into any style shoes—even "sensible" tie shoes or flats—can cause toe and heel problems if the shoes are too short. You should be able to press a thumb's width between the end of the shoe and the end of your longest toe, according to Phyllis Ragley, D.P.M., vice-president of the American Academy of Podiatric Sports Medicine who practices in Lawrence, Kansas. If you can't get your shoes on without a shoe horn, chances are that they're too small.

Rashes
Make Itchy Red Splotches Vanish

*Y*ou have an itch, so you scratch it—only to find that your skin has erupted in a streak of red bumps. Where did this mystery rash come from, and what can you do about it?

Rashes can come in many forms, including red, itchy patches, hives or even blisters. Depending on the cause, they may take a week or longer to heal. What's tricky about rashes is that they can be triggered by about a gazillion things. It helps if you can do a little detective work to determine what the cause of your rash is, so you can eliminate it from your life.

One way to sleuth out what caused your rash is to look at the location of the rash on your body. If it is caused by an internal trigger (such as a food, medication or virus), the rash will generally be more widespread and symmetrical. If the rash is caused by something external (like detergents or poison ivy), then it will be confined to the areas of skin exposed to the bothersome material, says Patricia Farris Walters, M.D., clinical assistant professor of dermatology at Tulane University School of Medicine in New Orleans and a spokesperson for the American Academy of Dermatology. Typical irritants that can raise rashes on women's skin include cosmetics, fragrances, hair dyes, harsh detergents, jewelry, poison ivy and rubber.

"It could be as simple as dry skin, or as complicated as a reaction to a medication that you're taking—in which case you need to call your doctor," explains Mary Ruth Buchness, M.D., chief of dermatology at St. Vincent's Hospital and Medical Center in New York City.

AN ARSENAL OF RASH REMEDIES

If a rash appears from some kind of trigger, you can deal with it accordingly. Here's what women doctors suggest.

Try a cool compress. Soak a washcloth or piece of gauze in cool water with Aveeno oatmeal preparation, made according to package directions, says Dr. Walters. To soothe itching and burning, hold the compress against the rash for about 15 minutes.

Heal the milky way. "Make a compress soaked in half milk and half water and apply it to the rash," suggests Amy Newburger, M.D., as-

WHEN TO SEE A DOCTOR

If you develop a rash and you are taking medication, call your doctor immediately. In some people medications, including antibiotics, can cause an allergic reaction in the form of serious rashes. Your doctor may recommend that you stop taking the drug or switch to something else.

You should also consult with a physician if a rash:

- Doesn't clear up within a week or so
- Is so painful and itchy that it keeps you awake at night
- Blisters and/or covers a large amount of your body
- Weeps or oozes
- Is accompanied by pus or swelling (or both)
- Is accompanied by a fever

If you scratch a lot, a rash can become infected. Signs of infection are yellowish or whitish fluid, swelling and warmth in the area.

You should also see a doctor if your rash is associated with other symptoms, such as joint pains, flulike symptoms, urinary tract irritation or stomach upset.

sistant clinical professor of dermatology at Columbia University College of Physicians and Surgeons in New York City and a dermatologist in Scarsdale, New York. There seems to be something in milk protein that is anti-inflammatory, she adds. "Just rinse off afterward, so that the milk doesn't turn bad. You don't want to smell like sour cream."

Soak in soda. Toss a half-cup of baking soda into a tub full of water and bathe in it to relieve your rash. "You could also make a paste from a spoonful of baking soda mixed with a bit of water and dab that on your rash to soothe your skin," says Dr. Walters.

Bewitch the itch. If the rashy area is not open and raw, witch hazel is wonderful to cool and soothe irritated skin, says Dr. Newburger. You can buy the clear liquid over the counter. Apply it to cotton balls and dab on your skin.

Pour on the tar. Skin preparations made with an ingredient called coal tar, which is an anti-itch medication, can provide tremendous rash relief, according to Dr. Buchness. You can find tar preparations over the counter at your local drugstore. "Pour some coal tar emulsion into a cool bath and soak in it or rub tar oil or gel onto your skin," she says. "The downside is that tar preparations are brown, and they can stain clothing.

Use them at night, and cover them with old pajamas. And put old sheets on your bed."

Use a cotton ball near your eyeballs. If a rash has developed around your eyes (maybe from an allergic reaction to a cosmetic or a cleaning solution), a safe way to soothe and cool the itch is to soak a cotton ball in cool skim milk or cool water and Aveeno oatmeal preparation and hold the cotton gently against your eyelids or skin, recommends Dr. Walters. "The eyelid skin is very sensitive, so only bland things should be applied."

Rule with Rhuligel. If you don't want to cover an already unsightly rash with pink calamine lotion, consider applying Rhuligel, a clear over-the-counter anti-itch gel. Not only is it invisible, but it also contains menthol and camphor, two skin-soothing ingredients, says Dr. Walters.

Let it breathe. Generally, you want to leave a rash uncovered, says Dr. Walters. However, if the rash is wet, oozing and blistering, you may want to cover it with a light gauze bandage to prevent an infection, or just so it doesn't run or get on your clothing, she suggests.

Pamper sore skin with pramoxine. If you want to apply a topical anesthetic to your skin to reduce pain and itching, look for lotions that contain the ingredient pramoxine, recommends Dr. Newburger. Look for the ingredient on the labels of products such as Aveeno Anti-Itch lotion, or Caladryl Clear lotion, she suggests.

Pop an antihistamine pill. Take an over-the-counter antihistamine pill at bedtime to quell swelling and itching, suggests Dr. Walters. Benadryl may make you drowsy, which can be an added benefit if the itch has been keeping you awake at night.

Steer clear of irritants. "Avoidance is the key to preventing future rashes," points out Dr. Walters.

(For practical ways to manage bikini bottom—associated with swimsuit wear—heat rash and posion ivy, see pages 49, 274 and 432.)

Raynaud's Disease
Warming Strategies for Cold Sensitivity

For women who live in cold climes, tingly fingers and numb toes are uncomfortable but to be expected. For anyone with Raynaud's disease, however, exposure to cold may be so painful that reaching into the freezer for a bag of peas can be unbearable. For these people a glitch in the body's circulatory system triggers a painful, super-spastic overreaction to cold that constricts blood vessels, especially in the fingers and toes.

"We know that Raynaud's is caused by a spasm of the blood vessels," says Kendra Kaye, M.D., clinical assistant professor of medicine at the University of Pennsylvania School of Medicine in Philadelphia. "What we don't know is why it happens."

Typically, Raynaud's causes color changes in the affected areas, most noticeably in the fingers. "A woman might see her fingertips turn white and then blue while she is in the cold. Later, when she warms up, her fingertips turn red. This is the classic color triad of Raynaud's," says Dr. Kaye.

Also, if you could look inside blood vessels affected by Raynaud's, you would see that the cells lining the vessel walls are noticeably thick, says Joan Merrill, M.D., assistant chief of rheumatology at St. Luke's–Roosevelt Hospital Center in New York City. The blood flow is slowed down, so that in severe cases, a spasm can cause blood flow to stop.

PRACTICAL STRATEGIES

Most strategies to prevent an attack of Raynaud's are focused on preventing a spasm in the blood vessels found in your fingers and toes, says Dr. Merrill. Here's what doctors suggest.

Put on your mitts. Slip on oven mitts whenever you need to reach in the freezer for a bag of peas or a tray of ice, says Dr. Merrill. The mitts may be a tad cumbersome, but they'll protect your fingers from the cold that can trigger a spasm.

Wear rubber gloves. Use rubber gloves whenever you immerse your hands in cold water to do delicate laundry or other household chores, says Dr. Merrill. Just make sure that they're a size or two larger than you normally wear. Otherwise, they can restrict your circulation and trigger a spasm.

Make a fist. Sometimes just moving from one room to a cooler one can be enough to trigger Raynaud's, says Dr. Merrill. To avoid a spasm, simply ball your hands into loose fists as you walk into the room. This allows your fingers to warm each other. Allow a few minutes for your body to acclimatize to the new temperature before releasing your fists.

Use an insulated cup. Just because you have Raynaud's does not mean that you have to give up ice-cold beverages, says Dr. Merrill. Just make sure that you put them in an insulated glass or a cup that has a handle.

Avoid air-conditioning. "A lot of women say that air-conditioning triggers their Raynaud's," says Dr. Merrill. Most women avoid air-conditioning as much as they can, but when they can't, they should ask to have the air conditioner turned down and sit as far away from its vents as possible.

Stock up on foot and hand warmers. "Keeping your fingers and toes warm when venturing outdoors is serious business for someone with Raynaud's," says Dr. Merrill. In addition to stocking up on mittens, gloves, socks, hats with ear flaps and knitted face masks, pick up several heat pouches—sold at sporting goods stores and hardware stores—and slip them into your gloves, pockets and boots.

Mobilize your fingers. A nasty side effect of Raynaud's is that your fingers can stiffen to the point that they become immovable, says Dr. Merrill. "But don't let the stiffness beat you. Twice a day, plunge your hands into a sink or basin of warm water and wiggle your fingers around until they move more freely."

Choose caffeine-free products. Whether it's in coffee, tea, cola or over-the-counter medication, caffeine can constrict blood vessels and exacerbate Raynaud's, says Dr. Kaye. Read product labels and try to avoid caffeine if you can.

WHEN TO SEE A DOCTOR

You should consult your doctor if you have Raynaud's and:
- Your hands swell.
- You notice hair loss.
- Your eyes feel dry.

Your doctor may prescribe oral medication to dilate blood vessels, helping to reduce spasms that cause pain and color changes.

Razor Burn
Care for Post-shaving Rashes

*Y*ou shave to make your skin look better—smooth, hair-free, sleek. So the last thing that you want is to whisk the razor over your legs and raise up an ugly red rash. Unfortunately, a lot of women do just that when they shave incorrectly. "They slap on soap and quickly shave over it, and end up with chafed, red skin—also known as razor burn," says Evelyn Placek, M.D., a dermatologist and doctor of internal medicine in private practice in Scarsdale, New York.

"Razor burn is actually a skin irritation," says Dr. Placek. "When you shave, you're basically peeling off part of your epidermis—the top layer of skin. The redness is a normal response to tissue injury. Blood flow increases to the area to heal the wound, and blood vessels dilate and become red."

Razor burn is hard to get rid of, says Patricia Farris Walters, M.D., clinical assistant professor of dermatology at Tulane University School of Medicine in New Orleans and a spokesperson for the American Academy of Dermatology. "Every time you shave again, you re-irritate your skin."

SMOOTH MOVES

One way to avoid razor burn is to stop shaving. If that's not your preferred option, women doctors offer these tips for taking the redness and itching out of shaving.

Reach for hydrocortisone. Reduce embarrassing redness by immediately applying a dab of 1 percent hydrocortisone cream to the area after you shave. "It will take the redness, sting and irritation right down," says Dr. Placek. Hydrocortisone constricts blood vessels, so less blood flows to the area—meaning less redness. "You probably need to do this only twice the first day, and symptoms should fade."

But don't use hydrocortisone daily. Any preparation containing cortisone should be used only as a short-term treatment, for a couple applications or a few days at most. "If you overuse cortisone, your skin could become habituated to it and actually become redder and more irritated when you stop using it," warns Dr. Placek. "So it's not meant to be applied every day." Plus, overuse of cortisone preparations can thin skin over time; blood vessels in the area may enlarge, and in your pubic area, you could even get stretch marks.

Lubricate skin after you shave. "A moisturizing body lotion will help reduce dryness and itchiness after shaving," says D'Anne Kleinsmith, M.D., a staff dermatologist at William Beaumont Hospital in Royal Oak, Michigan.

Shave after you bathe. Next time you shave, give irritated skin a break by making sure that it's well-hydrated before you graze a razor over it. "The best time to shave is after a shower or bath," says Dr. Placek. "Your skin won't be dry, and your hairs will soften and stand up, so shaving will be less traumatic."

Drop the soap. People with razor-sensitive skin should stick with a shaving cream that contains aloe or some other soothing ingredient, recommends Dr. Placek.

"Shaving cream is a real help," agrees Dr. Kleinsmith. "Put it on after you bathe, when your skin and hair are already soft. Then, leave the shaving cream on for another couple of minutes to soften your hair even more before you shave."

Shave it down. Shave hair in the direction that it grows—in a downward motion. "This won't irritate the hair follicles as much as if you're shaving upward against short, bristly hairs," says Dr. Walters.

Switch to a hair-dissolver cream. If you know that you're prone to razor bumps, consider using a lotion depilatory, which dissolves hair. "These lotions may be a little smelly and messy, but they're less traumatic to the hair follicles than scraping a razor over them," says Dr. Placek.

Most people tolerate depilatories very well, but some people are allergic, says Dr. Walters. If you notice a rash, irritation or burning sensation in reaction to a hair-removing lotion, rinse it off and don't use it again.

Zap bumps with acne preps. As a long-term treatment, topical acne preparations containing 2.5 or 5 percent benzoyl peroxide can help minimize razor bumps and lessen the chance that they will return. "There's actually a shaving cream called Benzashave, which contains benzoyl peroxide, and it can help minimize razor bumps. If you're prone, use it every time you shave," suggests Dr. Placek.

Replace your razor. "You get a close shave with double-edge razors and disposables—so close that they can really irritate your skin and traumatize hair follicles," says Dr. Walters. "And the duller they get, the more irritating they become—like a rake dragged over your skin." She

WHEN TO SEE A DOCTOR

If razor burn or bumps don't seem to heal in a few days, or if they look at all infected, see a doctor. Any signs of pus, increased swelling, heat in the area or throbbing are clues that infection may have set in.

Recurring razor bumps should probably be treated by a doctor, since repeat shaving will only make them worse.

advises that women toss a disposable razor and break out a new one after three or four uses or replace the blade after three or four uses in a nondisposable handle.

Go electric. "Sometimes I recommend that women switch to electric razors," says Dr. Walters. "It may give you a smoother, more even shave than a regular razor."

(For practical advice on removing bikini-line hair, see page 51.)

Rectal Itching
A Grown-Up Version of Diaper Rash

*I*n an era when women think nothing of chatting on national television about intimate secrets, like how they seduced their daughter's fiancé while under the influence of sugarless gum, here's a secret that only the bravest divulge: rectal itching.

Doctors call chronic rectal itching *pruritus ani*—Latin for anal itching. Rectal itching has many possible causes. And very often, it's chronic. Most often, rectal itching is associated with hemorrhoids, which affect about half of the population by age 50 and are common among pregnant women. Other possible causes include allergic reactions to scented soaps;

drinking coffee, tea or alcoholic beverages or eating citrus fruits and chocolate, which are common bowel irritants.

SOOTHING THE ITCH FOR GOOD

Here's what women doctors advise if you are bothered with chronic rectal itching.

Pick up petroleum jelly. You wake up and your rectum is itching, itching, itching. For quick relief a little bit of petroleum jelly carefully applied to the site of the itch will ease the irritation until you have time for the more lasting remedies that follow, says Robyn Karlstadt, M.D., a gastroenterologist at Graduate Hospital in Philadelphia.

Wipe until it's clean. If you routinely wipe only once after a bowel movement and then pull up your undies, your rectal area may not be clean. The result is itchy irritation. "It may take a couple of wipes, but make sure that you leave no trace of stool on the toilet paper," says Dr. Karlstadt.

Dampen your toilet paper. Unusually sticky stool can be hard to clean. "If you've wiped a few times, and your anal area still isn't clean, wet toilet paper may work better," says Dr. Karlstadt. Then pat dry with a fresh section of toilet paper.

Make sure that your bottom is dry. A wet bottom irritates the skin around your anus. The best way to keep it dry? "Baby yourself with baby powder," says Barbara Frank, M.D., gastroenterologist and clinical professor of medicine at Allegheny University of the Health Sciences MCP–Hahnemann School of Medicine in Philadelphia. Pat it on with a disposable cotton ball.

Lather up naturally. Deodorized or perfumed soap can irritate your rectum. To keep your rectum itch-free, choose unscented soaps, says Dr. Frank.

WHEN TO SEE A DOCTOR

Tried home remedies for two to four weeks, and your rectum still hurts? See your doctor.

Rectal itching may be associated with diabetes or incontinence. Have kids? They often spread pinworm, an infection that causes the skin around the anus to become irritated.

Repetitive Strain Injury

Stop Overuse Abuse

*I*f you do something over and over again, you'll get better at it, right? Maybe, maybe not. Women who experience repetitive strain injury know too well that years of performing a task over and over, whether it be keying data into a computer all day, ringing up cash-register sales day after day, or knitting for hours in the evenings, can cause long-term pain. Worse, this kind of injury can interfere with on-the-job performance or continued employment.

Repetitive strain injuries now account for more than 50 percent of all occupational illnesses reported in the United States. The most common of these injuries is carpal tunnel syndrome, in which wrist, arm, elbow and hand muscles hurt from overuse.

The carpal tunnel is indeed a tunnel; it is a small, rigid space with nerves and tendons running through it. Carpal tunnel syndrome can occur when frequent use of your wrist causes the tendons to swell and compress the nerve that runs to your hand. And you feel pain.

"The pain is often worst at night, with numbness and tingling, particularly in the thumb and index fingers. And you may have trouble gripping objects," says Diana Carr, M.D., an orthopedic surgeon in private practice in Sebring, Florida.

HORMONES AND YOUR WRIST HEALTH

More than half the cases of repetitive strain injury occur in women. Researchers say that women between the ages of 30 are 45 are at twice the risk—for various reasons. A higher percentage of them work at clerical and factory jobs requiring repetitive motion. Typists, grocery clerks and even women who knit and crochet are particularly vulnerable to repetitive strain injuries.

Compounding the problem is that in women, the carpal tunnel is smaller, so that it takes less swelling for the problem to occur, making women more susceptible to the compression that causes pain, Dr. Carr says.

466

"Also, fluid retention during pregnancy causes the carpal tunnel to swell," says Mary Ann Keenan, M.D., chairman of the Department of Orthopedic Surgery at the Albert Einstein Medical Center in Philadelphia. When the rest of the body swells, so do the fluids in the carpal tunnel.

Who would have thought that hormones would have anything to do with wrist pain? According to women doctors, fluid retention prompted by shifts in levels of the female hormone estrogen before menstruation and during menopause also may put women at risk for carpal tunnel syndrome.

FREEDOM FROM REPETITIVE STRAIN

Luckily, there are measures that can bring relief for most women.

Take mini-breaks. "If you can take a break from the activity that's causing you pain, do so," says Dr. Carr. If you do needlepoint to relax at night, and you work at a keyboard for a living, try to take a rest from your leisure activities until your wrists feel better. At the very least, take mini-breaks of a minute or so every half-hour a day, and if you can, periodically switch to a different activity, she suggests.

Use a wrist rest. "If you type at the computer, always use a wrist pad to soften the stress on your wrists," says Dr. Keenan. A wrist pad helps soften the blow of repetitive motion.

Sit properly. "Your wrists should be in a neutral position on the keyboard—that is, neither flexed up or down—with your elbows at a 90 degree angle," says Margot Miller, P.T., a physical therapist in Duluth, Minnesota.

Stretch. Periodically flexing and extending your wrist and arm muscles will help relieve stress on your pinched nerve, says Miller. To limber up, open and close your fingers for a few minutes or slowly bend your wrists back and forth a few times (or do both).

Splint your wrist at night. "One way to stop the pain is to wear a wrist splint—at night, or any time that you don't need to use your

WHEN TO SEE A DOCTOR

If, despite self-care strategies, you have constant pain that interferes with activities for more than a week, see a doctor. If you have repetitive strain injury, the sooner you're treated, the lower the odds that you'll have to have surgery.

wrist," says Dr. Keenan. That will keep your wrist steady and prohibit the movement that causes pain. They're available from drugstores without a prescription.

Bandage tennis elbow. So-called tennis elbow is actually a form of repetitive strain injury. "If you have tennis elbow, you can purchase a special pressure bandage from a drugstore or medical supply store, which you can wear over your forearm to take the strain off," says Dr. Keenan.

(For more information on practical ways to manage tennis-related pain, see page 537.)

Restless Legs Syndrome
Calm Crawly, Fidgety Legs

After sitting at her desk for an hour peering at rows of data on a computer screen, an odd sensation began to creep through Claudia's calves. She shifted her legs and tried to ignore it, but the urge to move kept coming back. Eventually, she gave up, leaned back in her chair and stretched, and the odd sensation—the one that she sometimes says feels like "ants crawling on my bones"—had disappeared.

Claudia is actually pretty lucky. The crawling ants feeling that she gets and her need to stretch are typical of restless legs syndrome—or what is also known as *anxietas tibiarum*, says Sheryl Siegel, M.D., assistant professor of neurology at New York Medical College in Valhalla, New York.

Restless legs can occur whenever someone is sitting or lying down. "We have no idea what causes restless legs," says Sarah Stolz, M.D., a neurologist at Providence Medical Center Sleep Disorders Center in Seattle. "But if you have it, it can make you miserable."

Pregnant women seem to have a one in ten chance of developing restless legs, says Dr. Stolz. People with nerve damage in their legs from diabetes or lumbar disk disease, for example, are also prone to restless legs. And some people with kidney disease who are unable to filter metabolic waste from their blood constantly feel the need to shift their legs 24 hours a day.

TRIAL AND ERROR

Since restless legs may have different causes, and no one treatment works for everyone, women doctors say that the only way to find relief is to try various tactics, then use what works.

Point your toes. If restless legs strike while you're sitting, point your toes and stretch both your legs from foot to hip, says Dr. Siegel.

Most people with restless legs try to resist the impulse to move their legs. But if you do, the urge to move will just build until nothing short of a day-long hike will satisfy the urge to move. Better to give in to the first impulse to move, she advises. You'll likely "travel" a shorter distance.

Get up. If restless legs strike after you have gone to bed, again, don't resist the urge to move, says Dr. Siegel. "Get out of bed and walk

---

WHAT WOMEN DOCTORS DO

Stretch, Walk, Read

Sheryl Siegel, M.D.

An assistant professor of neurology at New York Medical College in Valhalla, New York, Sheryl Siegel, M.D., gets restless legs once or twice a year. Here's what she does for relief.

"I only get minor symptoms—nothing like what some women experience," says Dr. Siegel. "So my routine is simple. I stretch my legs and walk up and down the stairs a few times. Then I pick up a book and read until I fall asleep."

As an alternative, Dr. Siegel recommends a technique called progressive muscle relaxation. Simply do this: Lie back with your arms at your sides and close your eyes. Breathe deeply, then exhale. Then, starting with your toes and ending with your scalp, tense and relax each muscle group, one at a time. Do this for at least five minutes.

WHEN TO SEE A DOCTOR

If your legs are so restless that the discomfort interferes with sleep, your job or other everyday activities, see your doctor. After ruling out any underlying problems, she may prescribe one of a variety of medications or other ways to try and control the problem.

Also, if you're currently being treated for kidney disease and experience a bothersome numbness or tingling in your feet, see your doctor.

up and down the hall a couple of times or, if you have stairs, up and down the stairs."

Focus on B vitamins and iron. Some scientists suspect that a deficiency of folate (a B vitamin) or iron—or both—may have something to do with the cause of restless legs. Dr. Stolz says that it makes sense to make sure that your diet has rich sources of both. Legumes, oranges and orange juice, brussels sprouts, spinach, asparagus and strawberries are good sources of folate. Steamed clams, lean beef, turkey, chicken, tofu, whole-grain bread and legumes provide a hefty serving of iron.

Try to get the Daily Value of both iron and folic acid (the supplement form of folate) every day, says Dr. Stolz—400 micrograms of folic acid and 18 milligrams of iron. It's a good idea to take a multivitamin/mineral supplement to be sure that you're getting the right amounts, but don't go overboard with megadoses. A supplement that contains the Daily Value amounts is sufficient.

Try hot or cold. Some women find that hot baths relieve restless legs, while others find that cold packs do the trick, says Dr. Stolz. She suggests that individual women experiment to see what works.

Avoid evening aerobic exercise. Although movement is important, try to schedule exercise that increases your heart rate for during the day rather than in the evening, says Dr. Siegel. Some women seem to experience restless legs more frequently after late exercise.

Relax. Once you've turned out the light and crawled between the sheets, try a relaxation exercise such as progressive muscle relaxation, says Dr. Siegel. "This is a two-step process: muscle relaxation followed by steady breathing." First, lie on your back with your arms at your sides and close your eyes. Take a deep breath and exhale. Then, tense and relax every muscle group you can identify, one at a time, starting with your toes and working all the way to your scalp. Then, start to count each inhalation and exhalation separately, so that on the first inhalation, you count "one," and on the first exhalation, you count "one" also. Count to eight, then start counting all over again. As thoughts or noises interrupt your breathing pattern, let them go and return to your counting and breathing. Do this for 5 to 20 minutes, depending on what you have time for.

Rosacea

Fight Flushing and Blushing

Elizabeth has fair, almost translucent skin that turns a glowing pink whenever she's hot, angry, embarrassed or somewhat tipsy.

But now, barely into her thirties, the pink is changing to red, the red is coming more often and small bumps, pimples and tiny broken blood vessels are appearing around Elizabeth's nose.

Elizabeth's doctor says that all the flushing she experienced was actually a prelude to rosacea, a skin condition in which blood vessels in the face tend to widen, engorge with blood and can turn your face red as a fire truck.

No one knows what really causes rosacea, although doctors have noticed that fair-skinned women of Irish or Celtic ancestry are genetically predisposed, says Karen S. Harkaway, M.D., clinical instructor of dermatology at the University of Pennsylvania School of Medicine and a dermatologist at Pennsylvania Hospital, both in Philadelphia.

What triggers the flush to begin with? "The big five are spicy foods, alcohol, emotional stress, heat and humidity," says Mary Lupo, M.D., associate clinical professor of dermatology at Tulane University School of Medicine in New Orleans.

Unfortunately, rosacea is a chronic condition that comes and goes, says Deborah S. Sarnoff, M.D., assistant clinical professor of dermatology at New York University in New York City. Doctors frequently treat rosacea with prescription antibiotics such as tetracycline, or Metrogel, a topical medication originally developed for parasitic infections.

STOP FLUSHING COLD

Sometimes medications don't work, says Dr. Sarnoff. So here's what you can do when the flush hits.

Apply a cold compress. Soak a cloth or paper towel in ice-cold water and apply it to the flushed areas of your face, says Dr. Harkaway. The cold will constrict the dilated blood vessels and halt the inflammatory process.

Use tinted makeup. If you're prone to frequent flare-ups, use a green-tinted under-foundation cover, available at beauty supply stores, for everyday wear, says Dr. Harkaway. The green combines with any red in your face and neutralizes it completely.

PREVENT FUTURE FLARE-UPS

Fortunately, keeping rosacea under control is frequently as simple as treating your skin gently and avoiding anything that's known to trigger a flush, doctors agree. Here's what women doctors suggest.

Find a gentle cleanser. Use a liquid facial cleanser that contains sodium lauryl sulfate or disodium lauryl sulfosuccinate, such as Skincare System's Gentle Purifying Cleanser, says Dr. Lupo. Both ingredients will clean your skin gently and without any stimulation that might cause flushing.

Soothe your skin with chamomile. Since chamomile is known to soothe rosacea-prone skin, Dr. Lupo suggests using cleansers, soaps and moisturizers containing chamomile, an herb related to the ragweed family. One caution though: If you are allergic to ragweed, you should avoid these cleansers.

Avoid abrasives. Any type of abrasion can cause a flush, says Dr. Lupo. So leave abrasive products such as scrubs, buff puffs or cleansing powders to others.

Keep wrinkle creams to a minimum. If you have rosacea and want to use an anti-aging cream that contains alpha hydroxy acids to prevent wrinkles, proceed cautiously, says Dr. Lupo. Read product labels carefully and only buy creams that keep the percentage of acid under 2.5 percent, she says. If package directions urge you to use the cream twice a day, don't push your luck. Use it once a day, tops. If there is any redness at all, discontinue using the product.

Gently apply a cucumber moisturizer. After you cleanse your skin (and also if you apply an alpha hydroxy acid preparation), smooth on moisturizers that contain cucumber extracts, says Dr. Lupo. Although no one knows why, cucumber lotions soothe rosacea-prone skin.

Select cosmetics for sensitive skin. Since the chemicals used in most cosmetics will irritate rosacea-prone skin, use only cosmetics that are labeled "for sensitive skin," says Dr. Lupo. Although not chemical-free, they usually have fewer and less-irritating chemicals than regular makeup.

Stay in the shade. "Stay out of the sun, period," says Dr. Lupo. "The sun will set off a flare-up"—and no cover-up or sunscreen will prevent it.

Use only a titanium dioxide sunscreen. Even in the shade, you're exposed to indirect sunlight, so use a sunscreen whenever you go outside, says Dr. Lupo. Avoid all the chemical sunscreens and stick to a sunscreen that lists titanium dioxide as its major ingredient. It's less irritating to rosacea-prone skin.

Stay cool. Since heat is a major cause of flare-ups, dress in layers of light clothes that you can peel off to keep your body cool, no matter where you are, says Dr. Lupo. And take tepid (not hot) baths and showers.

Avoid wool. If you have rosacea, says Dr. Lupo, you're better off avoiding wool—it tends to keep you too warm and seems to cause redness and rashes in those who have rosacea.

Choose cool food. Spicy food is known to make those with rosacea flush, so Dr. Lupo recommends that women with rosacea avoid it as much as possible. Avoid foods prepared with chili peppers, Tabasco sauce, horseradish and the like.

Runny Nose
Stifle the Sniffle and Drip

*Y*ou're carrying tissues. You're sniffling. You're blowing. You're pretty uncomfortable and not a little embarrassed about it. For when your nose is dripping as freely as a faucet, it's pretty hard to feel attractive, accomplished, professional or even very maternal.

"A runny nose is often associated with allergies," says Karin Pacheco, M.D., staff physician in the Division of Allergy and Immunology at the National Jewish Center for Immunology and Respiratory Medicine in Denver. "You can blame histamines—substances that your body produces in response to allergens."

SOLUTIONS YOU NEVER HEARD OF

If your nose runs chronically, see a doctor to find out why, suggests Dr. Pacheco. In the meantime, these tips will help you dry up.

Making love? Be prepared. According to Barbara P. Yawn, M.D., associate professor of clinical family medicine and community health at the University of Minnesota and director of research at the Olmsted Medical Center in Rochester, Minnesota, really good sex can make your nose run. "The same substances that dilate and relax your vagina when you're sexually aroused can also make your nose run," she says. Dr. Yawn's tip for preventing a sex-provoked runny nose? "Keep tissues on your night table."

Think red-hot foods. Eating hot, spicy foods to make your nose run more when it's already running may seem like an odd cure, but, says Carol Fleischman, M.D., staff physician at Allegheny University of the Health Sciences MCP–Hahnemann School of Medicine and at the Center for Women's Health, both in Philadelphia, it's a good way for your nose to rid itself of irritants. "I favor hot curries from Indian restaurants to end stuffy, runny noses fast." In a pinch, sprinkling generous amounts of red-pepper flakes on your food will achieve the same effect.

Use an inhaler. "Over-the-counter menthol inhalers can provide some relief for runny noses," says Dr. Yawn. "Blow your nose first, then use the inhaler as directed by your doctor."

Try a nose rub. "A dab of Vicks Vaporub near your nose can slow down a runny nose, provided that the skin around your nose isn't irritated," says Dr. Yawn.

THE DRUGSTORE ROUTE

If you get satisfactory results with at-home treatments, fine. If your nose is still running like a faucet, women doctors offer these alternatives.

Take an antihistamine. "An antihistamine can relieve runny noses caused by allergies," says Dr. Pacheco. "Actifed, Drixoral, Dimetapp or Tavist-D seem to be the ones most preferred by my patients."

In a pinch, spray. If you have to be dry-nosed and presentable for some occasion, use Afrin nasal spray at the last minute, says Dr. Pacheco. "But don't use it for more than three days, to avoid the rebound effect," she advises. In other words, when you stop using it, your symptoms return worse than ever.

Saggy Breasts
A Nonsurgical Lift

They've added to your sex appeal. They've given sustenance to a child. But now your formerly round, firm breasts are, at the unfair age of 40 or so, drooping toward your waist.

Besides being attractive, breasts are functional units of milk glands and fat supported by muscles of your chest. Unfortunately, over time, the ligaments from which your breasts are suspended stretch, and your breasts sag.

"Once you reach your forties, the skin becomes more lax, the milk ducts shrink and fat replaces the ducts," says Debra Price, M.D., clinical assistant professor of dermatology at the University of Miami School of Medicine and a dermatologist in South Miami.

WHAT WOMEN DOCTORS DO

Works Out Every Other Day

Debra Price, M.D.

Like a lot of women her age, Debra Price, M.D., wants to keep her breasts firm and youthful as long as possible. A clinical assistant professor of dermatology at the University of Miami School of Medicine and a dermatologist in South Miami, Dr. Price relies on exercise to counter the effects of gravity on breast tissue.

"I work out every other day," says Dr. Price. Her trainer, Bini Masin, an exercise physiologist in Coral Gables, Florida, recommends push-ups, in particular.

"The push-up is the best and most effective exercise to build the pectoral muscles in the chest that underlie the breast," says Masin.

Dr. Price also applies a suncreen when wearing chest-bearing clothes, like tank tops or swimsuits with a low neckline, to protect her breasts from the damaging effects of the sun.

"I always use a SPF (sun protection factor) number greater than 15," says Dr. Price. "But I really like the nonchemical sunblocks with titanium dioxide that reflect the sun's harmful rays— both ultraviolet A and B."

This process tends to occur earlier—or is more pronounced—in women who have had children and breastfed, according to Anita Cela, M.D., clinical assistant professor of dermatology at New York Hospital–Cornell Medical Center in New York City.

WHAT YOU CAN DO

Other than visiting a plastic surgeon, the only thing that you can do to prevent your breasts from sagging (or firm up already slack breasts) is to build up the pectoral muscles under your breasts and fill the sag with muscle, says Dr. Price.

Here's how to give your breasts a lift.

Try the fly. "To build more muscle, try what's called the dumbbell fly, using a pair of one- to three-pound weights," says Peggy Norwood-Keating, director of fitness at Duke University Diet and Fitness Center in Durham, North Carolina.

To start, pick up one weight in each hand, then lie back on the floor. Extend your arms out at shoulder level on the floor with your palms up, clutching your weights. The weights should be parallel to your body.

Draw both arms straight up together above your body, keeping your elbows slightly bent, so that the weights meet over your chest, says Norwood-Keating. Then, return the weights out to your sides at shoulder height, as if you were drawing a semicircle or half-moon over your body.

Repeat the exercise 12 to 15 times, then rest for 1½ minutes, says Norwood-Keating. Repeat the exercise a second time and rest once again. Then repeat the exercise for a third and final set.

The stronger you become, the more weight you'll be able to handle. This means that you should be able to gradually increase your weight (by one to two pounds) while decreasing repetitions (8 to 10) in order to work your muscles gradually, says Norwood-Keating. Your goal here is 8 to 10 repetitions in three sets.

Try a chest press. A variation on the fly that also builds chest muscle is the chest press, says Norwood-Keating. This time, pick up a five-pound dumbbell in each hand and lie back on the floor. Extend your arms and hold the dumbbells up in the air over your chest, parallel to your body. Then, bend your elbows and lower the dumbbells toward your chest, with your elbows out to the sides at shoulder level. Extend your arms straight back up over your chest and repeat the exercise 12 to 15 times. Rest for 1½ minutes, then do a second set of 12 to 15 repetitions. Rest again and do a third set.

As with the previous exercise, if doing this exercise as described gets easy, increase your weights by one or two pounds. Your goal, says Norwood-Keating, is the same as above: 8 to 10 repetitions in three sets with as much weight as you can safely and comfortably handle.

Round out your workout. All these exercises may be great for your chest, but you need to round out your workout with an exercise that strengthens your back muscles, says Norwood-Keating. Otherwise, you're likely to become round-shouldered and weaken your back. So pick up a five- to ten-pound weight in your left hand, then lean on a bench or a low, sturdy table by placing your right knee and right hand down on its surface. Your left foot should be on the floor.

Bend your left elbow, bring the weight up to your armpit and try to squeeze your left shoulder blade toward your spine. As you resist gravity, slowly lower the weight back down until your arm is fully extended. It won't be easy, but resist letting the weight fall by squeezing with your left shoulder blade as the weight returns to the starting positon, explains Norwood-Keating.

Repeat the exercise 12 to 15 times, rest for 1½ minutes, then do a second set of 12 to 15 repetitions. Rest again and do a third set.

Don't forget sunscreen. Since sun exposure can speed up the aging of the elastin fibers that keep your skin from sagging, make sure that you wear a sunscreen whenever you wear a sundress, tank top or bathing suit with a low neckline, says Dr. Price.

Many dermatologists recommend a sun protection factor, or SPF, of 15, she adds. Whatever you use, don't forget to reapply regularly.

Wear a bra. To prevent your breasts from sagging further, wear a bra. "It does help," says Petra Schneider, M.D., a plastic surgeon in private practice in Melbourne, Florida. "Wearing a bra puts less stress on your ligaments. The more you wear one during the day, the more it helps."

Wearing a bra is especially important if you jog, play tennis, do aerobics or participate in other forms of exercise that bounce your breasts. If you're a C cup or larger, look for sports bras with good support that control your breast movement, says Dr. Price. Some women find that nonelastic shoulder straps are best for minimizing movement. Sports bras are available in the lingerie department of some department stores or in sporting goods stores.

Scars

Get Rid of Acne Marks and Other Nicks

Scars usually represent unpleasant memories that most of us would rather forget—the time you fell off your bike and scraped your knee, the night you tripped and gashed your chin, the day the car door hit you in the cheek when you were unloading groceries, even the night before your junior prom, when you decided to pick a zit.

"A scar is a raised or indented section of fibrous tissue formed by the body's healing process in response to an injury that penetrates the skin," says Mary Stone, M.D., associate professor of dermatology at the University of Iowa in Iowa City.

If the injury penetrates only the top layer of skin—the epidermis—

the healing process may leave only a light, temporary mark, adds Deborah S. Sarnoff, M.D., assistant clinical professor of dermatology at New York University in New York City. But if the injury penetrates the body's deepest layer of skin—the dermis—then the body may form a scar.

Besides cuts, scrapes and burns, picking a pimple or scratching a chicken pox sore can also leave a scar (to say nothing of the scars left by surgical incisions).

CAMOUFLAGE AND PREVENTION

Women doctors offer these tricks for minimizing existing scars and preemptive strategies for preventing scars from forming in the future.

Send the scar under cover. If the scar is markedly lighter or redder than the rest of your skin, then any good foundation such as Dermablend or Covermark will do a good job of eliminating it, says Dr. Stone. It's best to check with the cosmetics salesperson at a local department store for help in selecting the right shade and applying it.

Apply a topical antibiotic. Once a wound is clean and bleeding has stopped, smear on an antibacterial ointment such as Bacitracin or Polysporin, says Dr. Sarnoff. Avoid Neosporin, since it is known to trigger an allergic response in a fairly large percent of the population.

Protect a wound. Contrary to what you may have heard in the past, letting cuts air-dry is not the best course, says Dr. Sarnoff. Air-drying kills extra tissue. "You get less damage to the skin if you keep it covered."

Instead, keep wounds moist by covering them with an adhesive bandage or other type of bandage right after you apply the antibiotic ointment, says Dr. Stone.

Keep the bandage on until the scab is fully formed, and make sure

WHEN TO SEE A DOCTOR

If you cut yourself deeply enough that a scar is likely to form, see a dermatologist within six to eight weeks of the injury, says D'Anne Kleinsmith, M.D., a staff dermatologist at William Beaumont Hospital in Royal Oak, Michigan. If the wound is on your face or another area that you rather not be scarred, a medical procedure called dermabrasion can prevent a scar from being as deep or noticeable, according to Dr. Kleinsmith.

that you rebandage the wound every time the bandage itself gets wet, says Dr. Sarnoff. Although a moist wound aids healing, a moist bandage may encourage bacterial growth.

Take vitamin C. Since vitamin C can speed wound healing, take a vitamin C supplement while your skin is healing, says Dr. Sarnoff. Although the Daily Value is 60 milligrams a day, Dr. Sarnoff suggests taking 500 milligrams of vitamin C a day, half in the morning and half at night.

Leave the scab alone. Although it's tempting to pick at a loose scab, resist the temptation, says Dr. Sarnoff. Picking at the scab or knocking if off sooner than it's ready to go can cause a scar.

Sciatica

Soothe Hot Needles of Pain

If you have sciatica pain, it hurts to stand. It hurts to sit. You can't even lift a half-gallon of milk without hot needles of pain shooting down your leg. And you're wondering what started it all.

Sciatica pain actually starts in your spine, says Leena I. Kauppila, M.D., a visiting researcher at Harvard Medical School. "The most common cause of sciatica is compression of one of the nerves in the spine," she explains. The nerve, which normally carries electrical impulses from your spine to your lower limb, has been pinched, squeezed or otherwise irritated. And the pain that you feel is the nerve's humble attempt to get somebody, somewhere, to figure out what's wrong and get the problem fixed. (It rarely affects both buttocks or both legs at the same time.)

Sometimes chemicals naturally produced by your body in response to an injury in your lower back will irritate a nerve, says Carol Hartigan, M.D., a physiatrist who specializes in spine rehabilitation at the Boston Back Center of New England Baptist Hospital and New England Spine Center, also in Boston. Other times, the gel-like contents of one of the circular disks of your spine will leak—frequently as a response to an injury—and press on a nerve.

In women over age 50, normal aging of the spine may cause bony projections to pinch or irritate a nerve, says Dr. Hartigan.

Or arthritis of the spine may pinch or irritate a nerve, says Mary Ann Keenan, M.D., chairman of the Department of Orthopedic Surgery at the Albert Einstein Medical Center in Philadelphia.

STRETCH IT, CINCH IT, ICE IT

Fortunately, sciatica pain usually disappears on its own within a month, says Dr. Hartigan. But a month is a long time to spend in pain. So meanwhile, here's what women doctors say that you can do to ease your discomfort.

Take a shower, then stretch. If a muscle strain, muscle spasm or other lower-back injury is responsible for sciatica, head for the shower, says Dr. Keenan.

Hold on to a grab bar or other sturdy structure so that you don't fall, then let the warm water run down over your body for five to ten minutes, with your back to the spray. As it does, gently lean forward from your waist until you reach a point just before it hurts. Hold that position for several seconds, says Dr. Keenan, then slowly straighten your body. Stand upright for a couple of seconds, then slowly lean back from the waist until you reach a point just before it hurts. Hold the position for several seconds, then slowly straighten once again.

Repeat the same gentle stretching movement to each side, says Dr. Keenan. By the time that you're finished, chances are good that you'll have quelled any muscle spasm that could be responsible for your pain.

Don't linger too long in the shower, and don't soak in a hot tub or bath or use a heating pad for longer than 30 minutes, cautions Dr. Keenan. Too much heat can actually exacerbate your pain by increasing swelling.

Try a gel pack. To help reduce pain and inflammation, Dr. Hartigan recommends applying a cold gel pack every few hours to whatever area hurts—your back, buttock or leg—for 10 to 15 minutes at a time. Gel packs are available at drugstores. (In a pinch, you can susbstitute a cold towel, soaked in ice water.)

Make a natural cushion. Buy a waist-cinching elastic back support from your local drugstore or medical supply house, says Dr. Keenan. The cincher pushes in your abdomen, which makes an internal cushion of air that soothes and protects nerves around your spine.

Stretch every 30 minutes. Movement encourages circulation and can reduce the inflammation associated with some damaged areas like

WHEN TO SEE A DOCTOR

Sciatica pain that lasts longer than four weeks should be checked by a doctor, says Carol Hartigan, M.D., a physiatrist who specializes in spine rehabilitation at the Boston Back Center of New England Baptist Hospital and the New England Spine Center, also in Boston.

It's rare, but if the problem turns out to be a herniated disk, your doctor may recommend a trial cortisone injection or even surgery to relieve pressure on a nerve. And by the way, spinal manipulation by a chiropractor or other practitioner should never be performed on someone with sciatica pain, warns Dr. Hartigan. It could make the problem worse. Be wary of massage as well. It can contribute to inflammation, which may intensify symptoms.

You should also check with your doctor if sciatica pain is accompanied by unexpected weight loss, fever, difficulty controlling your bowel or bladder or a feeling of numbness in your buttocks, rectum or vagina or if you are over the age of 50, she says.

disks, says Dr. Hartigan. So don't sit for prolonged periods when you have sciatica.

Take a walk every hour. Taking a three- to five-minute walk every hour will also speed healing, says Dr. Keenan.

Seasonal Affective Disorder

Light Therapy for the Winter Blues

A blue mood on a gray November day is normal. Four months of the winter doldrums, however, sounds suspiciously like an outright form of depression called seasonal affective disorder (SAD).

The depression associated with SAD can be oppressive—typically, all you want to do is eat, sleep and laze around. The problem does, in fact, arrive in winter, when daylight tapers off by late afternoon. It disappears in spring, when the light lingers longer. SAD is more common in northern, sun-spare places like Massachusetts than in sun-soaked southern locales like Florida. And it's considerably more common among women than men—three to four times as common.

Sleepiness and carbohydrate cravings are two additional markers of SAD. Symptoms of SAD (and their severity and duration) vary from person to person, says psychiatrist Ruth Ragucci, M.D., assistant clinical professor of psychiatry at Case Western Reserve University in Cleveland.

While some people with SAD are affected in late October and drag

Summer Sadness: It Happens

If you feel fine in winter but, come summer, lack energy and generally get irritable, you may have the summertime version of Seasonal Affective Disorder (SAD). Or you may switch from winter SAD-ness to the summer version with the change of seasons.

Scientists don't know what causes summer SAD, but they suspect that heat may play a role, says Ellen Leibenluft, M.D., a researcher in the clinical psychobiology branch of the National Institutes of Mental Health. In that case, low humidity, coolness and dark—say, staying indoors in an air-conditioned environment—may help.

483

WHEN TO SEE A DOCTOR

If you think you have Seasonal Affective Disorder (SAD), it's important to see your doctor to rule out other health problems—thyroid disorders, low blood sugar or viruses—that can mimic SAD's symptoms, says Ellen Leibenluft, M.D., a researcher in the clinical psychobiology branch of the National Institutes of Mental Health. Doctors advise seeing a doctor if:

- You can't function at normal capacity—can't concentrate, finish things as quickly as usual or get to work on time.
- You feel severely depressed.
- You need several extra hours of sleep every night.
- You have a hard time waking up in the morning.
- You can't control your eating.
- You have suicidal thoughts or thoughts of death.

If your doctor diagnoses SAD, she's likely to prescribe some kind of light therapy, says Dr. Leibenluft.

themselves through May, others succumb only when the days are at their shortest, in December and January. Both the light-sensitive hormone melatonin, which regulates our sleep pattern, as well as the hormone seratonin, which affects our mood pattern, may play a role, says Dr. Ragucci.

"We really don't know exactly what causes SAD," says Ellen Leibenluft, M.D., a researcher in the clinical psychobiology branch of the National Institutes of Mental Health. Hormones and other biochemical factors seem to play a part, because they vary between men and women or from individual to individual.

SOLAR THERAPY

The good news is that SAD is successfully and simply treated—with light. If you feel less enthusiastic or less productive during winter months, you can help yourself with these strategies.

Go for a walk at lunch. The sun's rays are strongest at noon, which may make it the best time to soak up some therapeutic daylight. Walking while you soak doubles the benefit, since the exercise will help stave off weight gain and possibly depression.

Research suggests that light need only enter your eyes (not soak through your skin) to have a beneficial effect, so you can still wear sunscreen.

Light up your home and office. "Most people feel better in a well-lit environment," says Dr. Ragucci. For some people, increasing regular household or office lighting will do.

Spend your winter vacation down south. "This has only a temporary effect, but most of the people who try it say they feel fine during those weeks," says Dr. Ragucci.

Graduate to light-box therapy. If increased exposure to more light—outdoor or indoor—doesn't help and SAD is casting a shadow over your winters, ask your doctor about a light box, says Dr. Leibenluft. She may recommend a bright light burning at 10,000 lux for 30 minutes to two hours a day. Dr. Ragucci estimates that three out of four people she treats respond to light-box therapy.

Plug in a dawn simulator. Even more convenient than a light box, this device is like having the sun at your bedside: Every morning around 4:00 A.M., rain or shine, it clicks on and, over the next two hours, emits light that gradually grows brighter, simulating sunrise. Doctors say that early trials with dawn simulators have been encouraging. Light boxes and dawn simulators are available from SunBox Company, 19217 Orbit Drive, Gaithersburg, MD 20879.

Shingles
Cool a Nerve Rash

On the surface, shingles may appear to be just a red, blistery rash, but there is much more to this serious nerve rash than meets the eye.

"Shingles is actually a reactivation of the chicken pox virus—meaning that it strikes only people who have had the chicken pox," says Mary Ruth Buchness, M.D., chief of dermatology at St. Vincent's Hospital and Medical Center in New York City. "The chicken pox virus never really goes away. It lies dormant in a nerve bundle in the spinal cord."

Then, during times of stress or illness, the virus can reactivate in certain people. It multiplies and travels down the nerve route to the skin.

"Wherever that nerve supplies sensation is where you will see the rash," says Amy Newburger, M.D., assistant clinical professor of dermatology at Columbia University College of Physicians and Surgeons in New York City and a dermatologist in Scarsdale, New York. This could be on your forehead, scalp, chest, down your shoulder and arm, on your trunk, on your buttock or down your leg.

The shingles rash is marked by blistery, water-filled bumps that sit on areas of reddened underlying skin. "Some people feel pain, tingling or discomfort in the area a few days before the blisters develop," says Susan C. Taylor, M.D., assistant clinical professor of medicine in the Department of Dermatology at the University of Pennsylvania School of Medicine in Philadelphia. The blisters will turn to pustules (bumps filled with pus) and then crust over, scab and heal—a process that can take up to three or four weeks. At that point the virus goes into remission, but it will always live dormant in your body. Shingles may or may not recur.

If you have shingles, realize that the blisters are filled with a contagious virus, which should not be touched by other people, especially if they have not had chicken pox. "Keep those areas covered," urges Dr. Newburger.

A HOST OF OPTIONS

If your doctor has confirmed that you have shingles, women doctors offer ways to relieve the pain and discomfort.

Baby yourself. Treat your body gently during an outbreak. "Do everything that you can to rest and avoid stressing the inflamed nerve route," advises Dr. Newburger. That means do not exercise; do not try to work through the pain. Give the rash time to heal. "Motion will increase inflammation of the nerve route, and you could end up with hefty scarring around the nerve—which means persistent pain—for six months, a year, maybe even forever. So take it easy," she warns.

Keep blisters wet to dry them up. Anything wet that you put on blisters will help dry them out, because as the liquid evaporates from your skin, it dries blisters along with it, says Dr. Buchness.

Calamine lotion works well. Discontinue the calamine after the blisters dry. Or use a compress made from cool water and Domeboro astringent solution. "Domeboro is an aluminum acetate preparation that helps dry blisters. It comes in the form of tablets or powder, which you mix with water to make a solution," explains Dr. Buchness.

Spill some milk. "Soak a washcloth in cold milk and hold it on the blisters," suggests Dr. Buchness. "There's something about milk that is soothing to blistery skin rashes."

Use antibacterial ointment. Once blisters crust over and start to scab, apply an antibacterial ointment to prevent infection, keep them soft, help them heal and reduce scarring, says Dr. Buchness.

Dr. Newburger recommends Bacitracin or Polysporin. Dr. Buchness advises avoiding ointments containing neomycin, since a fair number of people are allergic to it.

Put on a paste. To dry up blisters and soothe itching, make a paste from water mixed with baking powder and spread that on the shingles rash, suggests Dr. Taylor.

Try some pepper power. Zostrix, an over-the-counter cream preparation made from an ingredient in red chili peppers called capsaicin, is effective at relieving the pain of shingles, but *only after* your skin rash or blisters have healed, says Patricia Farris Walters, M.D., clinical assistant professor of dermatology at Tulane University School of Medicine in New Orleans and a spokesperson for the American Academy of Dermatology. "The medicine makes the nerve endings release their pain-causing chemicals. It causes nerve endings to keep firing until there is no chemical left," she says.

"Zostrix can sting and burn for a while when first applied," says

WHEN TO SEE A DOCTOR

Shingles is distinctively different from other kinds of rashes. With shingles, the rash is confined to either the left or the right side of your body and does not cross the midline.

If you think that you're developing shingles, get to a doctor immediately. "If you treat it within 48 hours of onset, you should be able to get the virus under control and minimize the risk of scarring around the nerve route," says Amy Newburger, M.D., assistant clinical professor of dermatology at Columbia University College of Physicians and Surgeons in New York City and a dermatologist in Scarsdale, New York. Studies suggest that if you start taking antiviral medication right away, you may be able to prevent the lingering, persistent nerve pain that often trails in the wake of shingles.

Dr. Walters. "But if you stick it out for a few days, you can really get relief." Apply a thin film of the cream three to four times a day for several days and as long as the pain is present.

Shoulder Pain
Help for Frozen or Stiff Shoulders

Shoulder pain is one of those mysterious hurts that sneaks up on your body after doing something that you haven't done for months (if ever), like washing and waxing the car or cutting the grass with a push mower for the first time all season.

In women, shoulder pain is most often a symptom of either tendinitis, muscle strain or something called adhesive capsulitis, commonly known as frozen shoulder, where the shoulder gets so stiff that you can't move it freely, says Stacie Grossfeld, M.D., an orthopedic surgeon at the University of Minnesota in Minneapolis.

Unfortunately, when you don't use your shoulder, it loses its flexibility and stiffens. "One day, after not using your shoulder muscles for months, you'll find that you literally can't reach back to grab your seat belt or unhook your bra," says Dr. Grossfeld.

Or your shoulder muscles can get pinched between the bones and ligaments in your back, a disorder called impingement that results from intense overhead activity, like throwing a softball or swinging a tennis racket, says Dr. Grossfeld.

STEER YOURSELF TOWARD RELIEF

Women doctors and physical therapists say that luckily, most shoulder pains can be eased by following these simple suggestions.

Give it a rest. "If your shoulder hurts, the first thing that you need to do is stop the activity that's causing the pain," says Dr. Grossfeld.

Reach for the ice. "Ice is the cheapest form of pain medicine there is with almost no side effects," Dr. Grossfeld says. Ice decreases inflam-

WHEN TO SEE A DOCTOR

If you try home remedies, but your pain doesn't improve after seven to ten days, see a doctor, says Stacie Grossfeld, M.D., an orthopedic surgeon at the University of Minnesota in Minneapolis.

If your shoulder pain results from a fall or a car accident, see a doctor immediately to rule out a fracture, she says.

mation. Wrap an ice pack or ice from the freezer in a towel and apply it to the site of pain for no more than 15 to 20 minutes every hour.

Allow yourself a painkiller. No need to be a martyr: An anti-inflammatory such as aspirin, ibuprofen or ketoprofen (Orudis) taken several times a day according to package directions will ease the pain and swelling, says Dr. Grossfeld.

Move it gently. Women doctors say that shoulder pain is a classic catch-22: Your shoulder hurts, so you don't want to use it, but if you don't use it, it's likely to get so stiff that you'll end up with a frozen shoulder, and then you won't be *able* to use it.

The solution? "Once your pain subsides, try gentle range-of-motion exercises," says Dr. Grossfeld.

Lynn Van Ost, P.T., a clinical specialist at the Sports Medicine Center in Philadelphia, suggests this exercise routine: Begin each exercise with your arm hanging down at your side. First, raise your arm straight in front of you until it is over your head (or go as far as you can without feeling any pain) and lower it back to the starting point. Then raise your arm out to the side and lower it. For the third exercise, keep your upper arm tucked against your body, but bend your elbow so that your forearm is in front of you. Rotate your forearm in toward your stomach and return to the starting position. Repeat the exercise again, rotating your arm away from you. Repeat each motion ten times before moving on to the next, and do the entire routine once or twice a day as long as you don't feel pain.

(For practical ways to manage tendinitis or muscle strain, see pages 537 and 383.)

Shyness
Baby Steps Build Confidence

Carol Burnett was once a shy kid who worried that her classmates wouldn't like her. Carly Simon was withdrawn and stuttered as a teenager. Barbara Walters was a quiet kid and even today acknowledges moments of self-doubt. Even Elizabeth Taylor says she's a bit on the shy side.

Shyness, it seems, is a pretty common commodity, even in show biz.

"A large percentage of people report some degree of shyness at some time in their lives," confirms Melinda Stanley, Ph.D., associate professor of psychiatry and behavioral sciences at the University of Texas Medical School in Houston.

WHAT MAKES PEOPLE SHY

As is so often the case, both genetic heritage and upbringing seem to determine whether we're shy or intrepid.

The problem with shyness is that it keeps you from speaking up, getting noticed and being heard, explains Myrna Shure, Ph.D., professor of psychology at Allegheny University of the Health Sciences in Philadelphia. And that can lead to depression, anxiety and loneliness.

TIPS FOR THE TIMID

Fortunately, most adults can also learn to manage and minimize shyness. You may still feel shy in some situations, but not as shy as often. Here are some options to try.

Check your assumptions. If you're the type who always tells herself, "I'm going to make a terrible impression," question the assumption, suggests Dr. Stanley. You haven't made terrible impressions before, have you? So isn't it irrational to think you will this time? Relax.

Breathe boldly. Dry mouth? Racing heart? To relax further, breathe slowly and deeply, says Dr. Stanley.

Play Barbara Walters. Not sure what to say? Pretend you are a journalist. Think of something that particularly interests you. Then make up a question about that interest. For example, "How do you feel about taking pictures in the park?" Now try answering the questions you just made up, out loud, suggests Dr. Shure.

Talk to the mirror first. To make it easier to talk to other people, talk to the mirror first. This will help you feel comfortable expressing your thoughts and feelings. Think of three to five questions you can ask and then answer, says Dr. Shure.

Set goals. "Promise yourself you'll say at least one thing to one person within the first minute of arriving," says Susan Heitler, Ph.D., a clinical psychologist in Denver and author of the audiotape *Anxiety: Friend or Foe?*. "Once you've said one thing, it's usually easier to say the next."

Give yourself time. "If you need more time, say to yourself, 'Okay, I need 30 minutes to warm up instead of three,'" says Leonora Stephens, M.D., a family systems psychiatrist and clinical associate professor of psychiatry at the University of Texas Southwestern Medical School in Dallas.

"Some people can jump into the middle of a group and are comfortable immediately. Others feel shy when they first walk into a gathering but are fine once they've had time to warm up," says Dr. Stephens.

Practice. "The more exposure you have to anxiety-producing situations, the easier they'll be for you," says Dr. Stanley. If, like many shy people, you're afraid to give presentations, keep at it. Join a public speaking club like Toastmasters where you can practice in a supportive atmosphere. If meeting new people makes your palms sweat, keep doing it. Attend work-related functions, social hours at church and similar get-togethers.

Side Stitch
Strike Out Piercing Pain

A side stitch isn't a life-and-death matter—just a sharp pain under the rib cage. The problem is, side stitches usually occur when we need to keep moving—sprinting to catch a bus, jogging around the park or trying to keep up with a new aerobics instructor.

What brings them on?

"The most common cause is either trapped gas in the intestine (in your abdomen) or a spasm in the diaphragm (a large muscle separating your abdomen and chest)," says Mona Shangold, M.D., co-author of *The Complete Sports Medicine Book for Women* and director of the Center for Sports Gynecology and Women's Health in Philadelphia.

When you're running or otherwise working your body pretty hard, most of your blood goes to the muscles involved in your activity—your arms and legs—and less goes to your diaphragm, explains Dr. Shangold. Pain is the diaphragm's way of alerting you to the problem.

BEFORE-AND-AFTER TACTICS

There is no way to tell if your side stitch is caused by a gas bubble or a diaphragm spasm, says Dr. Shangold. So here's what women doctors say you should do.

Breathe. Take a deep breath, purse your lips, tighten your abdomen and push all the air out of your lungs, says Dr. Shangold. Inhale and exhale nine more times in this way. If a gas bubble is causing your side stitch, breathing this way will move it on its way.

Slow down. If forced breathing doesn't stop the pain, the problem is probably a lack of blood to your diaphragm, says Dr. Shangold. Just slow down, and your body will automatically send your diaphragm more blood. The stitch should be gone within minutes.

Walk. If the stitch is still piercing your side once you've slowed down, try walking slowly for one minute, says Dr. Shangold. That should do the trick.

Eat lightly before a workout. To prevent a stitch in the first place, eat lightly before you exercise, suggests Angie Ahlemeyer, an exercise physiologist at Washington Sports and Family Medicine in Kirkland, Washington. Since eating a big meal can draw blood away from your diaphragm and toward your stomach, plan to eat meals at least two hours before exercising. A piece of fruit or a bagel are light snacks that can provide quick energy before a workout.

Sinus Problems
Relief for the Permanently Stuffy Nose

*M*alfunctioning sinuses cause all kinds of trouble. Like headaches and facial pain. Like coughs, congestion and post-nasal drip or permanently stuffy noses.

Chances are, you or someone close to you is all too familiar with the pressure, pain and stuffiness that are hallmarks of sinusitis (otherwise known as sinus trouble).

Sinus trouble comes in two varieties: acute and chronic. Both involve hollow cavities in the bone structures around your eyes and nose.

Acute sinusitis is typically short-lived and triggered by a cold or flu, and it is accompanied by facial pain, puslike discharge of mucus, congestion and sometimes even fever. Antibiotics are the usual treatment, and decongestants and home remedies can ease the symptoms.

Chronic sinusitis is milder but constant, and it's often traced to allergies and environmental pollutants.

OPEN UP CLOGGED SINUSES

Either way, you'll want to put sinusitis on the endangered list of your personal medical problems. Follow these suggestions from some top women doctors.

Install an air conditioner in your bedroom. "The first thing to do is rid your environment of the pollutants that can trigger sinus problems," says Barbara P. Yawn, M.D., associate professor of clinical family medicine and community health at the University of Minnesota in Minneapolis and director of research at the Olmsted Medical Center in Rochester, Minnesota. And remember to change the filter regularly.

"The little hairs inside your nose comb out airborne particles—smoke, pollen, molds and other pollutants. These pollutants irritate the lining of your nose and sinuses and cause swelling that results in feelings of pressure and stuffiness," says Dr. Yawn. "So do whatever it takes to avoid them."

Get someone else to clean. "Pass on doing dusty cleaning jobs if you can," says Dr. Yawn. "If you can't, wear a mask." Dr. Yawn also sug-

WHEN TO SEE A DOCTOR

If you've tried everything, and chronic sinus pain is making life insufferable, check with your doctor, says Barbara P. Yawn, M.D., associate professor of clinical family medicine and community health at the University of Minnesota in Minneapolis and director of research at the Olmsted Medical Center in Rochester, Minnesota. "Several treatment options can ease your discomfort quickly. Topical cortisone nasal sprays are very effective and have few side effects," she says.

Sinus symptoms that need a doctor's care include:
- Mucus discharge that is puslike, green, yellow or foul-smelling
- Persistant cough
- Fever
- Facial pain or headaches
- Toothaches

gests that you wear a mask when working with oven cleaners and other noxious chemicals.

Make yours a humid home. "The nasal hairs that filter out irritants work best when they are plumped up and moisture-rich," says Dr. Yawn. "So be sure to humidify the air that you breathe." Humidifiers in your home and office should do the trick. But there's a right way and a wrong way to humidify a room.

"The mist from a humidifier should fall close to your face," says Dr. Yawn. "If your humidifier is down on the floor dampening the rug, it's not doing your nose any good." She recommends using cool-mist humidifiers and cleaning them regularly.

Take a super-soaker shower. "Before bedtime, a nice long, hot shower will humidify you for a good night's sleep," says Dr. Yawn.

Drink up. Be sure to drink at least eight glasses of liquids a day, says Carol Fleischman, M.D., staff physician at Allegheny University of the Health Sciences MCP–Hahnemann School of Medicine and at the Center for Women's Health, both in Philadelphia. "You need internal as well as external humidity to keep nasal passages moist."

Don't rely on sprays and pills. "When you have chronic sinus problems, it's a mistake to rely on nasal sprays like Afrin or decongestant pills like Sudafed. Both will cause a rebound effect," says Dr. Yawn. In other words, they work temporarily, but over time, they make the problem worse. "If you're on a plane or in a situation where you just can't be stuffed up, short-term use of either a nasal spray or decongestant can provide temporary relief."

Sleep Deprivation
Get Your Rest and Feel Good Again

Constant daytime sleepiness is the hallmark of chronic sleep deprivation. But some of us are so accustomed to plodding by on too little sleep that we don't even recognize it.

"People may not realize what's going on until they go on vacation and allow themselves the sleep they need," says Margaret L. Moline, Ph.D., director of the New York Hospital–Cornell Medical Center Sleep-Wake Disorders Center in White Plains, New York. "They'll come back feeling great, so relaxed. We ask them how many hours they were sleeping, and they'll say eight hours. It turns out that they usually sleep only six hours."

MAKING UP A SLEEP DEFICIT

Sleep is like money: The longer you go without adequate supplies, the worse your situation gets.

"As the days go on, a sleep deficit accumulates like interest on an unpaid credit card balance," says Mary A. Carskadon, Ph.D., professor of psychiatry and human behavior at Brown University School of Medicine and head of the sleep research lab at E. P. Bradley Hospital, both in Providence, Rhode Island. "Say you don't get enough sleep on Sunday night. You may not feel the effects on Monday. But keep it up, and by Friday, you'll feel awful."

One night's insomnia won't hurt you, says Dr. Moline. But running up a sleep debt can take a heavy toll. You can't concentrate. Your memory is shot. You feel edgy. Your coordination suffers. You risk falling asleep on the job or driving and causing an accident. And you're also less adept at fighting off illness.

495

WHEN TO SEE A DOCTOR

If you're running up a sleep deficit, you may need medical help to resolve the problem, depending on the cause. See a doctor if:

- Night sweats from menopause awaken you and leave you exhausted come morning. Hormone replacement therapy may help, says Margaret L. Moline, Ph.D., director of the New York Hospital–Cornell Medical Center Sleep-Wake Disorders Center in White Plains, New York.
- Nighttime allergy symptoms or asthma wake you and wear you out. Control the allergies, and you'll sleep better.
- You work a night or rotating shift and are struggling with daytime sleepiness. Light therapy—exposure to bright, full-spectrum light—may help your body adjust.
- You snore and feel tired even after spending eight or so hours in bed. You may have a sleep disorder called sleep apnea. If so, your doctor may refer you to a nearby sleep disorders clinic.
- Your arms and legs twitch throughout the night. Called periodic limb movement, this tendency may not wake you fully but may still disrupt your sleep enough to leave you haggard come sunup, says Dr. Moline. A clinic can help.
- You have daytime sleepiness but don't know why.

If you've been shortchanging yourself an hour of sleep a night for a week, you don't need to sleep an extra seven hours, says Dr. Moline. But you do need to get a couple extra hours of sleep a couple of days in a row, she explains.

Try the insomnia remedies on page 317. If you're still not sleeping better, here's what to do.

Listen to your internal clock. You can get too little sleep if you go to bed too early *or* too late, says Sonia Ancoli-Israel, Ph.D., professor of psychiatry at the University of California, San Diego, School of Medicine and director of the sleep disorders clinic at the Veterans Administration Medical Center in San Diego. Go to bed when you feel tired—not before or after.

When you're a teenager, your body clock is set so that you tire around midnight and want to waken at 8:00 or 9:00 A.M. By your thirties, forties and fifties, you're getting sleepy closer to 10:00 or 11:00 P.M. and waking at 6:00 or 7:00 the next morning. In your sixties and seventies, an 8 o'clock bedtime sounds most appealing, and you're up by 4:00 or 5:00 come morning. (Contrary to popular belief, you don't need less sleep as you age, says Dr. Ancoli-Israel. You just tend to fall asleep and awaken earlier.)

Shift with your shift. If you work a night or rotating shift, you're forced to sleep during the day, when your body clock is set on alert, and that makes quality sleep harder to come by. Researchers say it could take up to three years to adjust to daytime bedtimes, and there are some people who never adjust. So those on rotating shifts may have it hardest of all.

If you work nights, ask for a permanent, not a rotating, shift if it's at all possible, says Dr. Moline. Or ask for a shift that rotates from days to evenings to nights rather than the reverse—it's easier than trying to adapt to a night-to-evening-to-day schedule.

Pregnant? Sleep on your side. Nine months is a long time to go without a good night's sleep. Yet many women find it difficult to get comfortable in bed when they're expecting, especially during those last few months of pregnancy. Obstetricians suggest sleeping on one side with a leg propped up on a pillow.

Slow Healing
Mend Cuts, Scrapes, Nicks and Bruises *Fast*

*D*oes it seem like the last cut you got took forever to heal? Was your bandage becoming a fashion accessory? The right kind of first-aid plays a big part in speed-healing, say the experts.

"Properly cleaning and dressing your wound should prevent infection and promote fast, healthy healing," says Libby Edwards, M.D., chief of dermatology in the Department of Internal Medicine at the Carolinas Medical Center in Charlotte, North Carolina, and clinical associate professor of dermatology at the Bowman Gray School of Medicine of Wake Forest University in Winston-Salem, North Carolina. In other words, a thorough but gentle approach is best.

OUT WITH THE BAD

If you've been skinned, scraped or cut, women doctors offer this advice.

Cleanse, don't scour. "The first thing you should do for cuts or scrapes is to wash the injury really well with plain soap and water," says Ann DiMaio, M.D., director of the pediatric emergency room at New York Hospital–Cornell Medical Center and associate professor of pediatrics at Cornell Medical Center in New York City.

Rinse, rinse, rinse. "The most important part is to rinse away the dead and injured tissue and the debris that may be in a wound. Bacteria thrive on dead tissue. You want to bring up the fresh, uninjured tissue that heals quickly," says Dr. DiMaio.

Rinsing avoids scarring, says Dr. DiMaio. "If you leave dirt in a wound, not only are you risking infection, you're risking a bad scar. The result is a tattoo effect—a scar pigmented by the dirt or debris left in it."

"The water temperature should be comfortable, but the force should be sufficient to wash the wound clean," says Dr. DiMaio.

Smear on an antibiotic cream. To prevent infection, try using an over-the-counter antibiotic cream like Bacitracin or Neosporin, says Dr. DiMaio.

Skip the heavy-duty antiseptics. "Many women think that the more a medication stings, the more effective it is at germ-killing," says Dr. Edwards. "But that's not the case. Antiseptics containing alcohol or Mercurochrome are irritating—they're caustic, they sting and they kill the good cells in addition to the germs," she says.

Cover it up. Once your wound is well-cleaned, cover it with a bandage and keep it moist with antibiotic cream, says Dr. Edwards. "Many women believe in letting a wound breathe," she says. "But then it will dry out and crack, not heal. Cover it, keep the bandage dry or change it after you bathe."

Immobilize the wound. If you have an extensive wound (like a nasty scrape) over an area that's constantly flexing (like the knee or wrist), "try to keep it immobilized until it heals," says Dr. DiMaio. Repeated flexing will keep the wound open and retard healing, she says.

NUTRITIONAL HEALING

"People who eat well heal faster than people who don't," says Dr. DiMaio. "So when you're recovering from a wound, injury or illness, pay special attention to your diet."

Have a turkey sandwich. To build and repair damaged tissue, your body needs protein—about 45 grams a day. That's the amount provided by seven ounces of lean fish, chicken or turkey.

Supplement with some A. "Vitamin A helps wounds heal," says Katherine Sherif, M.D., instructor of medicine at Allegheny University of the Health Sciences and on staff at the Institute for Women's Health, both in Phildelphia. "Take 10,000 IU a day (with food that contains some fat to make certain the vitamin A is properly absorbed), until the wound is healed."

Add zinc. "When it comes to wounds, zinc has very strong healing power," says Eleanore Young, R.D., Ph.D, a licensed dietitian and professor in the Department of Medicine at the University of Texas Health Sci-

WHEN TO SEE A DOCTOR

Healthy wounds show steady improvement each day, says Libby Edwards, M.D., chief of dermatology in the Department of Internal Medicine at the Carolinas Medical Center in Charlotte, North Carolina, and clinical associate professor of dermatology at the Bowman Gray School of Medicine of Wake Forest University in Winston-Salem, North Carolina. "After about four or five days, a wound should be noticeably smaller, less sore and less red; if it's not, see a doctor."

Women with diabetes are especially prone to infection, because the disease impedes circulation, which is essential for healthy healing. So if you have diabetes or any other chronic illness, watch for signs of infection.

Call your doctor if the wound is:
- Draining pus
- Very painful
- Extremely red and inflamed

Also, be careful about infection if you're on steroid medication, which suppresses the immune system, leaving your body less able to fight infections.

ence Center at San Antonio. "Women should be certain to get 12 milligrams of zinc a day."

Snoring

The His 'n' Hers Problem

A woman in Davis, California, snored so loudly that a neighbor had her arrested in the middle of the night under the city's new anti-noise statute.

"We think of snoring as being normal and sometimes even cute," says Kristyna M. Hartse, Ph.D., associate professor of psychiatry, human behavior and otolaryngology and director of the Sleep Disorders Center at St. Louis Health Sciences Center. "But there's nothing normal or cute about it."

According to Dr. Hartse and other sleep experts, loud snoring can disrupt good marriages or worsen bad ones.

Who snores more, men or women?

Men are more frequently dragged in for treatment by their wives, according to Nancy Collop, M.D., associate professor of pulmonary and critical care medicine and director of the Sleep Disorders Clinic at the Medical University of South Carolina in Charleston. But Dr. Collop doesn't attribute this to men snoring more than women. "It's possible that women snore as much and as loudly as men do, especially as they get older, but men seem to sleep more soundly than women, so they're less disturbed by a snoring spouse."

ROLL OVER, BEETHOVEN

To restore that loving—and restful—feeling, try these home remedies. All remedies apply to snorers of either sex.

Sleep on your side. "Snoring is usually worse when you sleep on your back," says Laurel Wiegand, M.D., associate professor of medicine in the Division of Pulmonary and Critical Care Medicine of the Department of Medicine at the Milton S. Hershey Medical Center at Pennsylvania State University in Hershey. "So try to get your snorer to sleep on his side, or to sleep stomach side down."

Sew a ball into some pj's. "Sew a pocket into the back of a pajama top or T-shirt and stuff it with a tennis ball," says Dr. Hartse. "That way, the snorer will find sleeping on his back too uncomfortable and roll to the side."

Keep earplugs handy. If your snorer bothers you only occasionally, try a pair of soft, foam ear plugs, suggests Dr. Wiegand. "Keep a pair on your night table and use them if your partner's snoring is keeping you awake."

Drop that drink. "Alcohol relaxes all the muscles in the throat that vibrate," says Dr. Wiegand. "And it's dose-related—the more you drink, the louder you'll snore."

Lose the pudge. "Losing just a few pounds can lessen snoring or even make it disappear," says Dr. Wiegand.

No butts. "Smoke may cause swelling and inflammation of the throat tissues, which, when swollen, are more likely to vibrate and produce snoring," says Dr. Wiegand.

WHEN TO SEE A DOCTOR

Snoring can be a symptom of sleep apnea, a breathing disturbance characterized by explosively loud snoring interspersed with pauses of silence. During those pauses, which can last for ten seconds or longer, the snorer actually stops breathing for dozens or hundreds of times each night. As a result, the snorer awakes feeling unrefreshed and exhausted. Worse, sleep apnea can lead to fatigue-related accidents.

"If you or your bed partner is very loud when snoring and doesn't respond to home remedies after a couple of weeks, see a sleep specialist for a complete evaluation," says Laurel Wiegand, M.D., associate professor of medicine in the Division of Pulmonary and Critical Care Medicine of the Department of Medicine at the Milton S. Hershey Medical Center at Pennsylvania State University in Hershey. "Today," adds Dr. Wiegand, "we have a number of effective options that can make ex-snorers out of most people."

Pick up a nasal splint. A product called Breathe works for some people. "These are little tapes that you place on the sides of your nose to keep your nostrils more open so that snoring will decrease. It's certainly worth a try," Dr. Wiegand says.

Try a nasal spray. If occasional snoring is caused by a cold, the snorer might give the bed partner some shut-eye by using a nasal spray or an over-the-counter decongestant before bedtime, suggests Dr. Wiegand. Be sure to use the medications according to package directions, she says.

Sore Feet

Easy Ways to Revive Tired, Aching Feet

*P*ity poor podiatrists. Just like waitresses, airline attendants and nurses, they're on their feet a lot.

"Some days, I see patients at heavily populated nursing homes, and that means I'm walking or standing almost all day long," says Teresa G. Conroy, D.P.M., a podiatrist in private practice in Philadelphia. She sidesteps pain with two important pieces of apparel: support hose and running shoes. "The stockings help keep my feet from swelling, and the shoes cushion my feet so they don't hurt," explains Dr. Conroy. "I recommend them to many of the women I treat."

It's true that preventive care is the best way to stop foot pain. No one should dismiss tired, aching feet as normal, even if you've been on your feet all day.

SOOTHING STEPS TO IMMEDIATE RELIEF

If your feet hurt, you'll instinctively take off your shoes. Here's what to do next.

Have a nice soak. Nothing beats soaking your feet in water as a quick fix for sore feet, says Cheryl Weiner, D.P.M., a podiatrist in Columbus, Ohio, and president of the American Association for Women Podiatrists. "It just plain makes aching feet feel better."

Some people prefer warm water, others cool water. Either is fine, says Dr. Weiner. Avoid very hot or very cold water, especially if you have diabetes, which can damage nerves in your feet, or circulation problems.

For an especially invigorating soak, says Dr. Weiner, draw two basins of water, one warm, one cool, and alternate between the two.

Get 'em up. If your feet are sore and swollen from a long day of sidewalk-pounding, lie down and prop your feet up so they are at least a foot or so above the level of your head, says Marika Molnar, P.T., director of West Side Dance Physical Therapy in New York City. "This position allows blood and other fluid that has pooled in your feet and lower legs to flow back toward your heart."

Treat your feet to a tennis-ball massage. This massage can be done with a Super Pinky (a solid rubber ball about the size of a tennis ball, but softer, which is available at some sporting goods stores) or with a tennis ball. "Stand and press your foot down on the ball. Working from the center of your heel, move down either side of your heel, then down to the ball of your foot," suggests Helen Drusine, a massage therapist who works with professional ballet and Broadway dancers in New York City. A massage like this helps release and relax muscles and connective tissue in the arch of your foot, spread the bones in the ball of your foot (called metatarsals) and energize nerves, says Drusine.

BE KIND TO YOUR FEET

In some cases, poor-fitting shoes play a role in sore feet. To buy shoes that fit—and fit well—here's what to do.

Shop for shoes late in the day. That's when your feet are at their largest, says Nancy Elftman, a certified orthotist/pedorthist (a profes-

WHEN TO SEE A DOCTOR

Lingering foot fatigue is often the result of poor biomechanics: Your foot may not move properly when you walk. If home-care tactics don't work, see a podiatrist, a doctor who specializes in foot care. She may prescribe orthotics, custom-made shoe inserts that can correct your gait. She can also check for dislocated or broken bones, including tiny stress fractures, and will diagnose and treat pinched nerves, inflamed tendons and other bone problems.

Make Yourself Comfortable

Marika Molnar, P.T.

All day long, Marika Molnar, P.T., director of West Side Dance Physical Therapy in New York City, administers to the city's hardworking ballerinas and Broadway dancers, helping them with exercises and treatments to heal their much-abused feet. So what does she do when her own feet hurt?

"I lie down with my hips and knees bent and put my feet up on a chair or bed to elevate my feet above my head," says Molnar. Then, breathing rhythmically, she gently and slowly rotates and flexes her ankles and feet to move the fluid out of her feet and back toward her heart. "I do this for about ten minutes, and it always makes my feet—and my legs—feel better," she says.

To strengthen your foot muscles, Molnar suggests standing in a doorway and, grasping the doorway, lifting one foot and balancing for about 30 seconds. Repeat with the other foot. "The muscles of your foot work to keep your weight balanced," she says.

sional shoe fitter) in La Verne, California.

If your feet swell considerably in the days before your period, you might want to have one especially comfortable pair of lace-on shoes for this time, adds Dr. Weiner.

Draw the perfect fit. Take a piece of paper and, standing with your full weight, trace your foot on it. Then make sure that any shoe you buy covers the tracing completely. If at any point the tracing extends beyond the shoe, it means that the shoe is too small or narrow, says Dr. Weiner.

Choose supportive shoes. If you strain your arches, your feet will ache all over, and your legs will feel crampy and tired, says Dr. Weiner. For good arch support, she says, wear high-tech sneakers—running or walking shoes. And if you're buying new shoes for work or dress, ask to see styles with good arch support. Running shoes also offer super shock absorption, so they're ideal for coddling arthritic or diabetic feet, adds Dr. Weiner.

Add support if you must. To improve arch support in nonathletic shoes, insert arch supports (available at sporting good stores and shoe repair shops), says Dr. Weiner. If achy legs still are troublesome, see your podiatrist. She might prescribe custom arch supports called orthotics.

Pad them. While most of our body parts accumulate fat as we age, our feet lose their fatty, shock-absorbing cushion. And the increased pressure on the bones in the ball and heel of a foot translates into pain.

To pad any shoe, insert firm rubber insoles, such as Sorbothane. "But make sure that adding insoles doesn't make your shoes too tight," says Dr. Weiner. For the best fit, buy a pair of insoles first, then insert them in whatever shoes you try on.

Retire the stilettos. "Never wear heels more than 1½ inches high," says Kathleen Stone, D.P.M., a podiatrist in private practice in Glendale, Arizona. Anything higher shifts your weight forward onto the ball of your foot, putting tremendous pressure on the tiny bones in that area. For many women, the result is pain, and sometimes permanent damage to the feet.

Sore Throat
Swallow without Pain

Sometimes you can pinpoint the exact moment when it starts. Awakening early for a frosty run or racing to a late-afternoon meeting, you swallow hard and whoa! What had been a natural reflex suddenly rings a dry and silent alarm. Your throat burns angrily, almost daring you to swallow again.

Dry heat, tobacco smoke, allergies, nasal infections, errant stomach acids and enthusiastic cheering can inflame and dry up the normally moist and smooth mucous membranes of your respiratory airway, setting the stage for a sore throat or other respiratory distress.

Infections can also trigger a sore throat. Sometimes even doctors have trouble determining which villain is most likely to blame for the parched tunnel of fire that used to be your healthy throat: a cold or flu virus, which just has to run its course, or a bacteria, like the well-known winter warrior, strep, or streptococcus.

WHAT WOMEN DOCTORS DO

Recipe for Sore-Throat Relief

Penelope Shar, M.D.

Bangor, Maine, is a popular winter destination for some least-loved members of the animal world: the viruses and bacteria that cause sore throats. When Penelope Shar, M.D., a Bangor internist in private practice, gets a sore-throat bug, she heads for her kitchen instead of reaching inside her medicine bag.

"I make a hot drink by mixing equal parts tea and lemon juice, plus enough honey to make it palatable. If you don't add enough honey, it tastes terrible," she says. "Then I heat it in the microwave. (About 2½ minutes per cup should do it.) It's really soothing."

Over-the-counter throat lozenges may be of use, but not for their medicinal properties, says Dr. Shar. If they're useful, it's because they stimulate saliva production and moisturize your throat while you suck on them. Dr. Shar prefers sugarless Ricola candies.

SELF-CARE WORKS

Antibiotic drugs haven't been conclusively proven to speed up the cure for common sore throats, and throat cultures aren't all that accurate. Nevertheless, if your doctor has pretty much ruled out strep throat or some other serious condition behind your symptoms, some doctors believe that it's best to slow down, get warm and cozy and baby your aching throat, just like they do. Here's what women doctors suggest.

Fill up your favorite mug. Warm liquids will not only feel good to your raw throat, but they will also help rehydrate your parched mucous membranes. Try to drink at least two quarts of beverages—preferably, caffeine-free—a day until you feel better. Perhaps this would be a good time to try some new herbal teas, hot lemonade or flavored decaffeinated coffees, says Penelope Shar, M.D., an internist in private practice in Bangor, Maine.

In fact, one woman doctor steers women away from antiseptic lozenges, or lozenges that numb the throat. They may contain ingredients that actually irritate your throat, according to Karen Rhew, M.D., of the National Institute on Deafness and Other Communication Disorders in Bethesda, Maryland.

In a pinch, candy will help. If you don't have any throat lozenges on hand, and you don't want to brave the cold and damp to get to the store, you can just as well use sugarless candy, says Dr. Shar.

Think zinc. Some people find that letting zinc gluconate tablets and lozenges dissolve on their tongues relieves sore throat discomfort. And according to a study conducted at the Clayton Foundation Biochemical Institute of the University of Texas at Austin, zinc gluconate is an effective reliever of sore throat. You can buy zinc gluconate tablets at health food stores. Follow package directions.

Swallow some crushed ice. Sometimes ice can cool the fire of your swallow, according to Dr. Rhew.

Add a pinch of salt. If your mother or grandmother fixed you a salt-water gargle whenever you had a sore throat as a kid, she was on the right

WHEN TO SEE A DOCTOR

A severe sore throat can signify more than a mild viral infection. "In younger women, I worry about mononucleosis," says Penelope Shar, M.D, an internist in private practice in Bangor, Maine. "In women of any age, I worry about strep throat." A serious streptococcus bacterial infection (strep throat) can lead, in rare cases, to rheumatic fever, kidney disease or pneumonia.

Call your doctor for an appointment if your sore throat isn't significantly better in five to seven days, or if you have any of the following symptoms.

- Severe, prolonged throat pain
- Swollen glands in your neck
- Trouble swallowing or opening your mouth
- A persistent lump in your throat or neck
- Hoarseness that lasts for more than two weeks
- Earache
- Blood in phlegm or saliva
- High fever (above 101°F)
- Joint pain
- Skin rash

If you can't swallow or have trouble breathing because of swelling of your airway, seek medical attention immediately, emphasizes Dr. Shar.

track. Dr. Shar says that gargling often with warm saltwater can ease the pain and restore moisture to irritated throat tissues. Mix a pinch of salt with a quarter-cup of warm water. Repeat four or fives times a day.

Warm your neck. Holding a hot-water bottle or warm (not hot) heating pad to your neck can further relieve the pain of a sore throat, according to Dr. Rhew.

Mist is a must. Just as your plants become revitalized with a good misting, your dry throat will thank you for using a cool-mist humidifier to moisten the hot, dry air of your home or office, says Dr. Shar.

Take acetaminophen. Tylenol or other painkillers containing acetaminophen are best for upper respiratory infections, Dr. Shar says.

(For practical ways to relieve coughing and laryngitis, see pages 147 and 339.)

Spider Veins
Hide Burst Blood Vessels

You have no idea when the quarter-size network of tiny red veins appeared on your left thigh. One day they weren't there, the next day they were. What are they, and where did they come from?

"Spider veins are very, very superficial veins that don't have any function," says Lenise Banse, M.D., a dermatologist and vein expert at the Northeast Family Dermatology Center in Clinton Township, Michigan, who easily identifies them from their description.

"They look like spiderwebs (or, sometimes, star bursts) and they can be caused by superficial injuries—anything from being hit by a tennis ball to being jumped on by a pet," she says.

You probably won't even remember when the injury occurred, adds Dr. Banse. It doesn't take an attention-grabbing accident with stabbing pain. And the veins can appear anywhere on your body.

Spider veins may be more likely to pop up during pregnancy, although no one knows exactly why.

CONCEAL AND CONQUER

"With spider veins, it seems as though if you're going to get them, you're going to get them," says Margaret A. Weiss, M.D., assistant professor of dermatology at the Johns Hopkins Medical Institutions in Baltimore. Once formed, spider veins tend to be permanent—unless you opt to have them removed by a dermatologist, by lasers or injection. Otherwise, your best recourse is to hide them—or discourage new ones from forming. Here's what women doctors suggest.

Look for cover. Spider veins are difficult to camouflage with makeup: You may need a heavy foundation like Dermablend, available in department stores, says Allison Vidimos, M.D., a staff dermatologist and vein expert at the Cleveland Clinic Foundation. Generally, says Dr. Vidimos, purplish spider veins are less obtrusive if they're covered with a green-tinted foundation.

That may sound weird, she adds, but the green tint combines with the purplish-red spider vein to create an optical illusion of flesh-colored tones. Salespeople are usually available to help you select the right shade.

Wear compression stockings. "Buy graduated compression stockings from a medical supply company," says Dr. Weiss. The stockings should fit tightly at the ankle and looser at the thigh. That makes it difficult for blood to pool in any weak veins and discourages the formation of spiders.

Avoid shiny support stockings from department stores, adds Dr. Weiss, because they won't work as well. Dressier support hose tend to look good but, she says, don't really do much for your veins.

Move around. Avoid standing in one place for more than a few minutes, suggests Dr. Weiss. Movement encourages venous blood to keep moving, while standing still encourages it to pool, which promotes spider veins.

Lunge and flex. If you must stand for long periods of time—perhaps you're employed as a cashier or a waitress, for example—Dr. Weiss suggests you periodically perform a stretch called a lunge.

Stand with your feet together, explains Dr. Weiss. Slide one foot about a foot forward, shift your weight to it, then bend your back leg at a 45-degree angle at the knee. Hold the position for a second, then stand up straight and return to your original position. Slide the other foot forward and repeat the exercise with the other knee. This movement will encourage blood to keep moving and not slow down long enough to fill out the troublesome veins, says Dr. Weiss.

Put your feet on the floor. If you have a job in which you sit a lot, sit up straight with your feet flat on the floor, suggests Dr. Weiss. Sitting with your legs crossed at the knees will increase pressure on the veins in your legs—and it may increase your chance of developing spider veins.

Split Ends
Heal Fractured Hair

*S*plit ends look like tiny frayed strands of thread, and they're usually caused by the intense temperatures of blow-dryers, curling irons and other styling devices that literally fracture the hair, explains Rebecca Caserio, M.D., clinical associate professor of dermatology at the University of Pittsburgh. The intense heat causes a strand of hair to crack at the tip and split vertically up the shaft.

PATCHWORK AND PREVENTION

Unfortunately, once your ends have started to split, the split can extend up the shaft unless you take action. So here's how you can heal split ends—and prevent healthy strands from splitting, too.

Give in to a trim. "In order to correct and eradicate split ends, you need a very sharp and precise snip," says Liz Cunnane, a consultant trichologist (a hair-care specialist) at Philip Kingsley Trichological Centre in New York City. "If it's not sharply cut, it starts fraying. It's almost like cutting rope. If you cut hair with a blunt instrument, splitting can start almost instantaneously," she says. You can buy haircutting scissors at beauty supply stores and drugstores.

If you have more than a few split ends, both Dr. Caserio and Cunnane recommend an allover trim.

Opt for hair thickeners. Use shampoos and conditioners containing hair thickeners, says Dr. Caserio. Most of these hair-thickening products—Thicket and Thick 'n' Hair, for example—contain waxes that add thickness, which increases diameter to each strand.

Air-dry your hair. Whenever possible, let your hair dry naturally to avoid re-sizzling your ends all over again, says Dr. Caserio.

Use thermal conditioners. If you must use a blow-dryer or hot rollers, spray a thermal styling conditioner such as HeatSafe on your hair while it's damp, says Wendy Resin, hair-care manager at the Neutrogena Corporation in Los Angeles. Then blow-dry or curl your hair as necessary. The spray-on conditioner will help protect and strengthen your hair.

Stick to the lowest setting. Set your blow-dryer on its lowest setting, says Dr. Caserio. The cooler the setting, the less heat damage.

Sports Widowhood
Living with a Sports Zombie

Some succumb on golf courses. Others meet their demise at bowling alleys. Many more give up the ghost in front of televisions while Sunday-night football blares over the airwaves.

Suddenly, men we've come to know and love show no signs of life—at least no signs of intelligent life. Transfixed by one sporting event or another, they turn into sports zombies, and, in so doing, turn us into sports widows.

Of course, women sometimes turn men into sports widowers, too. But that's less common, says Shirley Glass, Ph.D., a clinical psychologist and marital therapist in the Baltimore area.

"Men get a lot of vicarious enjoyment from watching competitive sports," says Dr. Glass. "Most men are more nostalgic and sentimental about playing and watching sports than women are."

Men are vulnerable to sports zombification for yet another reason. For some, the ball field, or game of the week, is a natural venue for spending time with male friends.

"Watching or playing sports can be one of the few ways men maintain their friendships with other men," explains Dr. Glass. "Men are more activity-oriented in their companionship and tend to relate to each other side by side—sitting side by side watching TV or standing side by side fishing—while women tend to relate to each other face to face."

POUTING WON'T HELP

If your guy's vital signs flat-line on the field or in front of the television set, here's what women doctors advise.

Try it. Striking the right balance between time apart and time with a sports zombie is easier if you like sports. If you can enjoy the occasional baseball game, the World Series is that much easier on your relationship.

Give his consuming passion a try, says Diana Adile Kirschner, Ph.D., a psychologist in private practice in Gwynedd Valley, Pennsylvania. When her husband started training for a triathlon, she decided to start exercising more as well. They ran and biked together. Though an injury tempered his interest, hers is still going strong.

WHAT WOMEN DOCTORS DO

Tennis, Anyone?

Shirley Glass, Ph.D.

Like a lot of women married to golf enthusiasts, Shirley Glass, Ph.D., a clinical psychologist and marital therapist in the Baltimore area, used to find her husband's twice-weekly golf games galling. And accompanying him to baseball games didn't thrill her. Eventually, she tried a different approach.

"I don't enjoy playing golf, but I do enjoy playing tennis, reading or going out with friends," says Dr. Glass. "So while he plays 18 holes, that's what I do.

"I even go to Baltimore Orioles games with my husband, as long as I have someone else to talk to," she adds.

If you wish for more shared activities with the man in your life and he resists, or you've talked it out and the situation isn't improving, you may need to see a professional trained in counseling couples, says Dr. Glass.

Of course, it helps if your zombie gives sports that interest you a try. You're a tennis devotee? He might become one, too.

Generate interest. If you can't get interested in the complexities of the game he loves, maybe you can get interested in the personalities.

"Read the sports page and get to know who the players are," Dr. Glass says. "Women are more relationally oriented. If you know stories about the players, you're likely to be more interested."

One woman dealt with her husband's die-hard enthusiasm for the New England Patriots by taking an interest in the coaching style of Bill Parcells and how he handled the team's promising star quarterback, Drew Bledsoe, idolized by her mate. As a new manager herself, the woman was interested in finding out more about how Parcells's coaching style translated into results on the football field.

Similarly, if you know he's competitive, pick a rival team and follow its performance. It's worth the effort just to see his reaction when you report on their relative standings.

Enjoy your time alone. Do whatever interests you while your partner indulges his yen for sports, suggest Dr. Glass and Irene Deitch, Ph.D., a psychologist, marriage and family therapist and professor of psychology at the College of Staten Island in New York.

"The notion of a woman being helpless at the hands of the man who has to devote all his time to making her happy is a sexist concept," says Dr. Deitch, who finishes *The New York Times* while her husband watches sports. "We want to move away from a 'dependency notion' to an empowering concept."

Air your grievances. If his sports appetite is so voracious that there's negligible time left for fun together, you need to talk, says Dr. Kirschner.

"If you feel hurt, the danger is that you'll allow yourself to drift away in a sea of resentment until there's real distance between you," she says.

Negotiate for equal (or nearly equal) time. "The ideal thing is to try to create a contract with your partner," Dr. Kirschner says. "You might say, 'I'm willing to support your watching this or playing that, but in return, I want you to do something for me.'" You could agree to make snacks for him and his buddies while they watch the Sunday night game, if he, in turn, agrees to cook you a special dinner Saturday night. Or, you might decide to spend every other Sunday doing something together and allow him the remaining Sundays with the Dallas Cowboys.

Sprains

Easy Does It

Sprains occur when you stretch or tear a ligament, a tough band of fibrous tissue that attaches one bone to another at a joint, such as the ankle or knee. You'll feel sharp pain, especially if you try to use the joint, and it may swell and turn black and blue.

SPEED HEALING

A sprain can take anywhere from two to eight weeks to heal completely. Rosemary Agostini, M.D., clinical assistant professor of orthopedics at the University of Washington School of Medicine and a sports medicine and family practice physician at the Virginia Mason Medical

513

WHEN TO SEE A DOCTOR

If you sprain your knee, ankle or another joint so badly that you experience extreme pain and cannot take even three steps on it, or if the injured joint looks disfigured, go to a hospital emergency room or an urgent care center, says Rosemary Agostini, M.D., clinical assistant professor of orthopedics at the University of Washington School of Medicine and a sports medicine and family practice physician at the Virginia Mason Medical Center, both in Seattle. It might be a fracture.

Center, both in Seattle, says that if you can take more than three steps, you may be able to care for the sprain yourself.

First, rest. "If it's painful, don't put weight on the injured joint," says Dr. Agostini.

Ice it, ice it, ice it. "Immediately ice a sprain to relieve the pain and decrease the swelling," says Dr. Agostini. Keep the ice on for 20 minutes and reapply three or four times a day until pain and swelling has decreased.

Make sure that you wrap the ice in a cloth so that it isn't in direct contact with your skin, and you don't end up with frostbite.

Elevate the sprained joint. To reduce pain and swelling, you should raise your sprained joint above heart level, says Dr. Agostini.

Bandage it. Wrapping your sprained joint with an Ace-type bandage will compress the area around your joint and decrease the swelling, says Dr. Agostini. The wrapping should be snug around the joint, but not so tight that your blood can't circulate freely.

Take a pain reliever. Anti-inflammatories such as aspirin and ibuprofen also will ease the pain, says Stacie Grossfeld, M.D., an orthopedic surgeon at the University of Minnesota in Minneapolis. Use the dosage recommended on the package or ask your physician. If you have a history of peptic ulcers, acetaminophen would be a more appropriate choice, she says.

Sties and Chalazia
Help for Pimples on Your Eyelids

*N*ext to a big zit on your nose, sties and chalazia (pimples on your eyelid) are among the most distressing of blemishes. Like pimples on your face, they show up at the most inconvenient times. Making matters worse, they tend to hurt.

Sties form when an eyelash follicle gets infected, perhaps because you used a contaminated mascara brush or because dandrufflike scales have clogged the follicle. You'll see a red, painful swelling like a little boil on the edge of your eyelid around the base of your eyelash, with a white head of pus on the swelling.

Chalazia form inside your eyelids when one or more oil glands get clogged, perhaps from makeup residue. Though often painless, chalazia can cause your eyelid to swell, itch and ache.

Each eyelid contains anywhere from 20 to 30 oil glands, and you can develop more than one chalazion at a time. Same for sties.

CLEAR UP THE BUMPS

Home treatment for both sties and chalazia is the same.

Drain with warm compresses. At the first sign of a sty or chalazion, place a warm, damp washcloth over your closed eyes for at least five min-

WHEN TO SEE A DOCTOR

A stubborn sty or chalazion calls for medical attention—you may actually have a cyst or other problem that should be taken care of. Same goes for recurrent sties, which sometimes signal diabetes.

More often than not, though, a sty is just a sty, and it can be drained. A chalazion can be removed. See a doctor if a sty or chalazion:

- Doesn't get better—or gets worse—after two days.
- Grows very quickly, despite compresses.
- Bleeds.

utes at a time, four times a day for two weeks, says Monica L. Monica, M.D., Ph.D., an ophthalmologist in New Orleans and a spokesperson for the American Academy of Ophthalmology. This will help the sty break open, or the chalazion to become absorbed, Dr. Monica says.

To keep the washcloth warm, wrap it around a hot baked potato or boiled egg. The washcloth will retain heat longer, says Monica Dweck, M.D., an ophthalmologist in Allentown, Pennsylvania, who specializes in eyelid problems.

Hands off. As with a pimple on your face, if you try to pop a sty, it may rupture beneath the surface, further aggravating matters, says Dr. Dweck.

Take a vacation from eye makeup. Let your eye heal (and your clogged oil glands clear) before you apply any eye makeup again. That means mascara, eyeliner or shadow. Otherwise, you may end up with several sties and chalazia instead of just one, says Dr. Dweck.

Stomachache
Pacify Your Cranky Tummy

You won't find "stomachache" in the medical dictionary. As a matter of fact, a stomachache is sort of a catchall term for a variety of all-too-familiar discomforts: knots, a dull ache, an acidy feeling. Maybe cramps and a little diarrhea or constipation just to make things interesting. And let's not forget nausea.

A stomachache can be all of these or just plain mid-body misery. And the possible causes are equally diverse and mysterious: gallstones, lactose intolerance, ulcers, heartburn, irritable bowel syndrome, stress, overeating. Or not eating enough. Or eating improperly prepared food in an unhygienic restaurant. (For more details, read about irritable bowel syndrome on page 322.)

HELP FOR PLAIN OLD STOMACH TROUBLE

If you have a stomachache, it helps to know what the problem is and, if needed, to get your doctor's advice. In general, though, there are a few things you can do that may soothe your sore tummy now.

Sip a soother. When your stomach feels a little calmer, try sipping uncaffeinated liquids such as water, peppermint or chamomile herb tea, flat ginger ale or chicken broth, says Wanda Filer, M.D., a family practice physician in York, Pennsylvania. "Try a few sips every five minutes." (Anything that includes caffeine—like coffee, regular tea and colas—irritates the stomach and digestive tract, she says.)

Eat daintily. When your stomach is irritated, it rebels against food. Whether the source of your stomachache is stress or indigestion, your body is on overload and needs to calm down. "If you feel better enough to eat a bit, stick to small, frequent, easy-to-digest foods such as cooked rice or dry crackers such as saltines or dry toast," says Dr. Filer. Digesting a heavy meal will make your stomach work too hard—not a good idea when it's already rebelling at the food that might have caused your tummy ache.

Shun lactose. Eliminate lactose-containing foods, another possible culprit, if you are sensitive to dairy products, suggests Marie L. Borum, M.D., assistant professor of medicine in the Division of Gastroenterology and Nutrition at George Washington University Medical Center in Washington, D.C.

Be a B-R-A-T. As your stomach feels better, you'll have more of an appetite, but the best way to make sure the ache is banished for good is to stick to a BRAT (bananas, rice, applesauce and dry toast) diet, says Dr. Filer. "Even on the BRAT plan, you should eat very little and add each new food gradually, so that your cranky stomach won't have to work too hard to digest it," she says.

Chew an antacid. If your pain is caused by too much acid in your stomach—a possibility if you have an ache on an empty stomach—over-the-counter antacids like Tums or Rolaids can relieve your ache, because they neutralize stomach acids, says Sheila Crowe, M.D., gastroenterologist and assistant professor of medicine in the Department of Internal Medicine in the Division of Gastroenterology at the University of Texas Medical Branch at Galveston.

Try an acid suppressor. Modern medicines called H_2 (histamine 2) blockers, such as Tagamet or Pepcid AC, which suppress acid at its source and keep it from irritating your stomach lining, are now available over the counter. "More powerful than antacids, acid suppressors are especially effective against heartburnlike pain," says Dr. Crowe. Pepto-

WHEN TO SEE A DOCTOR

Usually, stomachaches go away without any specific treatment. If they persist and don't respond to over-the-counter treatment, you should seek medical advice, says Sheila Crowe, M.D., a gastroenterologist and assistant professor of medicine in the Department of Internal Medicine in the Division of Gastroenterology at the University of Texas Medical Branch at Galveston. Also, if over-the-counter drugs only provide temporary relief, you may need prescription-strength drugs to treat underlying conditions such as gastro-esophageal reflux or peptic ulcers. If you do have a history of peptic ulcers, you should be checked for *Helicobacter pylori* infection, a bacteria that is associated with ulcer disease, she says. See a doctor right away if your stomachache is particularly severe or accompanied by fevers or blood in the stool. "It could be a sign of a more serious condition such as an ulcer, gallbladder inflammation or pancreatitis," says Dr. Crowe.

If your stomachache is accompanied by nausea and vomiting that doesn't go away after a few days, see your doctor to rule out other possible causes (such as pregnancy or a virus), says Wanda Filer, M.D., a family practice physician in York, Pennsylvania.

Bismol can also provide relief for some stomachaches, although the way this drug helps is less clear.

Loosen your belt. If your stomach is distended from IBS, you can loosen your belt. If you're tightly buttoned and belted up, try switching to comfortable, loose clothing, which can ease the pressure on your aching stomach, says Dr. Borum. (It's obvious only after you think of it.)

Stop. The best thing to do for any stomachache may be nothing except resting and relaxing, says Dr. Crowe. If you calm down, you'll help your stomach calm down, too.

Or pound the pavement. Stomach in knots over a conflict or hassle? For some women, exercise is the best medicine for a stress-related stomachache, Dr. Filer says. "Get up and walk away," she says. And regular exercise—that's at least 30 minutes of aerobic exercise such as walking or biking three days a week—is such a great stress reliever that you may get rid of tension stomachaches forever, Dr. Filer says.

Nix the coffee and alcohol. Coffee and alcohol also are well-known stomach irritants, says Dr. Filer. "I tell women who get stomachaches to stick to decaffeinated, nonalcoholic drinks," she says.

Kick that habit—please! Everyone has heard that smoking does a number on your lungs, but did you know that it's murder on your stomach? "Cigarettes and other tobacco products decrease the stomach lining's ability to defend itself against powerful acids that cause stomachaches," Dr. Filer says. So if you smoke, stop. And to protect yourself against chronic stomachaches, don't start again after you feel better, she says.

Stomach Cramps
At-Home Comfort Measures

*Y*ou hurt bad. You're doubled over, knotted up. You want to scream. You want to sleep. Anything to get rid of this pain.

"Stomach" cramps can (and often do) carom around your abdomen like a cue ball on a billiard table. Almost every woman has had cramps sometime. If you suffer from irritable bowel syndrome or lactose intolerance or even have the occasional bout of PMS, you know a cramp when it grips you. The exact diagnosis or cause of stomach cramps may or may not be obvious. It could be stress, or a virus, or something else.

TEA AND SYMPATHY

Stomach (or abdominal) cramps will go away on their own after a few hours or days. But you don't have to suffer that long. Women doctors offer these comfort measures.

Try a hot-water bottle. A cramp is really just a knotted muscle. "If stomach muscles are making you crampy, lying in bed with a hot-water bottle on your stomach may help ease the pain," says Wanda Filer, M.D., a family practice physician in York, Pennsylvania. A hot-water bottle is much safer than a heating pad, says Dr. Filer, because it cools down, while a heating pad stays hot and can burn you if you fall asleep or use it overnight.

WHEN TO SEE A DOCTOR

If stomach cramps are accompanied by nausea, vomiting, fever or blood in the stool, see a doctor to rule out more serious conditions such as ulcers, says Wanda Filer, M.D., a family practice physician in York, Pennsylvania.

Stick to the B-R-A-T diet. That's bananas, rice, applesauce and dry toast—foods that are easy to digest and won't hurt your tummy. "High-fiber foods like popcorn, nuts or cabbage can be hard to digest and make cramping worse," says Dr. Filer.

Drink plenty of water. If your cramping stems from constipation or diarrhea, the best way to ease the cramping is by drinking water, water and more water, say women doctors. Water gets the waste products moving through your intestines, which should ease your constipation. If you have diarrhea, drinking lots of water will keep you from becoming dehydrated.

Cook up a batch of chicken soup. "It works," says Dr. Filer. Nobody knows why, but chicken soup soothes stomach and abdominal cramps and cleans out the digestive system.

Avoid dairy. If you have diarrhea or lactose intolerance, you'll find that milk and other dairy products such as cheese and milk are hard to digest and often cause cramping. So until your cramps subside, go easy on the white stuff, says Dr. Filer.

Swallow some peppermint oil. If you have bowel spasms or trapped gas, peppermint oil stops the aching, says Tori Hudson, a naturopathic physician and professor at the National College of Naturopathic Medicine in Portland, Oregon. Peppermint oil is available in capsule form in health food stores. "Take one capsule two or three times a day between meals until your cramping goes away," says Dr. Hudson.

Or check out herbal teas. "Valerian, fennel, ginger, chamomile, rosemary, peppermint and lemon balm teas also relieve gas and stop spasms of mild stomach cramps," says Dr. Hudson.

Stress
Ease Out from Under It

*B*ack in the Stone Age, life was stressful. But probably not as stressful as it is today.

Sure, you had to run from the occasional saber-toothed tiger and put up with Neanderthal behavior. But your job as forager was secure. And you didn't have to worry about your kids quitting school or your husband straying—since there was no formal education and everyone believed the world ended at the horizon anyway.

MORE RESPONSIBILITY, LESS CONTROL

"Women are probably under more stress than ever before," says Camille Lloyd, Ph.D., professor in the Department of Psychiatry and Behavioral Sciences at the University of Texas Medical School at Houston. At work we have more responsibility but less job security. We're juggling demands made by our bosses, our kids and our spouses. Our relationships are less secure—consider the divorce rate. And we're less likely to have extended family and lifelong friends to lean on, since everyone relocates so often, says Dr. Lloyd.

Add it up, and too much responsibility, too little control and too few resources amount to too much stress, says Dr. Lloyd. Plus, women tend to absorb the stress felt by those who are close to them, compounding the problem.

"Research shows that women are more sensitive to the stress of people close to them," continues Dr. Lloyd. "If their husbands are under stress or their kids are under stress, they experience more stress themselves."

That's not healthy. Studies suggest that your body's physiological reaction to high levels of sustained stress—increased blood pressure, an outpouring of adrenaline and other changes—makes you more susceptible to serious disorders like heart disease.

You may also find yourself depressed, irritable, despairing or edgy, says Sharon Greenburg, Ph.D., a clinical psychologist in private practice in Chicago. Or you may find that you can't sleep, concentrate or recall things. You may get headaches.

WHEN TO SEE A DOCTOR

Stress can contribute to serious health problems, such as heart disease and alcohol abuse. Don't hesitate to talk to your doctor if you experience stress-related symptoms such as:

- A racing pulse
- Dizzy spells
- Severe headaches
- Chronic back or neck pain
- Anxiety
- Depression

If stress is driving you to drink or your drinking becomes a problem, you might also want to call Women for Sobriety at 1-800-333-1606 or your local chapter of Alcoholics Anonymous.

UNWIND, EASE UP, UNLOAD

The calming news is that there's plenty you can do to relieve stress. Here's some advice from the experts.

Take a moment to relax. Stress is most damaging if it's unrelenting. Even a few moments of relaxation can help considerably, says Susan Heitler, Ph.D., a clinical psychologist in Denver and author of the audiotape *Anxiety: Friend or Foe?*.

"Take mini breaks," she says. "If you're at work and start feeling stressed, get up and stretch or talk to a co-worker for a couple of minutes." If you're home, take a break in a quiet room.

Give yourself a longer break at least once every day, recommends Dr. Greenburg. "If you have children, set aside some time for yourself to read a magazine, watch television or simply do nothing at all." That time can be when the kids are napping, at school or playing by themselves, she says.

Talk it out. If you have more to do than you can realistically handle or too little control over your schedule to get things done, speak up, says Deborah Belle, Ed.D., associate professor of psychology at Boston University.

At work, talk to your boss. She may have no idea that you're overloaded, or that your assignments are so ambiguous that you spend an extra hour each day trying to figure out what's expected, says Dr. Belle. Or consult co-workers to find out if and how they've handled similar situations.

"If nothing else, you'll feel less powerless having spoken up—and that sense of control can significantly reduce the negative impact of stress," says Dr. Heitler.

At home, talk to your spouse.

"In relationships, poor communication is often a source of stress," says Rosalind Barnett, Ph.D., a clinical psychologist, visiting scholar at Radcliffe College in Cambridge, Massachusetts, and co-editor of *Gender and Stress*. "If you have concerns about your job, your partner, your kids—bring them up."

Go easy on yourself. "If you're in a job where expectations are unrealistic, you'll only feel more stressed if you tell yourself, 'I'm really in-

WHAT WOMEN DOCTORS DO

The Scarlet O'Hara Approach

Marian R. Stuart, Ph.D.

When Marian R. Stuart, Ph.D., finishes her teaching responsibilities as clinical professor of family medicine at the University of Medicine and Dentistry of New Jersey Robert Wood Johnson Medical School in New Brunswick, she endures a 45-minute commute in tear-out-your-hair traffic to her home office in Morristown, New Jersey. There, she sees patients for three hours before her day is finished.

An author, medical educator and practicing psychologist, Dr. Stuart's life is hardly stress-free. By 10:00 at night, she's pretty wound up, she says. But, taking a cue from her own books (Coping With the Stressed-Out People in Your Life and The Fifteen-Minute Hour: Applied Psychotherapy for the Primary Care Physician), Dr. Stuart knows how to turn off the pressure and give herself a break.

"First, I run a hot bath," she says, dipping into aromatherapy to suit her mood. She starts with a base of two ounces of sweet almond oil, which she found with the salad dressings at her local health food store. Then she adds 12 drops of lavender oil to calm and soothe, 6 drops of lemon oil and 4 drops of patchouli to spice her steam with a happy aura. "I rub it on my hands. It's fragrance is wonderful," she says.

Next, she might make herself a cup of a favorite herbal tea.

Lying in bed, she takes the time to breathe deeply, use mental imagery and conjure up whatever is bothering her. "I don't have to deal with that now. I'm going to let that go," she tells herself. "Tomorrow is another day."

competent,'" says Dr. Greenburg. "Instead, be objective. Tell yourself, 'I'm doing as much as anyone could—and more.'"

At home, accept the fact that you can't give the people you love everything, says Dr. Barnett. "So do the best job you can and be okay with that."

Off-load some chores. According to Dr. Barnett, studies find that women who work full-time outside the home still do more than half the housework, especially such tasks as buying groceries, meal preparation and cleanup and child rearing. Strive for a more even split.

Make room for Daddy. "Our research finds that, for many husbands, being with the kids actually felt like a reward after a hard day at the office," says Dr. Barnett. "When husbands and wives shared more equally, everyone felt less stress."

Think before you cut. "A common assumption is that every role you take on adds to your stress," says Dr. Belle. "But research actually suggests that people with many roles—worker, parent, spouse, community volunteer—fare better." Evidently, the satisfaction you get from one role can buffer the stress that you feel in another.

So before you give up your post as den mother, ask yourself what you're getting out of it, recommends Dr. Belle. It may be providing leadership opportunities that are lacking at work, for example. By the same token, the sense of satisfaction and mastery that you get at work could be the ideal antidote to the stress you feel raising a teenager with purple hair. More roles may also mean a wider stress-relieving social support network.

Exercise, a useful antidote. The satisfaction that you get from outside activities can counter pressures at both home and the office, says Dr. Lloyd. Activities that get you moving—tennis, volleyball, running, swimming, walking—are ideal. Why? Exercise burns off stress-related chemicals, and it strengthens your heart so that it can withstand the ravages of stress.

Stretch Marks
The Secret Formula

*P*regnancy is one of two causes of stretch marks. The other is weight gain.

"Stretch marks occur on the breasts, hips and stomach during pregnancy, plus other areas such as the thighs when you gain weight," says Margaret A. Weiss, M.D., assistant professor of dermatology at the Johns Hopkins Medical Institutions in Baltimore.

They're triggered when skin is stretched to the max, which occurs when growth is so rapid that your skin's elastic fibers break. And though it occurs less often, stretch marks can also be caused by some hormonal problems, certain diseases and medications, says Dr. Weiss.

WHAT WORKS

"Moisturizers, wrinkle cream and massage don't get rid of stretch marks," says Dr. Weiss. (For a possible exception, see "Vitamin Cream Works Wonders" on page 526.) And makeup doesn't cover them very well.

The best you can do is to minimize stretch marks, says Dr. Weiss. Firming any areas that have stretch marks—usually the thighs, hips and abdomen—makes stretch marks less apparent, she says. Women doctors suggest these exercises. (You can expect to see results in about two months.)

Start with 20 leg raises. One of the best exercises to work the hip and leg area, which is where stretch marks are most likely to occur, is a straight leg raise exercise, says Carol Garber, Ph.D., director of the Human Performance Lab at Brown University in Providence, Rhode Island.

To begin, lie down on the floor on your side, legs straight, one on top of the other. Then extend the arm that's floor-side down over your head and rest your head on your arm. Put your other hand flat on the floor in front of your waist. Keeping both legs straight and toes pointed straight ahead, raise your top leg from hip to toe as far as it will go, then lower it back to the floor.

"Don't just jerk your leg up in the air and let it fall back down," says Dr. Garber. "You can get injured if you raise it too quickly. Instead, raise and lower your leg in a slow, controlled motion.

"Begin with 8 to 10 leg raises on each side at least three times a week," says Dr. Garber. Then, as each exercise begins to seem easy, add a leg raise or two until you've worked your way up to 20 leg raises three times a week.

Do 20 inner-thigh exercises. To firm your inner thigh, lie down on the floor just as you did for the leg raises, says Dr. Garber. But this time, instead of raising your top leg, bend that knee and place your foot in front of your bottom leg, then try to raise the bottom leg up about six inches. Then lower the leg to the floor.

Begin with 8 to 10 bottom-leg raises on each side at least three

Vitamin Cream Works Wonders

Lisa Giannetto, M.D.

Lisa Giannetto, M.D., does not have a single stretch mark on her body. Yet the diminutive 35-year-old associate professor in the Department of Medicine and Community and Family Medicine at Duke University in Durham, North Carolina, has carried two babies to term within the past five years.

Not any stretch marks?

"Not one," she says cheerfully. "And since I'm only 95 pounds, I really stretched. I had a significant belly both times."

Her secret: a nonprescription fluid containing vitamin C, called Cellex-C Serum, formulated based upon research conducted at Duke University Medical Center.

Research suggests that the fluid will promote the development of collagen, a substance that gives your skin its elasticity, says Dr. Gianetto. And the result, as she can attest, is smooth, unmarked skin.

Her advice to pregnant women who want to avoid stretch marks: "From the moment you begin to show at about 6 to 12 weeks, apply vitamin C fluid to your abdomen every day. After your bath or shower, dry off, then put enough fluid in your hand to cover your hips and abdomen; rub your hands together and smooth the cream over your belly."

You don't have to be a doctor to get your hands on Cellex-C Serum fluid, although you can ask your doctor or dermatologist to order it for you. You can also order it directly from the Cellex-C Distribution Company by calling 1-800-423-5539.

times a week, says Dr. Garber. Then, as each exercise begins to seem easy, add a couple of bottom-leg raises until you've worked your way up to 20 bottom-leg raises three times a week.

Swing your legs. One incredibly simple exercise that firms the whole thigh is to sit in a chair with your feet flat on the floor, hands either by your sides or in your lap, then swing both legs up so that they're extended straight out in front of you at seat level, says Dr. Garber. Then swing them back down.

You can swing your legs whenever you feel like it—when you're on the phone or watching television, for example—or you can incorporate the exercise into your workout. Whichever you choose, your goal should be 20 swings three times a week.

Lift off. If you get bored with swinging, put your hands down at your sides to hold on to your chair and swing your legs up until they're fully extended. Then lift each leg, from foot to hip, about three to six inches, says Dr. Garber. Finally, lower your leg until both legs are straight out in front of you once again.

Start out with 8 to 10 lifts, then work your way up to 20 lifts three times a week.

Firm your butt. To firm your bottom, lie face-down on the floor, arms out at your shoulders, elbows bent and palms flat on the floor, says Dr. Garber. Now lift one leg, heel first, off the floor about three to six inches, then lower it back to the floor and repeat the lift with your other leg.

Start out by lifting each leg 8 to 10 times three times a week. Add a couple of lifts to each workout as they get easy. Your goal is 20 lifts three times a week.

Keep the scale steady. Since extra pounds create stretch marks, try to keep your weight on an even keel, says Dr. Weiss. To control calories, avoid high-fat foods, watch your portions and get more physically active. Walk instead of drive, take the stairs instead of an elevator, do your own yard work instead of hiring the neighbor's kid.

Sunburn

Cool Advice for Sun-Scorched Skin

*Y*ou just got home from a day on the beach, and your skin knows it. If you forgot your sunscreen and got burned—or if you slathered it on unevenly and you have a streak of red across your face or shoulders—you're paying for it now with burned skin. Ouch. Redness, pain, swelling, discomfort and maybe even blisters are the telltale signs of too much unprotected time in the sun.

Women who wear makeup and moisturizers with sunscreen in them have an advantage in preventing sunburn, says D'Anne Kleinsmith, M.D., a staff dermatologist at William Beaumont Hospital in Royal Oak, Michigan. Sunscreen protects against wrinkles and skin cancer, too, she notes.

When it comes to sunburn, higher amounts of a protective pigment called melanin give women with dark skin and hair a slight edge over

WHAT WOMEN DOCTORS DO

Protect Dark Skin, Too

Patricia Farris Walters, M.D.

When she was in college, Patricia Farris Walters, M.D., clinical assistant professor of dermatology at Tulane University School of Medicine in New Orleans and a spokesperson for the American Academy of Dermatology, went to Florida on midwinter break. A dark-skinned brunette of Greek-American descent, she thought that her dark coloring made her immune to the sun's harsh rays. Not so. After spending a day on the beach in the middle of the winter, she experienced the worst sunburn of her life. Here's her advice.

"My whole face blistered and peeled," she says. "I looked awful, and I was sick with fever and chills the whole night."

So she tells women, no matter what your coloring, protect your skin.

(By the way, don't let yourself be seduced into thinking that tanning booths are burn-proof alternatives to natural sun. You can get a bad burn at a tanning salon.)

WHEN TO SEE A DOCTOR

A sunburn isn't usually serious enough to call for medical attention—unless it starts to blister. That's because blistering sunburn could potentially develop into deeper wounds and open the door to infection. Your doctor may prescribe ointments or cortisone lotions to reduce redness and antibiotics to prevent infection.

"Also, if you're taking medications, check with a doctor *before* you spend time in the sun," says D'Anne Kleinsmith, M.D., a staff dermatologist at William Beaumont Hospital in Royal Oak, Michigan. "Common antibiotics such as tetracycline, sulfonamides and some medications for diabetes and high blood pressure can leave you much more sensitive to the same amount of light that other people wouldn't even react to, and you can get a bad sunburn," she says. This goes double for a drug called psoralen, prescribed for skin conditions including psoriasis and vitiligo. Used incorrectly, it can bring on severe sunburns, says Dr. Kleinsmith.

women with fair skin and blond, red or light brown hair—but not much. Anyone can get sunburn, says Patricia Farris Walters, M.D., clinical assistant professor of dermatology at Tulane University School of Medicine in New Orleans and a spokesperson for the American Academy of Dermatology. Also, certain medications can interact negatively with ultraviolet light (from the sun or tanning booths), causing more severe sunburn. Any drug containing hormones—for example, birth control pills and estrogen-replacement pills—can make women more sensitive to the sun, causing brownish, blotchy pigmentation on the face or sometimes redness and sensitivity, Dr. Kleinsmith adds.

HELP FOR THE RAW AND THE COOKED

If you're as red as a lobster and hurting from sunburn, women doctors offer these tips to help ease your misery.

Reach for pain relief. Dr. Walters suggests taking a couple of aspirin or ibuprofen (such as Advil) as you realize that you overdid it in the sun, even before you start feeling the burn. "Aspirin or ibuprofen offer sunburn relief in two ways," she says. They kill pain, and they also reduce inflammation and swelling.

"If you take them soon enough, aspirin or ibuprofen can help keep inflammation down and prevent a burn from getting worse," says Dr. Kleinsmith.

Continue taking two 200-milligram pills every 6 hours for 24 to 48 hours to keep inflammation down, suggests Evelyn Placek, M.D., a dermatologist and doctor of internal medicine in private practice in Scarsdale, New York.

Fashion a cool compress. The best way to soothe a sunburn is to apply cool water (not ice, which could traumatize irritated skin) as quickly as possible to prevent the sunburn from getting worse, advises Dr. Kleinsmith.

If the sunburn is in one small area, apply a compress made from a towel or washcloth soaked in cool water, suggests Dr. Placek.

Run a cool bath. If the sunburn covers most of your body, soak in a cool bath. "You probably don't want to take a cold shower, though, because the water beating on your sunburned skin will hurt," says Dr. Placek.

Step into an oatmeal bath. To relieve the itchiness of dried, sunburned skin, add a powdered oatmeal preparation such as Aveeno (available in drugstores) to a tub full of cool bathwater and slip in for a skin-soothing soak, suggests Dr. Walters.

Soothe on cortisone ointment. This anti-inflammatory salve can help keep down inflammation and swelling. For sunburned skin, use an ointment, not a cream. "Creams contain preservatives that can sting irritated or blistered skin," says Dr. Placek. "A few years ago, when I missed an area of my shoulder with sunblock, I got a minor sunburn, so I put on cortisone ointment, and it helped soothe and heal it," she says.

Swimmer's Ear
Not for Water-Lovers Only

If your ear aches and you pull on it, wiggle it or push on that little bump (called the tragus) in front of the ear canal and it really hurts, you don't have just any old earache. You have swimmer's ear, an inflammation of the external ear canal (known in medical circles as otitis externa).

Swimmer's ear usually occurs after water gets trapped in the ear following a swim, shower or even a shampoo. The damp, dark environment is ideal for bacterial and fungal growth.

At first your ear may feel blocked or itchy. At that point home remedies can help. Untreated, the ear canal will swell and possibly even shut. A milky or yellowish liquid may drain out, and it will hurt to touch your ear. At that point, you need medical treatment.

KEEPING EARS PROBLEM-FREE

For mild cases of swimmer's ear, women doctors offer these tried-and-true home remedies.

Whip up some eardrops. "Combine equal amounts of rubbing alcohol and white vinegar in a clean, empty eyedropper bottle," says Jennifer Derebery, M.D., assistant clinical professor of otolaryngology at the University of Southern California in Los Angeles. You can find eyedropper bottles at the drugstore; just ask the pharmacist.

"If you're sure that your eardrum has never been perforated (say, from an accident or previous ear infection), apply a few drops to each ear," says Dr. Derebery. "If it's just a mild infection, you may need no further treatment."

This home remedy works, says Dr. Derebery, because the alcohol kills the bacteria and evaporates the water; the vinegar changes the pH of

WHEN TO SEE A DOCTOR

The following symptoms need immediate attention, says Laura Orvidas, M.D., senior associate consultant and instructor in the Department of Otorhinolaryngology at the Mayo Clinic in Rochester, Minnesota.

- Drainage (especially a foul-smelling yellowish or milky discharge) from the ear
- Hearing loss
- Sudden, sharp pain in the ear

"Even in the absence of a fever, these symptoms indicate a serious infection that requires medical treatment," says Dr. Orvidas. "Your doctor will most likely prescribe an antibiotic and eardrops containing cortisone."

the external ear, making it less hospitable to bacteria and fungi, the "germs" that cause swimmer's ear.

To prevent future problems or if you have chronic swimmer's ear, Dr. Derebery recommends using the drops each time you swim or take a shower.

Try peroxide. Place a few drops of drugstore-variety peroxide in the ear, says Laura Orvidas, M.D., senior associate consultant and instructor in the Department of Otorhinolaryngology at the Mayo Clinic in Rochester, Minnesota. Its antibacterial action can quell minor cases of swimmer's ear.

Tachycardia
Rein In a Racing Heart

Everyone's heart beats faster when they dash for a bus or swerve out of the way of an oncoming car, jumping to well over 100 beats a minute compared to its normal average of 60 to 80 beats or so.

But if your heart simply starts zipping along without any apparent provocation, you may have tachycardia, a scary condition in which the heart temporarily races at a faster-than-normal pace, says Pamela Ouyang, M.D., associate professor of medicine at Johns Hopkins University School of Medicine and a cardiologist at the Johns Hopkins Bayview Medical Center, both in Baltimore. The whole episode may last only a few seconds, but for women with tachycardia, the fast beats are quite noticeable.

Here's what happens: Although the heart has a tiny group of cells that normally generate electrical signals to maintain the heart's rhythm, any part of the heart can generate these fast beats, say Dr. Ouyang. While temporary episodes of tachycardia aren't necessarily dangerous in themselves, in some people they could be a sign of heart disease, high blood pressure, cardiomyopathy (an abnormality of heart muscle) or even damaged heart valves. In many people, particularly those with no heart disease, tachycardia is often harmless in that it is unlikely to lead to a heart attack, says Dr. Ouyang.

For most people, tachycardia is nothing to get upset about. "Anxious people can often get benign—harmless—tachycardia," explains Dr. Ouyang. So can people who experience panic attacks—a frightening occurrence in which the individual's heartbeat accelerates for no known reason and they experience a sense of impending doom. (For details on handling panic attacks, see page 416.)

CALMING TECHNIQUES

Though all tachycardia should be evaluated by a doctor, here's what experts suggest you do if it's not related to serious problems.

Tighten tummy muscles. As soon as your heart starts to race, tighten your stomach muscles, advises Deborah L. Keefe, M.D., professor of medicine at Cornell Medical Center and a cardiologist at Memorial Sloan-Kettering Cancer Center, both in New York City. That will cause your abdominal muscles to put pressure on a group of nerves that will tell your heart's electrical system to slow down.

Chill. Take a deep, long breath and slowly let it out, suggests Dr. Keefe. Sometimes relaxation is all it takes to stop tachycardia. And deep breathing is frequently one of the fastest ways to relax.

Use common sense. Anything that speeds up the heart—caffeine and cigarettes, for example—can trigger a rapid heartbeat, says Dr. Ouyang. So common sense says that if you're prone to tachycardia, you should avoid any substance that might give your heart an extra kick.

WHEN TO SEE A DOCTOR

If your heart starts to race without any apparent reason, don't ignore the symptoms, says Pamela Ouyang, M.D., associate professor of medicine at Johns Hopkins University School of Medicine and a cardiologist at the Johns Hopkins Bayview Medical Center, both in Baltimore. Have it checked out, particularly if a racing heartbeat:

- Is accompanied by weakness, lightheadedness or shortness of breath
- Returns again and again, as opposed to occurring as an isolated episode

Temporomandibular Disorder and Jaw Pain
R and R for Your Aching Jaw

*O*ften referred to as TMJ syndrome, a temporomandibular disorder (TMD) is among the most vexing of problems: You can't open your mouth. Or you can't get it closed. Your jaw hurts so much that you're grimacing in pain. And it's making strange popping noises, like when you would crack your knuckles as a kid. And you have a Godzilla-size headache.

Also known as TMJDS, or temporomandibular joint disorder syndrome, TMD affects the jaw joint and the muscles that control chewing. Part of the reason TMD hurts is that many people who have it clench or grind their teeth—most often at night, but sometimes during the day. All that clenching and grinding can tire the jaw muscles and make you wince with pain.

If you have TMD, you might also experience severe headaches; pain in your neck, face or shoulders or clicking or grating sounds in your jaw. And you may notice that, suddenly, your upper and lower teeth no longer line up the way they used to.

The temporomandibular joint connects the lower jaw, or mandible, to the temporal bone, which is part of the skull (hence the name). When the temporomandibular joint is overstrained or injured, you hurt and can't use it as easily as when you're healthy and limber.

BLAME ESTROGEN

Women doctors say that TMD falls into three main categories. The most common form is characterized by discomfort or pain in the jaw, neck or shoulder muscles. Less common forms include a dislocated jaw or injury to the jawbone or joint diseases such as osteoarthritis or rheumatoid arthritis. A woman affected by TMD may have one or more of these conditions at the same time.

"Women are treated for TMD twice as often as men," says Donna

Massoth, D.D.S., Ph.D., a dentist and psychologist in the Department of Oral Medicine at the University of Washington in Seattle.

There may be a link with estrogen. A study of female baboons showed that they have receptors for the female hormone estrogen in the jaw—male baboon's don't. And, just as migraine headaches are linked to an increase in estrogen, the hormone also may be a factor in TMD.

BREATHE DEEP (AND LOSE THE CHEWING GUM)

For some individuals TMD pain tends to come and go. Not that TMD pain is easy to forget. Luckily, whatever the root of your TMD pain, women dentists offer these tips to help you ease the discomfort.

Try frozen corn and a hot washcloth. "Jaw pain can be relieved with ice," says Dr. Massoth. Apply an ice pack or a bag of frozen vegetables to your jaw for up to ten minutes an hour, repeating as necessary through the day.

In between icings, apply moist heat—that's a heating pad or washcloth—for 20 minutes at a time.

"Use ice for immediate, acute injury less than a day old. And use heat for older, chronic injuries. Heat will help increase circulation and relax your jaw muscles," says Barbara Rich, D.D.S., a dentist in Cherry Hill, New Jersey, and spokesperson for the Academy of General Dentistry.

Rest your jaw. As with any strained muscle or joint, the best remedy for an overtaxed jaw is rest, Dr. Rich says. "You can do that by avoiding chewy, crunchy foods like steak or French bread," she says. Also, don't cradle the phone between your neck and shoulder, and use good posture.

Stifle that yawn. Opening too wide can make your jaw hurt, says Dr. Rich. "So try not to open your mouth all the way. If you feel a yawn coming on, try to stifle it."

Go easy on that hoagie. Taking very large bites can also make your jaw hurt. To lessen the ache, take small bites. Hoagies, for example, are too big a target for an aching jaw.

Cut your food into smaller pieces and chew thoroughly and slowly to keep your jaw from aching, says Leanne Wilson, Ph.D., clinical psychologist in the Department of Oral Medicine at the University of Washington in Seattle.

Toss the chewing gum. Nervously chewing pencils, pens or chewing gum may aggravate TMD, says Dr. Wilson, so skip the chewing gum entirely and keep your writing utensils in your hand.

Massage your jaw. Gently massaging your jaw can increase the blood flow to the joint and help relieve pain.

WHEN TO SEE A DOCTOR

If you experience radiating pain in your face or mouth, painful clicking or popping in your jaw, or a sudden change in the way your teeth fit together, or if pain persists despite two weeks of self-help remedies, see a dentist.

Your dentist may suggest a bite plate, a plastic guard that fits over the upper or lower teeth, to reduce clenching or grinding and ease mucle tension. She may also suggest physical therapy and short-term use of muscle relaxants and anti-inflammatory drugs to help relieve TMD pain.

Breathe deep. "Stress and TMD are often intimately related," says Dr. Wilson. "Tension and stress can aggravate any physical ailment," she says. No surprise, then, that you're more likely to find yourself grinding your teeth before asking your boss for a raise than when you're relaxing in a sauna.

To calm yourself when you're tense and help your TMD pain subside faster, try taking a few deep breaths, says Dr. Wilson. Listening to a relaxation tape can help relax your muscles and mind even further.

Chip away at caffeine. Avoid caffeine, Dr. Massoth suggests. Caffeine wires up your nerves, which may increase muscle tension. And remember: Caffeine isn't found just in coffee, but in many teas and sodas as well as chocolate. Read labels for hidden sources of caffeine.

Stretch. "Once the severe pain of a TMD attack subsides, it's important to use your jaw muscles again," Dr. Wilson says. It's a natural tendency to baby a muscle that hurts, but if you stop opening your jaw, the muscles can tighten and end up hurting even more.

To keep your jaw limber, try this: Open as wide as you can without feeling pain, hold a few seconds, then slowly close halfway. Open again, hold a few seconds, then slowly close your mouth. Do this as often as 10 to 15 times a day, suggests Dr. Wilson. Any exercise program should be approved by your dentist, and if opening causes significantly more pain or locking or catching of the joint, it should be discontinued, she adds.

Tendinitis and Bursitis

Ease the Ouch of Playing Too Hard

*Y*ou're active. Tennis matches several times a week. Or regular step aerobics classes. Or maybe you can't get enough golf. Congratulations—you're avoiding the pitfalls of a sedentary lifestyle. But now your doctor says that you have tendinitis. Or bursitis. It's often the price women pay for doing too much too quickly.

"As the name implies, tendinitis develops when tendons, which connect muscle to bone, become inflamed," says Rosemary Agostini, M.D., clinical assistant professor of orthopedics at the University of Washington School of Medicine and sports medicine and family practice physician at the Virginia Mason Medical Center, both in Seattle. "So you feel pain."

Bursitis occurs when bursae, the fluid-filled sacs that decrease friction in the body's joints, become inflamed, Dr. Agostini says. If that occurs, you'll likely experience pain and swelling.

DIFFERENT AILMENTS, SAME REMEDIES

Tendinitis and bursitis are painful, but there are some steps that you can take right away to relieve the pain.

Stop doing what you're doing. It sounds obvious, but the last thing that you should do is try to work through the pain, as active sorts are apt to do. "Your joints are not supposed to hurt when you use them," says Dr. Agostini. "If they do, your body is trying to tell you something."

So if your shoulder hurts when you play tennis, cancel your matches until the pain subsides. Otherwise, it will only get worse, says Lynn Van Ost, P.T., a clinical specialist at the Sports Medicine Center in Philadelphia.

Make an appointment with ice. There's nothing like ice to decrease swelling and ease pain. Buy an ice pack in a drugstore or use ice from your freezer, says Dr. Agostini. Either way, wrap it in a cloth so that you don't end up with an indoor case of frostbite. Apply ice for no more than 20 minutes at a time, and repeat three or four times a day.

Elevate the joint. "If you can rest the painful joint above your heart level, you can often decrease the swelling," says Dr. Agostini. If your ankle hurts, elevate it by lying down and propping a pillow or two underneath it.

WHEN TO SEE A DOCTOR

If your tendinitis or bursitis gets worse after three or four days, or if it doesn't improve with home remedies, see your doctor for an evaluation or to rule out other conditions.

Take your medicine. An anti-inflammatory such as aspirin, ibuprofen or naproxen sodium (Aleve) taken according to package instructions will ease the pain and swelling, Dr. Agostini says.

STAYING IN THE GAME

Bursitis and tendinitis tend to flare up from time to time. So women experts recommend the following precautions to help keep these conditions at bay.

Move that joint. It's natural to want to avoid pain, but if you baby your shoulder by trying not to use it, you will get stiff, and you'll be more likely to hurt yourself again, says Van Ost.

After the initial pain subsides, "make sure to do some simple exercises to keep your joint flexible," says Van Ost. If you have shoulder pain brought on by tendinitis, for example, Van Ost recommends four movements that can help. Each begins with your arm hanging down at your side. First, raise your arm straight in front of you until it is over your head, and lower it back to the starting point. Then raise your arm out to the side and lower. For the third exercise, extend your arm to the side so that it's perpendicular to your body and rotate it toward yourself. Return to the starting position. The final exercise is similar to the third, but you rotate your arm away from you. Repeat each of the motions ten times before moving onto the next exercise. "Do the routine consistently one or two times a day, so that you maintain flexibility, but don't overuse or irritate the joint," says Van Ost.

Get stronger. Another good way to combat tendinitis and bursitis brought on by overusing a particular joint is to make sure that your limb is up to the tasks that you set for it, Dr. Agostini says.

Van Ost's advice: Try specific exercises designed for the joint that's aching. For example, if you have bursitis of the knee, try riding a stationary bicycle on medium pedal resistance, adjusted so that you have no knee discomfort, for five to ten minutes.

Do sport-specific stretches. Careful stretching prevents tightness and is important in treating both bursitis and tendinitis, Dr. Agostini says. Stretch for at least five to ten minutes after activity.

Cross-train. You love playing tennis, but hate tendinitis? You don't have to give up the sport you love, but you can vary your routine. "Take every other day off from tennis and go swimming or take a walk instead," says Van Ost.

Check your grip. If you play tennis, check your racket size. Sometimes women end up with tendinitis because they're playing with a racket that's too big or too small for them to grip comfortably. "To prevent overuse injuries, check with a qualified instructor or pro-shop staffer to make sure that you're using the right size racket," Dr. Agostini says.

Replace worn-out workout shoes. A worn-out, worn-down heel on a walking or running shoe can contribute to tendinitis, "so make sure that your footwear is comfortable and in good condition," says Dr. Agostini.

Tinnitus

Noises Only You Can Hear

Imagine listening to chirps, roars, whirring, buzzes or rings—annoying noises that only you can hear—over and over and over again. That's the devilish lot of people with tinnitus.

"Tinnitus—internal head noises with no external source—may accompany hearing loss," says Carol Flexer, Ph.D., an audiologist and professor of audiology at the School of Communicative Disorders at the University of Akron in Ohio.

People who have been exposed to noise regularly for most of their lives—musicians, carpenters and pilots, for example—are among those most commonly affected by tinnitus, says Laura Orvidas, M.D., senior associate consultant and instructor in the Department of Otorhinolaryngology at the Mayo Clinic in Rochester, Minnesota.

"And more and more young adults are complaining of tinnitus,"

WHEN TO SEE A DOCTOR

"Tinnitus is like a headache," says Anita T. Pikus, chief of clinical audiology at the National Institute of Deafness and Other Communication Disorders at the National Institutes of Health in Bethesda, Maryland. "Everyone experiences it, and there are many different causes—and many different treatments."

If you hear noises that others don't hear—like ringing, buzzing, roaring, whirring and so forth—make an appointment with an audiologist or an otolaryngologist. She will make a thorough evaluation and will, if necessary, refer you to the appropriate medical specialist.

says Kathy Peck, executive director of H.E.A.R. (Hearing, Education and Awareness for Rockers) in San Francisco. She predicts that teenagers who attend rock concerts regularly will likely experience tinnitus and other noise-induced hearing problems at earlier ages.

More than 200 prescription and over-the-counter drugs (including aspirin, quinine and some antibiotics) can trigger tinnitus as a possible side effect, says Gloria Reich, Ph.D., executive director of the American Tinnitus Association in Portland, Oregon. Tinnitus can also be caused or aggravated by cardiovascular disease, stress, allergies, an underactive thyroid or degeneration of bones in the middle ear.

Diagnosis is simple, say doctors.

"If you think that you have tinnitus, you have tinnitus," says Dr. Reich.

FOCUS ON CAUSE FIRST

Tinnitus is rarely a sign of anything serious or life-threatening. Nevertheless, you should have it checked out to rule out medical causes from the outset. "See an otolaryngologist (a medical doctor specializing in ear and related problems)," says Dr. Reich.

"Focus first on the cause, then on the treatment," says Dr. Reich. Otherwise, self-help measures may be of no avail.

If tinnitus is confirmed, here's what you can do.

Mask the noise. "Keep a radio tuned to static (between radio channels) on or a fan going at bedtime," says Dr. Reich. "Tinnitus is more noticeable when your surroundings are quiet. So masking tinnitus with other noises can help quite a bit."

Plug in a white-noise machine. If a whirring fan or radio static doesn't work, Dr. Flexer suggests special devices that play white noise— nondescript sounds that resemble static. Another helpful distraction includes playing a machine, tape or CD that recreates the sound of waves or wind, says Dr. Flexer. "These tinnitus maskers may relieve people of their tinnitus totally," says Dr. Flexer. "The theory is that white noise trains the nerves to stop sending messages when there's no noise stimulus."

Cut down on the coffee. "Caffeine is a stimulant, and stimulants can aggravate tinnitus," says Dr. Orvidas.

Nix cigarettes, salt, sugar and alcohol. For some, tinnitus abates when they stop smoking or reduce their salt or sugar consumption, says Dr. Orvidas. Drinking alcohol can exacerbate tinnitus.

Wear earplugs and noise protectors when exposed to loud noises. No matter what your tinnitus is related to, it's wise to prevent future damage, says Dr. Reich. "You can still enjoy the fireworks on July fourth," she adds. "Just be prepared for the noise with earplugs."

Give ginkgo a try. "Though some of the scientific studies appear contradictory, some evidence suggests that ginkgo may be effective in reducing tinnitus," says Dr. Reich. Ginkgo is a tree whose fan-shaped leaves have been used by the Chinese for thousands of years to cure a variety of ailments. Researchers theorize that ginkgo may help increase blood flow to the brain, which could improve tinnitus caused by circulatory problems.

"Some people have used ginkgo for tinnitus with promising results," says Dr. Reich. "Since the side effects are rare and few, it's safe to try," she says. Experts recommend 120 milligrams daily of a concentrated, standardized ginkgo extract called GBE (ginkgo biloba extract), purchased from an established health food store. Note, however, that if ginkgo works, it may take weeks or months to notice improvement.

Toothache
Subdue That Throb

*A*mong the Top 10 Pains Most Women Want to Avoid, a toothache has to rank right up there with Don Rickles.

Your tooth may ache for any number of reasons. Tooth decay—caused by acids from an accumulation of bacteria-laden plaque on your teeth and beneath your gums—is number one, says Carole Palmer, R.D., Ed.D., professor and co-head of the Division of Nutrition and Preventive Dentistry in the Department of General Dentistry at Tufts University School of Dental Medicine in Boston.

Women seem to have eating habits custom-made for the plaque attack. "Women tend to be snackers and nibblers," says Dr. Palmer. Each time a sugar or refined carbohydrate settles on your teeth (and that includes sweets, juice, milk, sweetened colas, breath mints and fruits), it provides a tasty meal for the bacteria that live in the plaque in your mouth. For the next 20 minutes or more, acid forms. If your teeth and gums are susceptible, you could be on your way to a cavity, gum disease or an abscess, all of which can cause a toothache.

NURSING YOUR ACHING TOOTHE

Women doctors unanimously agree: If you have a toothache, don't ignore the pain, hoping that it will get better. Pick up the phone, call your dentist and ask for an immediate appointment. The hints offered here are meant to get you through the night until you're safely in the dentist's chair and are not intended as a substitute for medical attention.

Floss. Sometimes a tiny piece of food, like a popcorn hull, can get trapped under your gum line, causing pain and an eventual abscess, says Heidi K. Hausauer, D.D.S., instructor of operative dentistry at the University of the Pacific Dental School in San Francisco and spokesperson for the Academy of General Dentistry.

Give it a chilly reception. An ice pack applied to the outside of your cheek might numb the region enough to give you some relief, says Caren Barnes, R.D.H., professor of clinical dentistry at the University of Alabama School of Dentistry in Birmingham. "But sometimes people

WHEN TO SEE A DOCTOR

No doubt about it: "Any time you have a toothache, you have to go to the dentist," says Caren Barnes, R.D.H., professor of clinical dentistry at the University of Alabama School of Dentistry in Birmingham.

Even if your pain subsides, don't cancel your appointment. The pulp of your tooth may have gone dead, while bacteria continue to multiply, with serious ramifications.

with toothaches are so temperature-sensitive, it's better just to leave the tooth alone."

Heat, too, may make a toothache worse, especially if it's a throbbing, pulsating pain caused by inflammation, says Carol Bibb, D.D.S., Ph.D., adjunct associate professor at the University of California, Los Angeles, School of Dentistry.

Walk away tooth pain. After her husband underwent root canal treatment, Dr. Bibb noticed him pacing around waiting for pain medication to take effect. In effect, she says, her husband was self-medicating without knowing it. "Exercise, or do whatever distracts you," says Dr. Bibb.

Twenty-five minutes or so of brisk walking, cycling or some other aerobic (heart-pumping) activity will trigger your brain to release natural feel-good substances called endorphins and supply a dose of pain relief, says practicing psychologist Marian R. Stuart, Ph.D., clinical professor of family medicine at the University of Medicine and Dentistry of New Jersey Robert Wood Johnson Medical School in New Brunswick.

(For practical tips on how to avoid toothache and gingivitis in the first place, see page 242.)

Tooth Discoloration
White Out Yellow Stains

*I*f you're like most adult women, the years have taken their toll on your pearly whites, tingeing your teeth with a yellowish hue.

"Women start to notice a change in the color of their teeth in their late thirties," says Fay Goldstep, D.D.S., a dentist in private practice in Markham, Ontario.

Some tooth discoloration can be traced to personal habits: Smoking yellows your teeth, and daily exposure to coffee, tea and cola drinks leaves behind brownish stains. There are also a whole variety of sometimes unexpected sources: tetracycline and other medications, severe attacks of certain childhood diseases such as measles or whooping cough, naturally super-fluoridated drinking water and even swimming frequently in a treated pool.

BRIGHTER TEETH CAN BE YOURS

If your teeth are less lustrous than you'd like, you're not alone. Dr. Goldstep estimates that three out of four women she treats in her dental practice express concern about the hue of their teeth and ask her advice about how to brighten them up.

Women dentists and other dental care professionals say that there are some things you can do at home to spiff up your smile, especially if your stains are superficial.

Chase your coffee with gum. Munch on a piece of sugarless gum after you've had your coffee or tea. Doing so will produce more saliva to swish away the darkening liquids before they have a chance to stain your teeth, says Carole Palmer, R.D., Ed.D., professor and co-head of the Division of Nutrition and Preventive Dentistry in the Department of General Dentistry at Tufts University School of Dental Medicine in Boston. Follow it up with a brushing and flossing, and you can keep ahead of the problem, she says.

Sip and smile. Dr. Palmer also suggests you stop by the office watercooler after eating or drinking a stain-producing food or beverage, like blueberries or coffee. Merely rinsing your mouth will help cleanse your teeth and prevent stains from accumulating, she says.

Don't rush when you brush. You'd be surprised how much cleaner your teeth can be by brushing effectively with a soft-bristled toothbrush and the proper technique, Dr. Palmer says. "People concentrate on how often they brush, without worrying about how effective they are," she says.

Start with your bottom teeth. Debbie Zehnder, R.D.H., a dental hygienist in suburban Philadelphia, tells women bothered by surface stains to put a pea-size drop of toothpaste on the brush, then start with the area that tends to accumulate the most tartar, which, for many people, seems to be the lower front teeth. "Most people start in with the molars, in the back, but if you tend to get more tartar buildup on your front teeth, this isn't the best method, because most of the toothpaste is gone or diluted," she says.

Skip the kits. Home bleaching kits sometimes require that you wear firm plastic molds that look a little like athletic mouth guards. But unlike those custom-fitted by your dentist, the over-the-counter variety can irritate your gums, says Dr. Goldstep.

Toss the butts. Common sense also says that if you smoke, your tooth-whitening tactics will be in vain. So if you quit, chances are you'll have prettier teeth, says Dr. Goldstep.

Tooth Grinding
Gnash No More

ost women who grind their teeth don't even know it—until their husbands tell them that they grind their teeth while they sleep, or their dentists see the wear and tear on their tooth surfaces.

Some women grind their teeth when they're nervous or concentrating hard at work. Maybe you clench your jaw in heavy traffic, or when your next-door neighbor does something that she knows will annoy you.

Tooth grinding (or bruxism, as it's known) isn't normal, says Geraldine Morrow, D.M.D., past president of the American Dental Associa-

WHEN TO SEE A DOCTOR

If your jaws ache in the morning, or if you get frequent headaches, and especially if your partner tells you that you're grinding your teeth at night, you should visit your dentist to see if you're damaging your teeth, says Geraldine Morrow, D.M.D., past president of the American Dental Association, a member of the American Association of Women Dentists and a dentist in Anchorage, Alaska.

A dentist or a medical doctor can treat tooth grinding (bruxism) with custom-fitted mouth appliances to protect your teeth while you sleep; relaxation therapies, including biofeedback, or (if needed) prescription medications.

tion, a member of the American Association of Women Dentists and a dentist in Anchorage, Alaska. And it's not good for you.

"Your teeth are not supposed to touch, except for fractions of seconds when you swallow," says Dr. Morrow.

WHY WOMEN GNASH THEIR TEETH

A study conducted at Duquesne University in Pittsburgh found that women who gnash their teeth tend to be hard-driving, impatient and worried. If you fit that description, the worn enamel on your teeth and your aching jaw may be telling you to relax a little and give yourself an emotional break.

Stress contributes to tooth grinding, but it isn't the only cause. Tooth and jaw misalignments may play a role. Whatever the cause, tooth grinding needs to be brought under control, or it can lead to serious problems, including headaches, jaw pain, fatigue, tooth sensitivity and wear, temporomandibular disorder, even changes in your facial appearance and bone loss.

MORE THAN AN ANNOYANCE

If your dentist has confirmed that you grind your teeth and should do something about it, women doctors offer these tips for kicking the habit.

Relax your jaw. "Consciously keep your jaws relaxed and your teeth apart," advises Dr. Morrow.

Follow the dots. Try this handy way to remind yourself to unclench your teeth, as suggested by Heidi K. Hausauer, D.D.S., instructor of operative dentistry at the University of the Pacific Dental School in San Francisco and spokesperson for the Academy of General Dentistry: Buy a sheet or two of orange dot stickers, available at stores that sell tablets and writing supplies. Paste them everywhere: on your mirror, your dashboard, your television and your refrigerator door. Every time you see one, says Dr. Hausauer, separate your teeth.

Huff and puff. "Exercise!" advises practicing psychologist Marian R. Stuart, Ph.D., clinical professor of family medicine at the University of Medicine and Dentistry of New Jersey Robert Wood Johnson Medical School in New Brunswick and co-author of *Coping with the Stressed-Out People in Your Life.* "It's good for stress, it clears your head, and if you do it for more than 25 minutes, it prompts your brain to release natural feel-good substances called endorphins." As an added benefit, endorphins act as pain relievers, too, for when your head and jaw are throbbing reminders of your night grinding.

Try herbal tea or warm milk before bedtime. Some research suggests that alcohol before bed can exacerbate your tooth grinding. Have a cup of relaxing herbal tea with honey or warm milk instead, Dr. Stuart suggests.

Shower yourself with relief. "Sore muscles respond to moist heat," says Carol Bibb, D.D.S., Ph.D., adjunct associate professor at the University of California, Los Angeles, School of Dentistry. Dr. Bibb says that stretching gently in the shower may make your jaw and neck feel better, as will a hot, moist compress.

(For practical ways to manage stress, see page 521. For information on temporomandibular disorder, see page 534.)

Tooth Sensitivity
Eat and Drink without Pain

*T*he annoying thing about tooth sensitivity is that even though it doesn't last long, its lightning bolt of pain strikes when you least expect it: sipping an ice-cold glass of lemonade on the front porch, sharing a cup of cappuccino with an old friend or laughing out loud as you ice-skate with your kids.

The trouble occurs when something riles the nerve endings of your teeth.

Remember how you learned in grade school that enamel is the hardest substance in the human body? Well, when the enamel gets worn away, through overly aggressive brushing, dental work, tooth grinding or acidic foods or drinks (such as lemons or soft drinks), you can expose a network of fluid-filled tunnels called dentin tubules that lead right into the nerve of your tooth.

What triggers the pain varies greatly from woman to woman, says Carole Palmer, R.D., Ed.D., professor and co-head of the Division of Nutrition and Preventive Dentistry in the Department of General Dentistry at Tufts University School of Dental Medicine in Boston. Sweets might make one woman jump out of her pumps, while hot or cold foods or tart or acidic foods might be the undoing of another, she says.

STOPGAP MEASURES FOR TOOTH PAIN

"The obvious solution is to stay away from what bothers you," says Dr. Palmer. "If hot and cold foods bother you, stay away from extremes."

Be sure to seek dental care to resolve the problem, since tooth sensitivity isn't normal, says Dr. Palmer. In the meantime, here are some ways that you can enjoy life's simple pleasures without the stabbing intrusion of unexpected pain.

Go easy with the toothbrush. All too often, women brush their teeth vigorously, as if they're scrubbing a floor, says Diane Schoen, dental hygienist, clinical assistant professor and coordinator of the Preventive Dentistry Program at the University of Medicine and Dentistry of New Jersey in Newark. Gentle and thorough is a better way to remove the

WHEN TO SEE A DOCTOR

If one of your teeth is extremely sensitive to either hot or cold pressure and the rest of your teeth aren't, you might have a cavity or a tooth fracture, says Mahvash Navazesh, D.M.D., associate professor and vice-chair in the Department of Dental Medicine and Public Health at the University of Southern California School of Dentistry in Los Angeles. In such a case, see your dentist.

If you have generalized tooth sensitivity that doesn't go away after a few weeks, see your dentist. She can give you a prescription fluoride treatment that you can apply at home to toughen up your tooth surfaces and, if necessary, she can bond your teeth to protect your nerve endings from external irritants, says Dr. Navazesh.

If your discomfort is more widespread because of habits like grinding or clenching, a dentist can fit you with a mouth guard to wear at night or make sure that you don't have an uneven tooth or filling that is exerting extra pressure on a nearby spot in your mouth, Dr. Navazesh says.

"Nobody should walk around with sensitive teeth on a regular basis," she says.

sticky buildup of plaque-ridden bacteria that you're trying to get rid of, she says. Proper technique, not elbow grease, is key.

Trade in your toothbrush for a softer model. "I generally recommend a soft brush for everyone, and extra soft for women who already have abrasion," says Schoen.

Switch toothpastes. Women commonly fall into the trap of buying toothpastes that promise to whiten and brighten their teeth to a sparkling sheen, says Geraldine Morrow, D.M.D., past president of the American Dental Association, a member of a American Association of Women Dentists and a dentist in Anchorage, Alaska. The problem with some of those toothpastes is that they are so abrasive and harsh that they can actually undermine the enamel on your teeth, says Dr. Morrow. Instead, choose a brand made for sensitive teeth (like Sensodyne). They contain one of two protective ingredients—strontium chloride or potassium nitrate—that over time will block painful sensations being sent to your tooth's nerves.

"These products work pretty well," says Caren Barnes, R.D.H., professor of clinical dentistry at the University of Alabama School of Dentistry in Birmingham.

Dab on some fluoride. The reason dentists apply a powerful fluoride gel to sensitive teeth is to toughen them. "At home, use a heavily fluoridated toothpaste, approved by the American Dental Association, and rub it into the sensitive areas of your teeth several times a day," says Dr. Morrow.

Watch what you eat. A diet soda with a lemon twist may save you some calories, but it could cost you your enamel. If your teeth are sensitive, limit your intake of highly acidic foods like tomatoes and citrus fruits and beverages like soft drinks, says Dr. Morrow. Drink skim milk or water instead.

Ulcers
New Causes, New Cures

The way digestion normally works, you chew and swallow your food, and it travels from your esophagus to your stomach. There the food is digested by hydrochloric acid and an enzyme called pepsin.

After that, food goes into the upper part of your small intestine (called the duodenum), where digestion continues.

When you have an ulcer, a sore forms in the lining of your stomach or duodenum, where acid eats away at your stomach lining. Though men traditionally were thought to develop more ulcers than women, the numbers are approximately equal, though no one knows for sure why, says Marie L. Borum, M.D., assistant professor of medicine in the Division of Gastroenterology and Nutrition at George Washington University Medical Center in Washington, D.C. Women are more likely to get stomach (gastric) ulcers; men are more likely to get duodenal ulcers (or ulcers in the duodenum).

The most common ulcer symptom is a gnawing or burning pain in the abdomen between the breastbone and the navel, occurring most often between meals and in the early morning hours.

THE INVASION OF THE SPIRAL-SHAPED BACTERIA

How and why does acid cause the inflammation that we call an ulcer? For years doctors thought that the acid erosion was caused by a rich diet, spicy foods, alcohol, smoking cigarettes or maybe stress. Now, research shows that a spiral-shaped bacteria called *Helicobacter pylori* (*H. pylori*) may also have a role in the development of ulcers.

Researchers know that *H. pylori* is an airborne bacteria, but they don't yet know where the bacteria come from or how infection occurs, says Melissa Palmer, M.D., a gastroenterologist in private practice in New York City. Researchers believe that ulcers develop when the bacteria penetrate the digestive tract's protective lining and settle in the stomach or small intestine, making the cell lining more susceptible to the damaging effects of acid and pepsin.

Ulcers not caused by *H. pylori* generally are caused by aspirin and nonsteroidal anti-inflammatory agents such as ibuprofen, says Barbara Frank, M.D., gastroenterologist and clinical professor of medicine at Allegheny University of the Health Sciences MCP–Hahnemann School of Medicine in Philadelphia.

Acid can be neutralized with antacid medication. Acid production can be reduced with over-the-counter H_2 (histamine 2) blockers, which suppress the release of histamines, such as Tagamet HB and Pepcid AC. Both suppress acid at the pathway where most of it is made (the "histamine pathway"), says Dr. Borum.

If you've been diagnosed with an ulcer, it's important that your doctor determine whether *H. pylori* is present. When *H. pylori* infection is certain, a course of antibiotic treatment is prescribed, in combination with drugs that suppress gastric acid, to heal ulcers while reducing risk of ulcer recurrence. The great news: "Antibiotic treatment cures ulcers, so there is no longer any such thing as a chronic ulcer," says Dr. Palmer. Evidence from the United States and Europe has shown that the use of antibiotics can heal ulcers caused by *H. pylori* and prevent their recurrence in about 90 percent of the cases.

CODDLE YOUR STOMACH

That said, women doctors say that there may be a few lifestyle changes that women diagnosed with ulcers can and should make to quicken the healing of an ulcer and lessen the chances of a flare-up.

Shun caffeine and citrus. These can slow the healing rate of existing ulcers, says Dr. Borum. Though experts no longer think that specific

WHEN TO SEE A DOCTOR

See your doctor if you experience:
- Severe pain between your breastbone and navel, especially between meals or early in the morning
- Blood in your stool
- Unexplained nausea
- Vomiting
- Weight loss
- Loss of appetite

Maybe you have an ulcer, and maybe you don't. A doctor can sort it out.

foods cause ulcers, you should still avoid foods that may aggravate symptoms, like coffee, citrus foods and juices.

For aches, pains or headaches, stick to acetaminophen. If you can avoid it, don't take aspirin, says Dr. Frank. That's because those ulcers not caused by *H. pylori* are now associated with aspirin and other nonsteroid painkillers such as ibuprofen.

Put out your butts. "Cigarette smoking increases your chances of getting an ulcer," Dr. Palmer says. Tobacco simultaneously impairs your digestive system's protective lining and stimulates the production of acid. Smoking also slows the healing of existing ulcers and contributes to their recurrence.

Drink Virgin Marys. "Alcohol inflames your stomach lining, which will irritate existing ulcers and may help cause them," says Dr. Palmer.

Underweight

Look Svelte, Not Scrawny

*W*hile most women find it all too easy to put on an extra ten pounds, others eat like mad and can't seem to gain.

If you're underweight, you're probably accustomed to envious comments from friends. And while some research indicates that slightly below average weight may lower your risk of heart disease, high cholesterol and diabetes, excessive thinness is another story.

"For women, the most important indicator that they're medically underweight is if they start having menstrual irregularities," says Mary Ellen Sweeney, M.D., obesity researcher at Emory University School of Medicine and an endocrinologist and director of the Lipid Metabolism Clinics at the Veterans Affairs Medical Center, both in Atlanta. This sometimes occurs in women who overexercise, particularly marathon runners. And estrogen levels drop when women don't eat enough to meet their needs.

Underweight women who don't menstruate have a hard time becoming pregnant later on, says Dr. Sweeney. And over time, low levels of estrogen can erode bone density, which can lead to osteoporosis (brittle bone disease).

WHEN TO SEE A DOCTOR

Some women are naturally thin and don't give it much thought. That's no cause for alarm. But others have an intense fear of gaining weight or becoming fat, even though they already weigh less than normal. If you fit this description, you may be developing an eating disorder, says Bonnie Worthington-Roberts, Ph.D., professor in the Nutritional Sciences Program at the University of Washington in Seattle. See your doctor or contact the National Association of Anorexia Nervosa and Associated Disorders, Box 7, Highland Park, Illinois 60035.

Also, any unintentional weight loss of more than ten pounds warrants medical attention.

Say Yes to Sweet Treats

Bonnie Worthington-Roberts, Ph.D.

Blame it on what she calls a busy metabolism. Bonnie Worthington-Roberts, Ph.D., professor in the Nutritional Sciences Program at the University of Washington in Seattle, knows how hard it is to gain weight, because she's been trying to put on pounds herself. Her method? Indulging herself with sweet treats once she has eaten her "real" meals.

"I'm five feet five inches and weigh 116 pounds," says Dr. Worthington-Roberts. "I'm kind of bony in spots, and I'd just like to fill out a little. So I'm trying to gain five to ten pounds.

"Once I've done the nutritious thing, then I go for the ice cream. For the past five months I've been really digging into pie and cake and ice cream."

Dr. Worthington-Roberts has several pounds to go, so she figures that gaining the weight will take some time. "Meanwhile, this stuff is fun to eat."

INDULGE WISELY

If you think that you could use some extra weight, here are some suggestions from women doctors.

Indulge in a little fat. "Everyone is bent on eating less fat, but less fat usually gives you fewer calories," says Bonnie Worthington-Roberts, Ph.D., professor in the Nutritional Sciences Program at the University of Washington in Seattle. "If your blood cholesterol is within normal limits, you can be less rigorous about fat."

So start with a bean-grain-vegetable diet, but then go ahead and add a pat of butter to your baked potato, and say yes to that rich dessert, Dr. Worthington-Roberts says. Just make sure to keep the fat to no more than 40 percent of your diet, or 600 calories if you're trying to take in 1,500 calories a day.

Try a liquid supplement. Liquid food supplements such as Ensure or Sustacal, available in supermarkets and drugstores, contain about 250 calories per can and are usually fortified with a good portion of all the essential vitamins and minerals. "One can is a whopping dose of good nutrition," says Dr. Worthington-Roberts.

Optimally, supplements should be used as just that—additions, rather than substitutes, for regular meals, says Dr. Worthington-Roberts. But if you just can't eat breakfast, a supplement is better than no food at all, because it will get needed calories into your body.

Build up with weights. If you feel weak and scrawny, a weight-training program can help you get stronger, says Kathleen Little, Ph.D., exercise physiologist and professor at the University of North Carolina at Chapel Hill. She suggests working out with barbells or dumbbells or—if you have access to a gym—weight-resistance equipment, two or three times a week for 30 minutes.

Unwanted Hair
At-Home Removal Options

A full head of hair is to be envied. But luxuriant growth of hair on your upper lip has considerably less appeal. And many women consider even normal amounts of underarm or leg hair fashionably unacceptable.

"Hair always seems to grow where it's not supposed to and disappears from where you want it to grow," says Allison Vidimos, M.D., a staff dermatologist at the Cleveland Clinic Foundation.

SHAVE OR WAX?

If a little extra hair doesn't bother you, fine. Otherwise, here's what experts consider the most effective ways to get rid of unwanted hair.

Ready, set, shave. "Shaving is the easiest way to remove hair," says Dr. Vidimos. Using an electric shaver is a cinch. But a double-edged razor will give you a closer shave. To use a razor, wash the area to be shaved, then apply a shaving foam or gel to lubricate your skin and ready your unwanted hair for removal. When you're finished, rinse well, pat dry and apply a soothing moisturizer. (For special directions on shaving your bikini line, see page 51.)

555

WHEN TO SEE A DOCTOR

"If you never had unwanted hair in unusual places and new, coarse hair pops up on your upper lip, chin, cheeks, center of your chest or above your normal pubic line, it's time to check with a doctor," says Allison Vidimos, M.D., a staff dermatologist at the Cleveland Clinic Foundation.

Abnormal hair growth, accompanied by irregular menstrual periods, thinning scalp hair, acne, deepening of the voice, increased muscle strength, increased sex drive or an enlarged clitoris can suggest a number of conditions, including a temporary hormone imbalance or an inherited adrenal gland condition, says Dr. Vidimos. Frequently, all that's necessary is to rebalance your hormones.

Repeat as needed. Shaved hair will start to grow back within a day or two, so if you opt for shaving, you'll have to shave a couple of times a week or more, says Dr. Vidimos. To avoid shaving-related rashes, bumps or irritation, be sure to use a fresh blade after three or four shaves.

Pick up a waxing kit. Waxing takes more time and preparation, and it isn't quite as painless as shaving, but your hair won't grow in as quickly, because the entire hair is removed from the follicle. But don't try hot waxing, says Dr. Vidimos. Hot waxing is tricky and, applied inexpertly, can harm your skin. For home use, she recommends the precut wax strips sold in over-the-counter hair-removal kits at your local drugstore.

Take a soapless shower. When you're ready to wax, take a warm shower, says Sam McKee (a woman), vice-president of product development in the Sally Hansen division of Del Laboratories in Farmington, New York. Use no soap and apply no moisturizers afterward—they interfere with applying the wax. Dry yourself thoroughly with a towel.

Powder up. If you plan to wax your legs or underarms, sprinkle talcum powder on the area to be waxed, says Natasha Salman, a face treatment and waxing specialist at Elizabeth Arden's Red Door Salon in New York City. It will help the wax grab hold of your hair and remove it more efficiently.

Study the box. For best results and to prevent potential problems with waxing, read and follow the directions, says McKee.

Work with your hair, not against it. Press the wax strips on your skin in the direction in which your hair grows, says McKee. If you're waxing your lower leg, for example, start at your knee, then continue down your leg to your ankle.

Rub, rub, rub. To warm the wax and make it stick better, rub the wax strip with your hands for several minutes after it's applied, suggests McKee.

Strip against the grain. Once the wax has hardened—it takes about ten minutes—pull the strips off against the direction in which your hair grows, says McKee. Otherwise, not all the hair will come off.

Apply a soothing lotion (or ice). Most over-the-counter hair-removal kits contain a lotion with a topical anesthetic such as benzocaine, plus skin soothers such as vitamin E and collagen, to ease postwaxing pain, says Dr. Vidimos. You can also reduce pain by appling cold compresses for 10 to 15 minutes, she says.

If the area remains irritated, says Salman, smooth on a combination of calamine lotion and zinc oxide, such as Elizabeth Arden's Soothing Lotion, available at most major department stores.

"An over-the-counter hydrocortisone cream may also help relieve red, irritated skin," says Dr. Vidimos.

Wait to rewax. Wait until your hair is around a quarter-inch long before you wax it once again, says Salman—about four weeks. If you rewax too soon, there won't be enough hair for the wax to grab onto.

THE CHEMICAL ROUTE

Depilatories are hair-removal creams and lotions that use strong chemicals to dissolve hair. As with waxing, hair takes a few weeks to grow back after you use a depilatory, so you don't need to use it as often.

For pleasing results, experts offer these tips.

Select the right product for the job. Be sure to select a product formulated for the area that needs hair removal, says McKee. Use a facial depilatory if you're removing hair from your face, for example, or an underarm depilatory if that's where you're working. Manufacturers are careful to vary the strength of depilatories to various parts of the body on which they're used and various types of hair (fine, normal or coarse). So using the right product will reduce your chances of irritation.

Test a small area. Depilatories may cause an irritant reaction, cautions Dr. Vidimos. So before you use a depilatory for the first time, smear a quarter-size amount of the preparation on your forearm, let it sit for the amount of time specified on the package (usually three minutes) and wipe it off. Wait 24 hours. If any itching, redness or irritation develops, don't use the product. If nothing happens, proceed.

Apply and wait. Apply the depilatory and let it set for about three minutes (or according to package directions). To remove the cream, scrub the area with a washcloth or body sponge for about three minutes, says McKee. Scrubbing removes hair along with the cream.

Rinse and moisturize. To remove every trace of a chemical hair remover, says McKee, rinse the area well, then moisturize your skin with your favorite skin lotion.

Urinary Tract Infections
Ease the Urgent, Burning Pain

*Y*ou need to go to the bathroom. Again. When you go, hardly any urine trickles out. And when it does, it burns. Within half an hour you get the urge again, so you go again—with the same results.

So it goes with a urinary tract infection (UTI). Bacteria enter the urethra, or urine tube, that enters the bladder, and set up shop. If the infection is limited to the urethra, it's called urethritis. More often than not, the infection travels farther up the tract and into the bladder, which is called cystitis (or, simply, a bladder infection). Unless treated promptly, a bladder infection can move to the kidneys, leading to a more serious condition called pyelonephritis.

Although a woman can have a UTI without knowing it, common signs and symptoms include pain and a burning sensation when urinating, urinating frequently, voiding just a few drops at a time or passing blood in the urine.

"Most women get one or two urinary tract infections at some time in their lives, and for the most part, physicians don't really know what causes them," notes Linda Brubaker, M.D., director of the Section of Urogynecology and Reconstructive Pelvic Surgery at Rush-Presbyterian–

St. Luke's Medical Center in Chicago.

"In these women the cells that line the urethra are stickier, making it easier for the bacteria to adhere," explains Kimberly A. Workowski, M.D., assistant professor of medicine in the Division of Infectious Diseases at Emory University in Atlanta.

Women who use certain birth control methods, such as spermicides containing nonoxynol-9, are also at higher risk for UTIs. "This ingredient alters the bacterial balance in the vagina, allowing growth of *E. coli*, the bacteria that causes most UTIs," says Dr. Brubaker. Nonoxynol-9 is found in spermicidal jellies, spermicidal foams or inserts and condoms with spermicidal lubricant.

ANTIBACTERIAL STRATEGIES

If a urine culture indicates that you have a UTI, your doctor will probably prescribe antibiotics. In addition to taking the medication, here's what you can do to relieve symptoms and prevent future recurrences.

Fix yourself a baking soda cocktail. "At the first sign of symptoms, mix half a teaspoon of baking soda in an eight-ounce glass of water and drink it," says Kristene E. Whitmore, M.D., chief of urology and director of the Incontinence Center at Graduate Hospital in Philadelphia. The baking soda raises the pH (acid-base balance) of irritating, acidic urine.

Drink water, on the hour. Drink one glass of water every hour for eight hours, continues Dr. Whitmore.

"Drinking a lot of fluids will increase urine flow," explains Dr. Workowski. "This will wash out the bacteria that are attempting to adhere to the cells lining your urethra. Drinking plenty of water will also help dilute and flush out the substances that are causing the irritation. Drink enough water so that your urine is clear. Aim for at least eight or ten glasses of water a day."

"Hydration is the best thing that you can do for a UTI," adds Dr. Whitmore. "Drinking water is fashionable, it's good for you and women I treat say that it's more effective than drug treatment."

Carry a bike bottle with you. So suggests Jean Kallhoff, advanced registered nurse practitioner at the Urology Clinic at the University of Washington Medical Center in Seattle. "It's handy, it's easy to carry and it reminds women to drink water throughout the day."

Reach for cranberry juice. "According to a study in the *Journal of the American Medical Association*, cranberry juice can prevent bacteria from sticking to cells that line the urinary tract," says Dr. Workowski.

WHEN TO SEE A DOCTOR

If you have more than two urinary tract infections (or what you think are urinary tract infections) in 6 months, or more than three episodes in 12 months, see a doctor, says Kristene E. Whitmore, M.D., chief of urology and director of the Incontinence Center at Graduate Hospital in Philadelphia.

"It's critical that we get the message out to women that if they have recurrent symptoms, they need to check with their doctors and ask for a urine culture," says Linda Brubaker, M.D., director of the Section of Urogynecology and Reconstructive Pelvic Surgery at Rush-Presbyterian–St. Luke's Medical Center in Chicago. "Just because you have symptoms, it does not mean that you have an infection. There's a difference between having inflammation in your urethra, which can cause sensitivity and irritation, and having a bacterial infection. I've seen women who were eating antibiotics by the pound for years, and they never had an infection to begin with. Many women think that they have a bladder infection every month, but they don't."

Women doctors say that you should always consult a physician if you experience any of the following symptoms.
- Blood in your urine
- Chills
- Nausea
- Vomiting
- Lower-back pain

You should also see a doctor if you've been diagnosed with a urinary tract infection and the symptoms don't start clearing up within two days.

"Plenty of anecdotal evidence says that cranberry juice works," adds Dr. Whitmore. "I know it works for my patients."

Dilute the juice. Women doctors caution that in some women with urinary tract sensitivity, cranberry juice can act as an irritant. "Some of my patients get worse when they drink a lot of cranberry juice," warns Dr. Brubaker. "That might be because of its high acid content." Dr. Whitmore suggests diluting the juice. If that doesn't help, stop drinking the juice altogether, says Dr. Brubaker.

Nix other offenders. Whether you have a simple irritation or an infected urinary tract, the last thing that you need are known bladder irritants. The most notorious bladder irritants are citrus, tomatoes, aged cheeses, chocolate, spicy foods, caffeine, alcohol and nicotine, says Dr. Whitmore.

For certain individuals, anything carbonated—especially beer or soda—may irritate your bladder and make you go more frequently or urgently, says Kallhoff.

Vitamin C supplements may also be a problem, says Dr. Brubaker.

Avoid artificial sweeteners. "Artificial sweeteners are among the worst offenders," says Dr. Whitmore. So if you have a UTI, avoid them.

Apply soothing heat. To ease the pain sometimes associated with urinary tract problems, place a heating pad on your lower abdominal area, says Dr. Workowski.

Wear skirts, loose pants and knee-highs. "If you have an infection, wearing tight undergarments and jeans forces the bacteria that normally line your vaginal area up into your urine tube," says Dr. Workowski. If you have an irritation, constrictive clothing can cause pain and discomfort, because it presses against the already inflamed urethral opening.

Toss out douches and sprays. Feminine hygiene sprays may irritate the urinary tract, say doctors.

Uterine Prolapse
Win the Battle against Gravity

*Y*ou might call uterine prolapse women's number one health secret. A prolapsed uterus occurs when the uterus loses the battle against gravity and descends into the vagina. And women are understandably reticent about mentioning the problem, even to their closest friends.

"Women don't talk to their friends about this one," says Linda Brubaker, M.D., director of the Section of Urogynecology and Reconstructive Pelvic Surgery at Rush-Presbyterian–St. Luke's Medical Center in

WHEN TO SEE A DOCTOR

The following symptoms may signal uterine prolapse and merit a visit to your physician:

- Pain or a sensation of heaviness or fullness in the lower abdomen
- Lower-back pain
- The sensation of "sitting on a ball"
- Pelvic pressure while standing, which is reduced when you're lying down

In extreme cases, women doctors say that you may actually see the uterus protruding through the vaginal opening.

Your doctor may recommend a pessary, a diaphragm-like plastic or rubber or silicone ring device inserted into the vagina and positioned against the cervix to provide support for a mildly prolapsed uterus. If you use one, you need to visit your doctor every few months to make sure that it's clean and in place.

Chicago. "They talk about their funny periods, they talk about their breast cancer, but they can't talk about the fact that their innards are starting to hang out through their vagina. There aren't any support groups for this. They feel, 'Oh dear, I'm really different from anybody else.' There's a real sense of vulnerability."

Uterine prolapse isn't the same as a retroverted, or tipped, uterus that tips back toward the rectum, a position that is perfectly normal in up to one-third of women. But even uterine prolapse is actually pretty common—even if you've never heard of it.

In a mild case of uterine prolapse, just a portion of the organ has descended. In an extreme case the uterus has fallen so far that you can actually see it protruding from your vagina. Making matters worse, the condition rarely occurs in isolation, because the uterus lives in the same neighborhood and shares a support muscle system with the vagina, bladder and rectum. When the uterus shifts, its neighbors can get bent out of shape, too. The bladder, for instance, can get dragged down or squeezed, which leads to incontinence problems.

Uterine prolapse is primarily a consequence of childbirth, "especially if a woman had to push for hours," says Yvonne S. Thornton, M.D., visiting associate physician at the Rockefeller University Hospital in New York

City and director of Perinatal Diagnostic Testing Center at Morristown Memorial Hospital in New Jersey. "The baby's head ends up acting as a kind of a battering ram against the perineal muscle between the vagina and the anus, stressing it along with the ligaments that support the uterus."

HOLD ON TO YOUR UTERUS

About one out of every ten women will have surgery for some type of prolapse some time in her life, says Dr. Brubaker. While you and your doctor determine the best course of treatment, here are a few things that women doctors say you can do to keep the problem from getting worse—or maybe even from developing in the first place.

Do Kegel exercises. "It's very unusual to see a woman with extremely strong pelvic muscles who has uterine prolapse," says Dr. Brubaker. The uterus and other pelvic structures—like the bladder—are held in place by muscles. When these muscles are weak or damaged, the job of supporting the uterus falls to the connective muscle ligaments. They, too, can get damaged and prolapse can result. So can bladder incontinence—accidental urine leaks.

"Think of your uterus as an ocean liner tied up at a dock," suggests Dr. Brubaker. "The water that's holding that ocean liner up is the muscle, and then you have these ropes—the ligaments—tying it to the dock. Those ropes can't hold it to the dock without the water."

Build strong pelvic-floor muscles by doing Kegel exercises today and every day of your life, advises Dr. Thornton. Kegels (named after the doctor who invented the exercise) use the muscles that control urination. Kegel exercises can help strengthen the pelvic-floor muscles. To do them, urinate little by little. Contract and release your pelvic-floor muscles 10 times slowly. Once you understand the process, you can practice doing Kegels when you're not urinating. Try to work your way up to 300 Kegels a day.

"Every so often, contract the muscles as hard as you can and hold for for a count of five to ten seconds or as long as you can," says Dr. Thornton. "Repeat 100 to 200 times a day. You don't have to do them all at once. Break it up into 30 in the morning, another 30 midmorning and so on. The rule of thumb is to be repetitive throughout the day, while you're sitting in your car waiting for a stoplight or pushing papers on your desk."

No heavy lifting. Hoisting heavy loads—like a 25-pound toddler or bag of cat kitter—"may exceed the physiologic limits of the ligaments," tearing them and worsening prolapse, says Dr. Brubaker. "Occupational stresses, like carrying around heavy trays of food in a job as a waitress, exceed the limits."

When you must lift things, says Dr. Thornton, "at least do it the right way. Squat down and use the muscles of your legs, not your back or abdomen."

And if you've had surgery for prolapse, you must continue to swear off heavy lifting at least for a few months to give yourself time to heal, says Dr. Brubaker.

Live smoke-free. You wouldn't think that swearing off cigarettes would have anything to do with keeping your uterus in shape, but it does.

"Coughing from smoking increases interabdominal pressure," says Dr. Thornton. "So women who smoke tend to have an increased incidence of uterine prolapse," says Dr. Thornton. Conversely, quitting does your uterus a favor.

Use the missionary position. Many women with uterine prolapse don't feel as sexually desirable because they think that, during sex, their partner is going to feel their uterus in their vagina, says Dr. Brubaker. Relax. The forces of gravity pull your uterus down only when you're standing up, she says. When you lie down, it pretty much moves back to its original position.

"Most men can't detect that the uterus is in the wrong place," Dr. Brubaker says.

Vaginitis

Secrets to Permanent Relief

Chances are, you've probably experienced an episode of vaginitis in some form at one time or another. Maybe it was bacterial vaginosis, the most common type, occurring when microorganisms that normally live there get out of their usual harmonious balance, allowing an overgrowth of certain types. Maybe it was a yeast infection. Or perhaps it was trichomonas vaginalis, caused by the sexually transmitted trichomonad parasite.

WHEN TO SEE A DOCTOR

Vaginitis refers to a number of different problems, all of which are easy to cure. But women doctors say that the correct treatment depends on getting the right diagnosis. Untreated vaginitis can lead to pelvic inflammatory disease, which can result in infertility. See your doctor if you notice any of the following:

- Pain or itching in your vagina and in the area of your vulva, the lips outside your vagina
- Reddening of your vulva
- Pain that is especially noticeable when you urinate or during sex, or pain that worsens upon urination or during sexual intercourse
- Greenish-yellow, frothy and foul-smelling discharge (which suggests trichomoniasis, a sexually transmitted organism)
- Foul-smelling, thin, white or blood-streaked discharge (which may signal atrophic vaginitis)
- Heavy, white, thick and odorless vaginal discharge (which could mean a yeast infection)
- White or gray and fishy smelling vaginal discharge (which suggests bacterial vaginosis)

You should also be screened for bacterial vaginosis if you're pregnant, as it is a common, but preventable, cause of prematurely delivering an undersized baby.

A FORMULA FOR SUCCESS

If you've been newly diagnosed with vaginitis, and your doctor has ruled out a yeast infection, she has probably ordered a course of antibiotics. Here's what else women doctors say that you can do to make yourself more comfortable during your recovery and protect yourself against recurrences. (For information on treating yeast infection, see page 580.)

Take all of your medicine. "By taking antibiotics, you can suppress the infection very quickly after two or three days," says Vesna Skul, M.D., assistant professor of medicine at Rush Medical College of Rush University and medical director of Rush Center for Women's Medicine, both in Chicago. "At that point, your tendency may be to back off and stop your medication. But if you do, the infection is more likely to return." So don't skip the last few pills if symptoms subside or save them just in case you get a repeat attack. Take all the pills. And read the labels for precautions that may apply to you.

Moisturize. The dry, easily irritated genital tissues that characterize atrophic vaginitis—a common occurrence after menopause—can easily be moisturized with a product like Replens, says Marilynne McKay, M.D., professor of dermatology and obstetrics/gynecology at Emory University School of Medicine in Atlanta. Apply once or twice a day.

Apply cold. "If you're really miserable with swelling and itching, cool compresses are often very helpful," says Dr. McKay. Lay a cold washcloth across the affected area. "Coolness causes blood vessels to constrict, which makes you less red and swollen."

Try tea. "A plain tea bag soaked in water, cooled in the refrigerator, and applied externally can relieve itching," says Kathleen McIntyre-Seltman, M.D., professor of medicine in the Department of Obstetrics/Gynecology at the University of Pittsburgh School of Medicine. "The tannin in tea can be very soothing."

Take a warm bath. A shallow sitz bath or an ordinary bath can be very soothing to irritated genital tissues, says Dr. McKay. And skip the soap. "Soap leaches out the skin's natural oils—the body's natural lipid barrier against germs," she says. (So does bubble bath.) This makes you more susceptible to infection, including vaginal infections.

Scrub your tub. Bathtubs are regular germ storage sites. Be sure to clean and disinfect yours regularly to keep bacteria and mold under control, says Dr. Skul.

Practice good toilet hygiene. Wipe from front to back after a visit to the toilet to avoid transferring germs from your rectal area forward to your genital area, advises Dr. McKay. Finish up with a final clean wipe to make sure that you've done a thorough job.

Rinse underwear and panty hose well. Wearing underclothes or panty hose with detergent residue can irritate tissues already stinging from vaginitis, says Dr. McKay.

Eat yogurt. Studies have shown, says Dr. Skul, that an eight-ounce serving of yogurt containing live cultures once a day helps women with recurrent bacterial vaginosis get better with fewer courses of antibiotics. The acidophilus bacteria that it contains help create a more normal bacterial environment.

Varicose Veins

Something New for Aching Legs

*A*t the beach you wear ankle-length cover-ups. At work you wear mid-calf skirts and dresses with dark hose or boots. At parties you dare to wear an above-the-knee skirt—with bright tights or panty hose.

And at home you wear pants, pants and pants.

What are you trying to hide? A bulging blue varicose vein that snakes along your calf almost from ankle to knee.

"Varicose veins are like a pair of stretched-out panty hose," says Lenise Banse, M.D., a dermatologist and vein expert at the Northeast Family Dermatology Center in Clinton Township, Michigan. They're stretched and baggy—the veins, not the hose—because the valves in your legs just aren't doing their job.

The problem, says Dr. Banse, is physiology. Arteries, which have muscles along their walls to push the blood along, take blood away from the heart. Veins, not aided by muscles, return the blood to the heart.

To compensate for the fact that blood returning to the heart is going against gravity, the veins have valves every so often that act like a set of French doors. They open one way only—up, toward the heart. A valve opens, the blood goes through and the valve closes.

"But sometimes those valves start opening in the opposite direction," says Dr. Banse. "The blood reverses direction and flows back toward the feet, pressure on the veins increases and the veins become stretched, or varicose."

What puts you at risk?

"Genetics, mostly," says Toby Shaw, M.D., associate professor of dermatology at Allegheny University of the Health Sciences MCP--Hahnemann School of Medicine in Philadelphia. If your mother had varicose veins, you probably have them, too. But estrogen production, pregnancy, being constantly on your feet and aging play a part as well.

THROB NO MORE

Fortunately, nobody has to put up with unsightly veins that make your legs feel tired and heavy, says Dr. Banse. Here's what doctors suggest

567

When to See a Doctor

Usually, varicose veins are unsightly and uncomfortable but not worrisome—unless they lead to a blood clot, says Lenise Banse, M.D., a dermatologist and vein expert at the Northeast Family Dermatology Center in Clinton Township, Michigan. See your doctor if you develop either of these warning signs.

• Leg pain occurs when you elevate your legs.
• Leg pain wakes you up at night.

you do to minimize discomfort and keep varicose veins from worsening.

Tighten up. Pull on a pair of support panty hose, says Dr. Banse. This will keep your veins tight so they can't stretch out. Tights are even better, she adds—especially the Lycra exercise tights that go so well with long tunics and sweaters.

Enlist the support of compression hose. "If you're on your feet all day, buy stockings that provide 20 to 30 millimeters of pressure," says Dr. Shaw. The numbers are on the package. Look for them at your local drugstore.

Pull panty hose on while you're still in bed. Whether you use regular support hose or compression support hose, "keep the stockings by your bed at night and put them on before you get out of bed in the morning, before gravity pulls blood through the valves to pool," says Dr. Shaw.

Free your thighs. Avoid garments that constrict at the groin, says Dr. Banse. Tight girdles and regular panty hose—which do not have the graduated, structured give of support hose—put pressure on leg veins and encourage them to stretch.

Stick a pillow under your feet. When sitting, elevate your legs three to six inches higher than your hips to take the pressure off your veins and relieve that heavy, achy feeling, says Dr. Shaw. At night, sleep with one pillow under your head and two under your feet.

Flex, flex, flex. Veins contain no muscles to help you push blood back to your heart, but the skeletal muscles in your legs can give you an extra hand, says Dr. Banse. "So take a break every hour and walk around. Any kind of movement that flexes and contracts the leg muscles so they can 'milk' the veins will discourage the veins from stretching."

Vomiting

Quiet a Heaving Tummy

Kids, it seems, throw up periodically for no good reason. Cats seem to throw up regularly just to stay in practice. But grown-up women rarely throw up, unless they're pregnant.

But it happens.

Vomiting is your body's way of divesting itself of a bad investment. So if you suddenly throw up and you're not expecting, it can usually be traced to either contaminated food or overindulgence in alcohol. So while it's little consolation if you find yourself hunched over the toilet bowl, chances are that if you're vomiting, it's good for you.

HELPING NATURE DO ITS JOB

If you're pregnant and vomiting, read about morning sickness on page 376. If you're not pregnant, here's what women doctors say healthy adults can do to ease the queasies and feel better faster.

Give your stomach a rest. "Don't eat or drink anything for several

WHEN TO SEE A DOCTOR

If you're vomiting up blood, see a doctor immediately. It may be a sign of internal bleeding.

And don't eat or drink anything, says Sheila Crowe, M.D., gastroenterologist and assistant professor of medicine in the Department of Internal Medicine in the Division of Gastroenterology at the University of Texas Medical Branch at Galveston.

Otherwise, nausea and vomiting usually clear within a day. If you're still throwing up, see a doctor. You may have food poisoning or another serious illness, Dr. Crowe says.

Continued vomiting may signal a condition such as viral or bacterial infections, ulcers or even diabetes.

hours after you vomit," says Sheila Crowe, M.D., gastroenterologist and assistant professor of medicine in the Department of Internal Medicine in the Division of Gastroenterology at the University of Texas Medical Branch at Galveston.

Then, drink fluids, but don't plan to eat a lot for the first eight hours, says Wanda Filer, M.D., a family practice physician in York, Pennsylvania. Then see how you can handle a bland diet for the next couple of hours. Try eating a banana, cooked rice, dry toast or an apple.

Sip clear fluids. As your vomiting subsides and your insides calm down, try to sip clear, caffeine-free liquids such as water, flat soda, chicken bouillion or Gatorade-type fluid-replacement drinks to help you replenish the fluids you lost when you were heaving up your insides, says Dr. Crowe.

Sip, don't gulp. "Your stomach is still so delicate that if you take normal mouthfuls, you may not be able to keep fluids down, so take small sips every five minutes or so," Dr. Filer says.

Gargle. It's a good idea to gargle with salt and water or a mouthwash after vomiting, Dr. Crowe says. "It gets rid of the bitter aftertaste and rinses away stomach acid, which can erode tooth enamel."

Warts

Painless but Unsightly

Warts are typically tough, flesh-colored little bumps on your skin caused by what's known as the human papillomavirus. Though usually harmless, these growths can appear anywhere on your face or body. But, say women doctors, they show up most frequently on the hands and feet.

Warts vary in appearance. Some are raised and rough, others are flat and smooth and some can even look reddish or blackened, because of tiny, blocked-off blood vessels trapped within the wart, says Suzanne M. Levine, D.P.M., clinical assistant podiatrist at Cornell Medical Center in New York City. "Some people are susceptible to warts all over their bod-

WHEN TO SEE A DOCTOR

If you've tried over-the-counter products and your wart doesn't improve within a month or two, it's time to visit your family doctor or a dermatologist, says D'Anne Kleinsmith, M.D., a staff dermatologist at William Beaumont Hospital in Royal Oak, Michigan. The wart can be removed with a topically applied chemical—liquid nitrogen—surgery or laser.

Women should also see a doctor immediately for treatment if they notice warts on their legs. "Even if you have just one wart on your leg, it is easy to spread it with your razor. One nick of the skin will open up the wart, and the virus will spread," cautions Dr. Kleinsmith.

Warts on your face should always be treated by a dermatologist, because the skin on your face is too delicate and visible to risk trying home treatments.

ies, because their immune systems aren't effective at fighting off the wart virus," she says.

Warts are contagious, says Karen K. Deasey, M.D., chief of dermatology at Bryn Mawr Hospital in Pennsylvania. So if you have a wart on your finger and pick at your face, you can get warts on your face, too.

It's not as common, but you can also get warts from others via hand-to-hand contact, says Dr. Deasey.

By the way, genital warts are caused by a different strain of the virus, and are usually passed through genital contact, says D'Anne Kleinsmith, M.D., a staff dermatologist at William Beaumont Hospital in Royal Oak, Michigan.

DECLARE WAR ON WARTS

A wart may disappear on its own. But if it lingers, and you find it disfiguring or you're afraid of it spreading, you can try taking matters into your own hands. Here are women doctors' tips on how to declare war on warts.

Keep it dry. "Thoroughly towel-dry your hands (or whatever body part has the wart) after washing," says Dr. Levine. "The wart virus loves a moist environment, so if you keep it dry, you'll reduce its chance of spreading."

571

Visit your local drugstore. Check out the wart remedy section in your drugstore, says Dr. Deasey. You'll find that wart preparations come in the form of patches, films, polishes and liquids. The most effective wart treatments typically contain salicylic acid, which erodes away the wart.

Use a dropper-type product. "I recommend liquid treatments that you apply to the wart with a dropper. Then you cover it with a Band-Aid-type bandage, leave it on overnight and wash it off in the morning," says Dr. Kleinsmith. "Duofilm and Occlusal are two good treatments that come with droppers."

Follow directions to the letter. "Wart medicines can irritate healthy skin nearby as well, so you have to follow directions carefully," cautions Dr. Deasey.

Be patient. "You have to use the product every day for up to six to eight weeks," says Dr. Deasey. "Do it and do it and do it until it works."

Ace it with vitamin A. "There is substantial evidence that vitamin A helps build your immune system and fight warts," says Dr. Levine. Good food sources of vitamin A include carrots, sweet peas, squash and leafy green vegetables.

(For practical ways to manage genital warts and plantar warts, see pages 240 and 430.)

Wedding Ring Dermatitis

Save the Ring, and Your Skin

*I*f your wedding band is making your skin sore and scratchy, that doesn't mean that you're allergic to your marriage. When you wear a ring every day around the clock, the skin underneath stays moist and doesn't have a chance to air out, which makes it more susceptible to irritations and allergies (contact dermatitis).

WHEN TO SEE A DOCTOR

If you have a chronic case of wedding ring dermatitis that seems to be lasting as long as your marriage (or longer), see a doctor—preferably, a dermatologist, advises Kristin Leiferman, M.D., professor of dermatology at the Mayo Medical School in Rochester, Minnesota. She can prescribe medication that can help. But more important, she can test your skin to determine what's causing the problem, and that may include testing your ring to find out if you are truly allergic to your ring.

"Most people wear their rings tight enough to stay put, which causes pressure against the skin and sets it up for problems," explains Kristin Leiferman, M.D., professor of dermatology at the Mayo Medical School in Rochester, Minnesota.

The result is a surprisingly common condition that dermatologists refer to as wedding ring dermatitis, in which the skin under the ring gets temporarily red, sore and itchy.

Most likely, you've developed a skin irritation to soap or debris that gets trapped under your ring and ground into your skin, especially if you wear a wide band, says Dr. Leiferman.

The problem is common among women who have their hands in water a lot, notes Amy Newburger, M.D., assistant clinical professor of dermatology at Columbia University College of Physicians and Surgeons in New York City and a dermatologist in Scarsdale, New York. "Liquid soaps are particularly irritating if not removed from the skin," explains Leiferman.

It's rare, but women doctors say that you could be allergic to the jewelry itself, even if it's an expensive gold ring.

SALVAGE EFFORTS

Before you relegate your ring to your jewelry case, women doctors suggest that you try these tactics.

Soak your skin. Take your ring or rings off and carefully set them aside so that you don't lose them down the drain. Then thoroughly rinse the skin under the rings, paying special attention to the areas between your fingers, where debris and soap can get trapped, says Dr. Leiferman. "Generally, a good rinsing with water is all that you need."

Rinse your ring. Put the stopper in the drain, and then rinse off the ring, making sure to clean the smooth underside that comes in contact with your skin. Wash away any residues of soap or debris, says Dr. Leiferman.

"If you soak your rings with jewelry cleaner, be especially careful to rinse the rings well with water," says Dr. Leiferman. Ring cleaners typically contain ammonia, a chemical that can dry and irritate skin, she says.

Give your ring finger a rest. Take your ring off at night to allow your skin a chance to air out and heal, suggests Dr. Leiferman.

"If you have severe contact dermatitis, you may even have to stop wearing your ring for a week or two until the irritation resolves," says Mary Ruth Buchness, M.D., chief of dermatology at St. Vincent's Hospital and Medical Center in New York City.

Heal with hydrocortisone. Rub hydrocortisone cream into your skin for a few nights while your ring is off, to reduce inflammation and redness, suggests Dr. Buchness.

Moisturize your hands. Keep the skin of your hands—particularly the area under the ring—supple by applying a bland, fragrance-free moisturizer several times a day, especially after washing. Not only will the moisturizer create a protective barrier against irritating debris, but it will also improve the skin condition. "If your skin is in good shape, it's not going to break down as easily, and it will heal faster if it does become irritated," explains Dr. Leiferman.

Try anti-itch medicines. To soothe irritated skin, apply over-the-counter anti-itch medications that contain the ingredients camphor or menthol (or both), suggests Dr. Buchness. "These ingredients are topical anesthetics, which relieve itch and pain."

Wear rubber gloves. To avoid future outbreaks, wear gloves when washing dishes, handling detergents or doing housework, to protect your hands from moisture and irritation, suggests Patricia Farris Walters, M.D., clinical assistant professor of dermatology at Tulane University School of Medicine in New Orleans and a spokesperson for the American Academy of Dermatology.

Windburn

Chapped Skin from a Dry Breeze

*Y*ou don't have to be a ski or sailing enthusiast to suffer windburn. "Whenever your skin is exposed to severe wind, it loses moisture quickly and becomes dry and chafed, especially if it's cold," says Patricia Farris Walters, M.D., clinical assistant professor of dermatology at Tulane University School of Medicine in New Orleans and a spokesperson for the American Academy of Dermatology. "The physical friction of the wind also agitates dry skin." Frequently, windburn comes hand in hand with sunburn, so skin gets a double whammy of dryness and redness.

With skiing you're often at high altitudes, where the air is very thin and dry, which adds to skin chapping, says D'Anne Kleinsmith, M.D., a staff dermatologist at William Beaumont Hospital in Royal Oak, Michigan.

TIPS FOR TENDER HIDES

Here's how to soothe dry, parched skin and put the moisture back, according to women doctors.

Cozy up to a warm compress. "First, gently try to warm the area to take away the sting," suggests Evelyn Placek, M.D., a dermatologist and doctor of internal medicine in private practice in Scarsdale, New York.

Get inside to a warm area and put a lukewarm compress (a washcloth soaked in warm water) on your skin. "Don't make water too hot, because that will dry your skin even more and remove oils from the surface," she says.

Wash with TLC. Cleanse tender skin with warm—not hot—water, and a rich, creamy, gentle soap that won't dry it, such as Basis, Dove, Oil of Olay liquid cleanser or Cetaphil liquid, recommends Dr. Kleinsmith. Handle your skin gently without rubbing. And don't overwash, because water strips away the oil that your skin needs to hold in moisture, she advises.

Use a heavy-duty moisturizer. Right after washing, while your skin is still damp, put on a moisturizer to help seal in and add back moisture. "Vaseline, or other pure petroleum jelly, is an even better bet than moisturizers, which can contain irritating ingredients," says Dr. Placek.

"A thin coat of petroleum jelly goes a long way," says Dr. Walters. "It's soothing and protective."

If you're acne-prone, however, choose a moisture cream that's labeled "noncomedogenic" (non-acne-forming) instead of Vaseline or generic petroleum jelly, which may actually worsen or exacerbate acne, says Dr. Kleinsmith.

Reapply. Whatever you choose to use, reapply it two or three times a day until your windburn is healed, says Dr. Placek.

Boost healing with antibiotic ointment. "Bacitracin, Polysporin or some other topical antibiotic ointment in a petrolatum base will help fight infection while it soothes and heals skin," says Dr. Placek.

Go for a vitamin D ointment. Aquaphor Healing Ointment, available by the tube at drug stores, can also help heal windburn. "It's a combination of the antibiotic Polysporin and a vitamin D ingredient, Panthenol, which soothes chapped, dry skin," says Dr. Placek. And it comes in a mild, pure, petrolatum and mineral oil ointment, which soothes and hydrates skin.

The vitamin D and antibiotic ointments can be combined for extra protection and healing, she notes.

Coat irritated skin with cortisone. An over-the-counter preparation of cortisone ointment will help reduce inflammation and redness. "Use ointment, not cream, which contains preservatives that can sting tender skin," suggests Dr. Walters.

Wrinkles

Best Defense against Crinkles and Creases

There has never been a shortage of products that cosmetic manufacturers claimed could stop or erase wrinkles but didn't live up to their promises.

Now, there are plenty of options to choose from, many of which have the blessing of women dermatologists.

TWO KINDS OF WRINKLES

A short refresher course on how wrinkles form in the first place will help you determine your best strategy against wrinkles.

"There are two types of skin aging, intrinsic and extrinsic, and both contribute to wrinkling," says dermatologist Ellen Gendler, M.D., director of New York University's Center for Skin Health and Appearance in New York City. Intrinsic aging is something that happens as the genes we've inherited from our parents trigger a reduction of two connective fibers, collagen and elastin. Collagen supports the skin and elastin gives it flexibility. Together collagen and elastin give skin its structure and tone. After age 30, connective fibers start to break down, and the skin starts to become more lax.

Extrinsic aging is aging that comes from environmental factors, especially sun damage, says Dr. Gendler.

"If you want to know how much genetics contributes to skin aging and how much is caused by the sun, just look down at the top of your forearm, then flip it over and check out the underside," suggests Anita Cela, M.D., clinical assistant professor of dermatology at New York Hospital–Cornell Medical Center in New York City.

"Genetics is responsible for the skin on the underside," says Dr. Cela. "Sun exposure is responsible for the skin on top." In particular, ultraviolet A and B, the invisible rays of the sun, penetrate below the skin surface and encourage wrinkles, because they damage connective fibers. These are the same rays that stimulate production of melanin and produce a tan, a look that is, ironically enough, pursued in the interest of looking young and sexy.

SMOOTHING THINGS OVER

It's not enough to try and fix what's already wrong with your skin. You also need to think about the future and try to prevent more damage from occurring.

Fortunately, "we have the power to prevent most of what we don't like about our skin," says Debra Price, M.D., clinical assistant professor of dermatology at the University of Miami School of Medicine and a dermatologist in South Miami. Here's how.

Shop for a product with AHAs. To erase fine wrinkles and prevent more from forming, make alpha hydroxy acids (AHAs) the foundation of your daily skin-care regimen, suggests Eileen Lambroza, M.D., clinical instructor of dermatology at New York Hospital–Cornell Medical Center.

What Women Doctors Do

A Regimen That Works

Ellen Gendler, M.D.

Every morning, dermatologist Ellen Gendler, M.D., director of New York University's Center for Skin Health and Appearance in New York City, practices what she preaches.

She does everything that she can to make sure that she won't face the day—or any other day—with wrinkles.

Dr. Gendler's routine includes:

- Washing her face with a foaming cleanser
- Smoothing on an alpha hydroxy acid lotion that removes old cells and uncovers new ones
- Stroking on a sunscreen that also doubles as a moisturizer
- Applying her makeup

"I use my sunscreen as a moisturizer, so I just apply makeup over that," she says.

These acids are derived from sugarcane, fruit and milk. They loosen old wrinkled cells on the skin's surface, peel them off, then uncover the younger, fresher cells underneath. They also plump the skin's surface—in essence, filling in the "dents" that you see as wrinkles. In lotion or cream form, AHAs also act as excellent moisturizers.

Glycolic acid (made from sugarcane) is the most widely used alpha hydroxy acid. Sold in different strengths according to the percentage of acids that they contain, AHAs are also available as gels. Gels are for younger women who do not need the moisturizing properties of lotions, lotions are for those who need a lightweight moisturizer and creams are for those who need a heavier moisturizer to keep their skin from drying out and causing tiny lines just from the dryness, says Dr. Lambroza.

The same AHAs are used in inexpensive products found at discount drugstores as the more elaborately packaged and expensive products found in department stores, says Dr. Lambroza.

Test first. To start using AHAs, smear a drop of a 5 percent AHA preparation on a small section of skin under your jaw, says Dr. Lambroza. If there is no sign of redness or irritation by the next day, the next morning you can wash your face, pat it dry, apply the AHA preparation to your face, then apply your usual sunscreen.

Do the eye area last. Smooth the AHA preparation over your entire face, but no closer to your eyes than the length of your eyelashes, says Dr. Lambroza. "I recommend that you do your face first and your eye area last, so that you don't apply too much to your eye area," she says. "You can use it underneath your eyes, but not on your eyelids. And be sure to follow up with a moisturizing eye cream."

Repeat daily. If no redness or irritation occurs, begin using the preparation once a day, says Dr. Lambroza. You may experience some tingling as the AHAs begin to work, but the tingling should subside within a few minutes. If no irritation develops after several days, you can increase your use of AHAs to twice a day: once in the morning and once at night, says Dr. Lambroza.

NO MORE LINES, EVER

Women doctors say that unless you take steps to protect your face against wrinkle-forming forces, your antiwrinkle efforts will be less than optimally effective. Here's what women doctors advise.

Double up on sunscreen. "I generally recommend that women use two sunscreens at the same time if they plan on spending the day outdoors," says Dr. Gendler.

Sun protection factor, or SPF, only refers to the product's ability to screen ultraviolet B (UVB) rays. But UVB rays only penetrate the top layers of skin. You also need to protect against ultraviolet A (UVA) rays, which penetrate to the deeper layers of skin, also causing wrinkles.

There are not many products that specifically protect you from UVA. The best product available is called Shade UVA Guard, says Dr. Gendler. It also has an SPF of 15 to guard against UVB rays. For day-to-day use it's all you need. But if you're going to be spending lots of time in the sun, apply a second sunscreen with a higher SPF over top to give you added UVB protection.

If you go swimming or participate in outdoor sports that make you sweat, adds Dr. Price, use a waterproof SPF sunscreen and reapply it every 1½ hours.

Forget tanning booths. Tanning salons should be called wrinkling salons. Tanning parlor operators and tanning equipment manufacturers claim that tanning booths and tanning beds give a "safe tan." The truth is, tanning equipment produces rays that can cause premature wrinkling of the skin and skin cancer, says Allison Vidimos, M.D., a staff dermatologist at the Cleveland Clinic Foundation. No woman who values her skin should set foot inside a tanning booth.

Keep your weight steady. Gaining and losing even small amounts of weight can create fine wrinkles by the constant stretching and tightening of skin, says Margaret A. Weiss, M.D., assistant professor of dermatology at the Johns Hopkins Medical Institutions in Baltimore. So try to get your weight down and keep it down.

(For effective ways to banish crow's-feet, see page 149. For ways to minimize frown lines, see page 234.)

Yeast Infections
Tame Vexing Vaginal Fungus

Sooner or later, most women get yeast infections, says Janet Mc-Combs, Pharm.D., clinical assistant professor at the University of Georgia College of Pharmacy in Athens. And it's easy to see why, say other women doctors.

"The vaginal milieu is a delicate ecosystem that is easily unbalanced by insult," says May M. Wakamatsu, M.D., instructor of obstetrics and gynecology and reproductive biology at Harvard Medical School. A variety of microscopic organisms normally reside as peaceful neighbors in the vagina, among them the yeastlike fungus *Candida albicans*. But "insults" such as taking antibiotics for other conditions can kill off certain flora and leave *Candida* to go on a rampage. This results in *Candida* vaginitis, or a yeast infection, the second most common form of vaginitis experienced by women.

As any woman who has had a yeast infection—or several—can avow, the symptoms are the pits: itching in a place that's not polite to scratch, burning during urination and sometimes a thick, white discharge.

PROPER AT-HOME CARE

If your doctor has confirmed that what you have is a yeast infection and not some other form of vaginitis, antiyeast medications are usually

WHEN TO SEE A DOCTOR

If you've been visited by the Yeast Beast within the past two months and recognize the symptoms, women doctors say that it's okay to self-treat with an over-the-counter yeast medication such as Gyne-Lotrimin or Monistat 7. Otherwise, see your doctor for proper diagnosis and initial treatment if you experience:

- A white vaginal discharge with a yeasty odor, similar to cottage cheese in texture and appearance
- Itching and irritation in the vulvar folds, in the area outside your vagina or both
- Pain during urination
- Pain during sexual intercourse

Also, you should see your doctor if self-treatment doesn't work. You could be having a more serious episode of the infection or a different infection altogether. A Pap smear, visual exam and other simple tests can sort it out.

necessary. But success depends on you. (For tips on soothing vaginitis in general, see page 564.)

Take every last pill. Be sure to take your full course of whatever antibiotic that your doctor has prescribed, says Kathleen McIntyre-Seltman, M.D., professor of medicine in the Department of Obstetrics/Gynecology at the University of Pittsburgh School of Medicine. Cutting treatment short just because you feel better invites a recurrence, since you've only wiped out some of the fungus.

Use a nonprescription remedy. "For the average yeast infection, over-the-counter antiyeast suppositories and creams (such as Gyne-Lotrimin or Monistat 7) are very effective," says Dr. McIntyre-Seltman. "If you've had an infection before and recognize the symptoms, go ahead and use one."

Lean back and apply. To reduce leakage from your vagina, use suppositories and creams at bedtime, suggests Janet Engle, Pharm. D., clinical associate professor of pharmacy practice at the University of Illinois at Chicago. Place the applicator as far into your vagina as possible by inserting it while squatting slightly or, even better, while lying on your back with your knees bent and pulled toward your chest.

Wear a sanitary pad or panty liner during treatment to protect your clothing, suggests Dr. McCombs.

NONDRUG STRATEGIES FOR THE YEAST BEAST

Over and above proper use of at-home medications, women doctors say that there are quite a few other things that you can do to get more comfortable and deter a recurrence.

Try a vinegar douche. Flushing your vagina with a dilute solution of vinegar and water occasionally—no more than once a week—may help prevent yeast infection recurrences. "This makes the vagina a little more acidic, which is bad for yeast." Mix two tablespoons of white vinegar with one quart of water and use a standard douching bulb, available at drugstores.

Women doctors advise against using commercial douches—or douching any more often than once a week. Douching kills off "good" *lactobacilli* bacteria in the vagina, leaving *Candida* to run wild, says Dr. McIntyre-Seltman.

Apply yogurt. Some people believe that yogurt, which contains bacteria that are cousins to the "good" bacteria in the vagina, may help the good bacteria repopulate, says Dr. McIntyre-Seltman. If you are going to try this remedy, be sure to use plain, unsweetened yogurt containing live cultures and apply it to your vaginal opening at bedtime.

Eat yogurt. In one study, women with recurring yeast infections who ate yogurt every day had fewer yeast infections, says Vesna Skul, M.D., assistant professor of medicine at Rush Medical College of Rush University and medical director of Rush Center for Women's Medicine, both in Chicago, and infections that they did get retreated quickly. "Yogurt gives women a double benefit: It's a low-fat, high-protein, high-calcium food, and the *lactobaccilus acidophilus* bacteria it contains helps create a more normal bacterial environment." She tells the women she treats to eat a daily eight ounces of yogurt containing live yogurt cultures.

Crunch on carrots. According to doctors in the Department of Obstetrics and Gynecology at Albert Einstein College of Medicine of Yeshiva University in New York City, eating carrots and other foods rich in beta-carotene—a natural substance that's converted into vitamin A in the body—may offer protection against yeast infections. In one study, vaginal cells in women with yeast infections had significantly lower levels of beta-carotene than the vaginal cells in women who did not have yeast infections. The doctors theorize that benefit may be due to beta-carotene's ability to boost the immune system.

Besides carrots, spinach, broccoli, sweet potatoes and apricots all contain plentiful amounts of beta-carotene.

Clothe in cotton. "*Candida* likes moist, warm environments to grow in," says Dr. Skul. Keep dry and cool by wearing cotton underwear, loose clothing and panty hose with a cotton crotch, she suggests.

Add cornstarch. "Sprinkling a little cornstarch in your groin area helps absorb moisture," says Kimberly A. Workowski, M.D., assistant professor of medicine in the Division of Infectious Diseases at Emory University in Atlanta.

Exercise without restraint. Tight exercise clothes, says Dr. McKay, invite yeast infections on two counts: You're usually sweating in them, and their tightness interferes with cooling air circulation. "A pair of running shorts is better than running tights, because air can circulate in them," she says. And look for sportswear with an open, rather than tight, weave.

Ditch your wet swimsuit. Walking around in a clingy wet swimsuit is an invitation to yeast proliferation, says Kristene E. Whitmore, M.D., chief of urology and director of the Incontinence Center at Graduate Hospital in Philadelphia. "Buy two identical swimsuits," she suggests. "After a dip, rinse your suit in clear water and put on the dry suit. No one needs to know that you changed suits."

Lay off the sweets. "Woman who have diabetes and who eat too much sugar—which they shouldn't be doing anyway—will probably get more yeast infections," says Mary Lang Carney, M.D., medical director of the Center for Women's Health at St. Francis Hospital in Evanston, Illinois. "Their blood sugar levels rise, and all their tissues have more sugar in them. When there's more sugar anywhere, yeast have a great feast and multiply like mad."

Index

NOTE: <u>Underscored</u> page references indicate boxed text.

586

C

_G_

_K_

𝒰

𝒱